Computer-Aided Otorhinolaryngology– Head and Neck Surgery

Computer-Aided Otorhinolaryngology– Head and Neck Surgery

edited by

MARTIN J. CITARDI, M.D., F.A.C.S.

Cleveland Clinic Foundation
Cleveland, Ohio

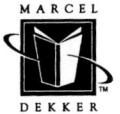

MARCEL DEKKER, INC. NEW YORK · BASEL

ISBN: 0-8247-0641-2

This book is printed on acid-free paper.

Headquarters
Marcel Dekker, Inc.
270 Madison Avenue, New York, NY 10016
tel: 212-696-9000; fax: 212-685-4540

Eastern Hemisphere Distribution
Marcel Dekker AG
Hutgasse 4, Postfach 812, CH-4001 Basel, Switzerland
tel: 41-61-261-8482; fax: 41-61-261-8896

World Wide Web
http://www.dekker.com

The publisher offers discounts on this book when ordered in bulk quantities. For more information, write to Special Sales/Professional Marketing at the headquarters address above.

Copyright © 2002 by Marcel Dekker, Inc. All Rights Reserved.

Neither this book nor any part may be reproduced or transmitted in any form or by any means, electronic or mechanical, including photocopying, microfilming, and recording, or by any information storage and retrieval system, without permission in writing from the publisher.

Current printing (last digit):
10 9 8 7 6 5 4 3 2 1

PRINTED IN THE UNITED STATES OF AMERICA

For my mother, Gloria, whose memory I shall never abandon.

To my father, Martin, for his guidance and example.

To my wife, Laura, for her inspiring love, boundless understanding, continuous support, and endless patience.

Note on CD-ROM: *The enclosed CD-ROM contains digital copies of the figures that appear in the printed text. The images are in JPG format and can be seen using an image viewer on a PC with a CD-ROM drive. Almost all of these images are in color. The JPG files are sorted into folders corresponding to chapters in the book. The figures in the printed book and on the CD-ROM have the same numbers; for instance, Figure 1.1 on the CD-ROM is the digital version of Figure 1.1 in the text.*

Chapter 25 also contains references to four movies, which are digital files in the folder for Chapter 25 on this CD-ROM. These files, which are in AVI format, may be viewed on a PC with a CD-ROM drive and a media viewer such as Windows Media Player 6 or greater (Microsoft Corporation, Redmond, Washington, http://www. microsoft.com/windows/windowsmedia/EN/default.asp).

Preface

Although numerous books about topics in otorhinolaryngology–head and neck surgery have been published over the years, few, if any at all, directly address clinical applications of computer-based technologies. Of course, some texts discuss computers, but the number of references is small and the references themselves are typically indirect and inconsequential. In light of the enormous impact of computers on medical care (as well as communications, manufacturing, entertainment, etc.), this deficiency seems surprising.

Computer-Aided Otorhinolaryngology–Head and Neck Surgery seeks to fill the gap left by these other publications. This book focuses on the applications of semiconductor-based technologies within clinical otorhinolaryngology–head and neck surgery. Of course, this text describes present technology; however, this is really a small part of the book. The real focus is on the principles of computer-aided surgery. This approach recognizes current challenges and technological limitations and proposes solutions and strategies based on semiconductor-derived systems. Many of the chapters also present visions of clinical care in the distant and not-so-distant future. In these ways, *Computer-Aided Otorhinolaryngology–Head and Neck Surgery* provides a framework for discussions that will guide future developments. This book may also serve as a guide for the further integration of this technology into healthcare delivery.

The primary audience for the book is practicing otolaryngologists who have an interest in computer-aided surgery or are exploring potential applications for computer-aided surgery in their clinical practices. Of course, resident physicians may also find this book very useful. In addition, this book contains information that nurses and other healthcare professionals may need as computer-aided surgery technologies become more prevalent in healthcare delivery. Finally, it is hoped that engineers and other individuals from the commercial sector will learn about the views of practicing physicians who have contributed to this text. The perspectives portrayed in each of the chapters can provide guidance for future technological development and adaptations.

Martin J. Citardi, M.D., F.A.C.S.

Contents

Preface	v
Contributors	xi

1. New Paradigm 1
   Martin J. Citardi

2. Historical Perspective 15
   Jack B. Anon, Ludger Klimek, and Ralph Mösges

3. Surgical Navigation Technology: Optical and Electromagnetic Tracking 31
   Ralph B. Metson

4. Principles of Registration 49
   Martin J. Citardi

5. Intraoperative Magnetic Resonance Imaging 73
   Neil Bhattacharyya, Marvin P. Fried, and Liangge Hsu

6. Internet-Enabled Surgery 91
   Ronald B. Kuppersmith

7. Virtual Reality and Surgical Simulation 99
   Charles V. Edmond, Jr.

8. Digital Imaging in Otorhinolaryngology—Head and Neck Surgery 117
   Eiji Yanagisawa, John K. Joe, and Ray Yanagisawa

9. The Neuroradiology Perspective on Computer-Aided Surgery 135
   S. James Zinreich

10. Moving Stereotaxis Beyond the Dura: A Neurosurgical Perspective on Computer-Aided Otorhinolaryngology 161
    Richard D. Bucholz and Keith A. Laycock

11. Role of Computer-Aided Surgery in Functional Endoscopic Surgery 185
    Stephanie A. Joe and David W. Kennedy

12. Image-Guided Functional Endoscopic Sinus Surgery 201
    Martin J. Citardi

13. Computer-Aided Revision Sinus Surgery 223
    Michael J. Sillers and Christy R. Buckman

14. Computer-Aided Frontal Sinus Surgery 243
    Frederick A. Kuhn and James N. Palmer

15. Computer-Aided Transsphenoidal Hypophysectomy 263
    Winston C. Vaughan

16. Computer-Aided Surgery Applications for Sinonasal Tumors and Anterior Cranial Base Surgery 277
    Roy R. Casiano and Ricardo L. Carrau

17. Computer-Aided Otologic and Neurotologic Surgery 297
    Eric W. Sargent

18. Computer-Aided Tumor Modeling and Visualization 311
    Gregory J. Wiet, Don Stredney, and Petra Schmalbrock

19. Head and Neck Virtual Endoscopy 329
    William B. Armstrong and Thong H. Nguyen

Contents

20.	Computer-Aided Facial Plastic Surgery *Daniel G. Becker, Madeleine A. Spatola, and Samuel S. Becker*	361
21.	Software-Enabled Cephalometrics *Martin J. Citardi and Mimi S. Kokoska*	377
22.	Computer-Aided Craniofacial Surgery *Alex A. Kane, Lun-Jou Lo, and Jeffrey L. Marsh*	395
23.	Computer-Aided Soft Tissue Surgery *Joseph M. Rosen and Marcus K. Simpson*	421
24.	Computer-Aided Reduction of Maxillofacial Fractures *Mimi S. Kokoska and Martin J. Citardi*	443
25.	Future Directions *Martin J. Citardi*	463

Index   *473*

Contributors

Jack B. Anon, M.D., F.A.C.S.   Associate Clinical Professor, Department of Otolaryngology, University of Pittsburgh School of Medicine, Pittsburgh, Pennsylvania

William B. Armstrong, M.D.   Adjunct Assistant Professor and Vice Chair, Department of Otolaryngology–Head and Neck Surgery, University of California, Irvine, Orange, and Chief, Otolaryngology Section, Veterans Affairs Medical Center, Long Beach, California

Daniel G. Becker, M.D.   Assistant Professor, Department of Otolaryngology–Head and Neck Surgery, University of Pennsylvania, Philadelphia, Pennsylvania

Samuel S. Becker, M.F.A.   University of California at San Francisco Medical Center, San Francisco, California

Neil Bhattacharyya, M.D., F.A.C.S.   Division of Otolaryngology, Brigham and Women's Hospital, and Department of Otology and Laryngology, Harvard Medical School, Boston, Massachusetts

Richard D. Bucholz, M.D., F.A.C.S.   Jean H. Bakewell Section of Image Guided Surgery, Division of Neurological Surgery, Department of Surgery, Saint Louis University School of Medicine, St. Louis, Missouri

xi

Christy R. Buckman, M.D. Assistant Professor, Division of Otolaryngology/Head and Neck Surgery, Department of Surgery, University of Alabama—Birmingham, Birmingham, Alabama

Ricardo L. Carrau, M.D., F.A.C.S. Associate Professor, Department of Otolaryngology, University of Pittsburgh Medical Center, Pittsburgh, Pennsylvania

Roy R. Casiano, M.D., F.A.C.S. Professor, Department of Otolaryngology, University of Miami School of Medicine, Miami, Florida

Martin J. Citardi, M.D., F.A.C.S. Department of Otolaryngology and Communicative Disorders, Cleveland Clinic Foundation, Cleveland, Ohio

Charles V. Edmond, Jr., M.D., F.A.C.S. Clinical Assistant Professor, Department of Otolaryngology–Head and Neck Surgery, University of Washington, Seattle, Washington

Marvin P. Fried, M.D. Professor and University Chairman, Department of Otolaryngology, Albert Einstein College of Medicine and Montefiore Medical Center, Bronx, New York

Liangge Hsu, M.D. Staff Neuroradiologist, Department of Radiology, Brigham and Women's Hospital, Harvard Medical School, Boston, Massachusetts

John K. Joe, M.D. Clinical Fellow, Head and Neck Oncology, Memorial Sloan-Kettering Cancer Center, New York, New York

Stephanie A. Joe, M.D. Lecturer and Clinical Fellow, Department of Otolarynogology–Head and Neck Surgery, University of Pennsylvania Health System, Philadelphia, Pennsylvania

Alex A. Kane, M.D. Assistant Professor, Division of Plastic and Reconstructive Surgery, Department of Surgery, Washington University School of Medicine, St. Louis, Missouri

David W. Kennedy, M.D., F.R.C.S.I. Professor and Chair, Department of Otorhinolarynogology–Head and Neck Surgery, University of Pennsylvania Health System, Philadelphia, Pennsylvania

Ludger Klimek, M.D., Ph.D. Professor of Rhinology and Allergy, Department of Otolaryngology,University of Heidelberg, Weisbaden, Germany

Contributors

Mimi S. Kokoska, M.D. Department of Otolaryngology–Head and Neck Surgery, Indiana University School of Medicine, Indianapolis, Indiana

Frederick A. Kuhn, M.D., F.A.C.S. Director, Georgia Nasal & Sinus Institute, Savannah, Georgia

Ronald B. Kuppersmith, M.D. Section of Otolaryngology–Head and Neck Surgery, Virginia Mason Medical Center, Seattle, Washington

Keith A. Laycock, Ph.D. Jean H. Bakewell Section of Image Guided Surgery, Division of Neurological Surgery, Department of Surgery, Saint Louis University School of Medicine, St. Louis, Missouri

Lun-Jou Lo, M.D. Associate Professor, Department of Plastic and Reconstructive Surgery, Chang Gung Memorial Hospital and Chang Gung Medical College, Taipei, Taiwan

Jeffrey L. Marsh, M.D. Appoline Blair St. Louis Children's Hospital Professor of Surgery, Professor of Radiology in Research, and Professor of Pediatrics in Surgery, Department of Plastic Surgery, Washington University School of Medicine and St. Louis Children's Hospital, St. Louis, Missouri

Ralph B. Metson, M.D. Associate Clinical Professor, Department of Otology and Laryngology, Harvard Medical School, and Department of Otolaryngology, Massachusetts Eye and Ear Infirmary, Boston, Massachusetts

Ralph Mösges, M.D., M.S.E.E. Professor of Otolaryngology, University of Cologne, Cologne, Germany

Thong H. Nguyen, M.D. Associate Clinical Professor, Department of Radiology, University of California, Irvine, Orange, and Chief, MRI and Neuroradiology, Veterans Affairs Medical Center, Long Beach, California

James N. Palmer, M.D. Assistant Professor, Department of Otorhinolaryngology–Head and Neck Surgery, University of Pennsylvania Health System, Philadelphia, Pennsylvania

Joseph M. Rosen, M.D. Division of Plastic and Reconstructive Surgery, Dartmouth-Hitchcock Medical Center and Dartmouth College, Hanover, Lebanon, New Hampshire

Eric W. Sargent, M.D., F.A.C.S. Michigan Ear Institute, Farmington Hills, Michigan

Petra Schmalbrock, Ph.D. Assistant Professor, Department of Radiology, The Ohio State University College of Medicine and Public Health, Columbus, Ohio

Michael J. Sillers, M.D., F.A.C.S. Associate Professor, Division of Otolaryngology/Head and Neck Surgery, Department of Surgery, University of Alabama—Birmingham, Birmingham, Alabama

Marcus K. Simpson Research Assistant, Dartmouth College, Hanover, New Hampshire

Madeleine A. Spatola, M.A. Thomas Jefferson University Medical School, Philadelphia, Pennsylvania

Don Stredney Director, Interface Laboratory, and Senior Research Scientist, Biomedical Applications, Ohio Supercomputer Center (OSC), Columbus, Ohio

Winston C. Vaughan, M.D. Associate Professor, Stanford Sinus Center, Division of Otolaryngology–Head and Neck Surgery, Stanford University, Stanford, California

Gregory J. Wiet, M.D. Assistant Professor, Division of Pediatric Otolaryngology, Department of Otolaryngology, The Ohio State University College of Medicine and Public Health, and Chief, Department of Otolaryngology, Columbus Children's Hospital, Columbus, Ohio

Eiji Yanagisawa, M.D., F.A.C.S. Clinical Professor, Section of Otolaryngology, Yale University School of Medicine and Attending Otolaryngologist, Yale–New Haven Hospital and Hospital of St. Raphael, New Haven, Connecticut

Ray Yanagisawa, B.A. Woodbridge, Connecticut

S. James Zinreich, M.D. Associate Professor, Radiology/Otolaryngology–Head and Neck Surgery, Department of Radiology, Johns Hopkins Medical Institutions, Baltimore, Maryland

1

New Paradigm

Martin J. Citardi, M.D., F.A.C.S.
Cleveland Clinic Foundation, Cleveland, Ohio

1.1 INTRODUCTION

Throughout history, progress in medicine has reflected the technological improvements in the civilization that medicine serves. That observation is intuitively correct; after all, physicians can only utilize the tools available to them. For instance, the discoveries that led to the Industrial Revolution also supported the foundation of modern medicine. Today the Digital Age is supplanting the Industrial Age, and digital technologies (namely, computer-based systems and communications and all of their different manifestations) are similarly guiding a new era in medicine.

The impact of the Digital Age upon medicine cannot be underestimated. Because the underlying technology advances at an increasing rate, the importance of computers in medicine will certainly expand dramatically. In recognition of these changes, physicians have begun to adopt this technology and even integrate it into the delivery of patient care. The application of digital technology to the diagnosis and treatment of disease has begun to revolutionize medicine.

For the surgical fields, the Digital Age is already reshaping how surgery is practiced. To understand these changes, one must assess the constituent processes that underlie the surgical care of patients.

1.2 PATIENT CARE MODEL

At the most elemental level, surgeons complete distinct, albeit related processes as they care for patients (Figure 1.1):

Data Collection. During the data collection phase, the surgeon performs a variety of maneuvers to collect relevant information. Traditional methods include a detailed history and physical examination. Today, testing methods, such as diagnostic imaging, are also performed.

Diagnosis. Next, the surgeon must review the information and establish a diagnosis. The collective knowledge base of medicine and the surgeon's clinical intuition guides this process.

Planning. After a diagnosis has been established, the surgeon formulates a plan of treatment. Planning incorporates information from medicine's knowledge base. In addition, the surgeon's professional experiences influence planning. Of course, all planning is tailored to the particular patient's care.

Execution. During the next phase, the surgeon then implements the plan of treatment. For surgeons, this typically involves a surgical procedure that reflects available medical technology.

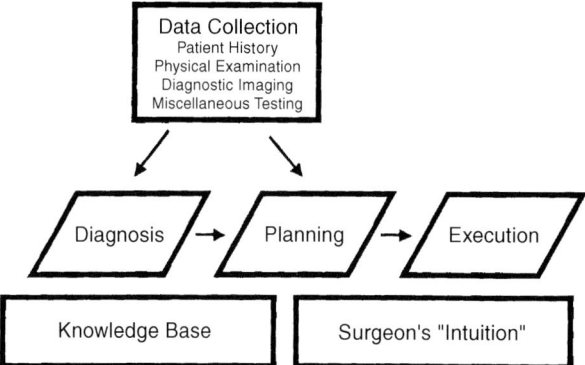

FIGURE 1.1 The surgical care of patients encompasses four distinct processes. During data collection, the surgeon collects relevant clinical information through routine history and physical examination, diagnostic imaging, and other testing modalities. Next, a formal diagnosis is established, and treatment planning commences. Finally, the treatment is instituted during the remaining phase. Each phase need not be sequential. In fact, data collection leads directly to the diagnosis and planning phases, and the execution phase is monitored via additional data collection. Each phase relies upon the knowledge base of medicine and the surgeon's clinical intuition.

New Paradigm

It is important to realize that these various phases of surgical practice are not necessarily performed sequentially. Commonly, these cognitive processes occur simultaneously. Information acquired during the data collection phase directly influences both the diagnosis and planning phases. Furthermore, the surgeon will continuously reassess new information during the execution phase. In this way, data collection is a continuous process that occurs throughout the delivery of care. In addition, the planning and execution phases are typically simultaneous in a feedback loop that permits modification of the treatment plan in response to new information. Of course, this new data may be specific to a particular patient (i.e., clinical information). Alternatively, the new information that is added to the collective knowledge base of medicine may impact the treatment plan.

Two critical components influence the phases of data collection, diagnosis, planning, and execution. First, the knowledge base of medicine provides the fundamental information about the various disease processes, testing modalities, procedures, etc. The knowledge base has been increasing rapidly; in fact, the explosive growth of the biological sciences and medicine is actually accelerating. Second, the surgeon's intuition guides him or her through the process of patient care delivery. For each patient encounter, the surgeon relies upon previous personal observations and experiences. In a sense, this "fuzzy logic" combines both deductive and inductive reasoning. By its very nature, it is difficult to characterize, but its impact is undeniable—it supplies the so-called art in the art of medicine.

The surgical care of patients reflects the prevailing technology of the time in which the care is delivered. First, imagine medicine in the preindustrial age. The planning phases consisted mostly of history and physical examination. Modalities such as radiography were unavailable, and the knowledge base was small. Available treatment options were limited. The technology provided by the Industrial Revolution revolutionized this. Diagnostic testing, such as radiography, was introduced, and the information in the knowledge base increased dramatically. Other technological advances, such as the introduction of general anesthesia, greatly increased the treatment options.

For surgeons, the technological impact of the past 150 years is perhaps best seen in diagnostic imaging. Without even plain radiography, physicians could only infer the status of internal body parts. In the late nineteenth century, the discovery of x-rays and their application to medicine began to give physicians the ability to assess issues in vivo that they could not directly observe. The significance of this change cannot be underestimated. Strategies that extended the usefulness of radiography were developed. For instance, the administration of contrast for barium enemas or upper gastrointestinal (GI) series permitted the observation of soft-tissue pathology that standard plain films do not. Similarly, arteriography provided detailed vascular anatomy that would otherwise be unknown (unless a formal surgical exploration was performed). Later, diagnostic radiography technology was adapted for therapeutic interventions (such as transarterial embolization). Finally, in the last third of the twentieth century, computed tomography (CT) and magnetic resonance (MR) were introduced; these diagnostic imaging modalities provide information that plain x-ray films simply cannot. As CT and MR became widely available and as physicians became familiar with them, they dramatically altered the delivery of care to patients.

The technological advances in diagnostic imaging have dramatically altered the data collection, diagnosis, planning, and execution phases of surgical care. CT and MR (and even advanced plain film radiography) provide better information for diagnosis; this information was heretofore unavailable. Furthermore, this information facilitates the creation of a more realistic surgical plan.

All of theses advances provide the surgeon with additional information, which the surgeon must then assemble for diagnosis and treatment. Better images only provide better information; the understanding of their significance requires a difficult cognitive process. After creation of the treatment plan, the surgeon must then implement this plan. This requires further extrapolation from the original data. Each step in this process introduces potential sources of error and may overlook critical information that may not be readily apparent.

As the available information for patient evaluation has grown, the complexity of treatment methods has also grown dramatically. Techniques such as minimally invasive procedures demand exquisite technical expertise.

It is for these numerous reasons, that the surgeon needs better tools for the management of this information. Computer-aided surgery (CAS) answers this need.

1.3 TERMINOLOGY

The term computer-aided surgery first appeared in the German scientific literature in 1986 [1]. Over the subsequent 15 years, a variety of other terms have appeared. Some authors have referred to *computer-assisted surgery*, and in the United States and Japan, the phrase *image-guided surgery* has been applied to surgical navigation in endoscopic sinus surgery. This abundance of terminology has led to some fragmentation of the field; however, *computer-aided surgery* (CAS) has emerged as the preferred term.

The problem with terminology was readily apparent in the early and mid-1990s. At that time, interest in the area was beginning to grow significantly. It was in this context that the International Society for Computer-Aided Surgery (ISCAS, *www.iscas.org* or *http://igs.slu.edu*) was established in 1996. The society created an organized forum for the exchange of ideas and the support of technological and clinical development. By its choice of name, ISCAS also promoted a term for the various manifestations of the underlying technologies.

ISCAS has proposed a rather broad definition for CAS [2]: ''The scope of Computer-Aided Surgery encompasses all fields within surgery, as well as biomedical imaging and instrumentation, and digital technology employed as an adjunct to imaging in diagnosis, therapeutics, and surgery. Topics featured include frameless as well as conventional stereotactic procedures, surgery guided by ultrasound, image-guided focal irradiation, robotic surgery, and other therapeutic interventions that are performed with the use of digital imaging technology.'' The unifying theme in each of these applications of CAS is that they are all semiconductor-based. The basic advances in semiconductor technology—which are driving the transition to the Digital Age—underlie CAS in all its specific applications. The increasing prevalence of computers and communications in the nonmedical world is reflected in the medical world.

The other terms, such as computer-assisted surgery, or image-guided surgery, are probably best used to describe specific areas within CAS. For instance, computer-assisted surgery encompasses surgical robotics, which is only a small part of the entire discipline of CAS. Similarly, image-guided surgery refers to intraoperative surgical navigation, but not to areas such as telesurgery. CAS includes both computer-assisted surgery and image-guided surgery. The converse statements that computer-assisted surgery includes CAS and that image-guided surgery includes CAS are simply inaccurate.

1.4 SCOPE OF CAS

Admittedly, the scope of CAS is quite broad. Today, many surgeons would state that intraoperative surgical navigation is CAS. Such conclusions overlook other important technologies, including, but not limited to robotics, telesurgery, virtual reality, computer-based simulations/modeling, and internet-based applications.

CAS has huge implications for the processes that constitute contemporary surgical care. Information management—which is obviously facilitated by computers—occurs throughout the various phases of surgical care. Surgeons must manipulate information from two sources. First, the knowledge base of medicine is continuously expanding. Second, patient information that is specific to a particular patient must be systematically organized and critical reviewed. Computers, which after all are simply complex information appliances, contribute to all aspects of this information management. Desktop and laptop computers, personal digital assistants, and network appliances are just some of the devices that are impacting this area. The Internet, which provides a decentralized but easily accessible store of vast quantities of information, has also emerged as important information management tool.

Furthermore, these technologies provide organization for the vast quantities of information. Without such organization, the information may become meaningless; with such information, the hidden patterns (that would otherwise go unnoticed) may become apparent. In this way, the structure provided by these various information management technologies may positively influence patient care.

Computer-enabled therapeutics fuses computer-based technologies into treatment modalities. A variety of telesurgery platforms have been proposed over the years. The early systems showed considerable promise; however, their expense was considerable and their use was extremely cumbersome. Newer applications, which rely upon digital imaging and communications (i.e., the Internet) show considerable promise. Robotic-assisted surgery devices are now under development; such devices will likely enhance surgical precision. Such robotics also may permit procedures that would otherwise be impossible. Virtual reality display systems may present imaging data to surgeons in ways that facilitate minimally invasive procedures with lower morbidity and higher success rates. Computer-based models depict three-dimensional anatomy and pathology. The quality of the resultant images has improved dramatically over the recent years. Now such models are beginning to be used for surgical simulations.

Intraoperative surgical navigation is probably the most widely utilized CAS therapeutic application. Through surgical navigation, the operating surgeon can directly relate preoperative imaging data (namely CT or MR) with intraoperative anatomy. This remarkable technology relies upon technology that permits tracking of surgical instruments with millimetric or even submillimetric accuracy.

These surgical navigation systems share a number of common components (Figure 1.2):

> *Computer workstation.* Early CAS systems relied upon relatively complex computer workstations that were optimized for image processing; however, more recently, PC-based computers have been used. Most CAS systems rely upon the UNIX operating system, although Windows 98, Windows NT, and Windows 2000 are increasingly common. Obviously, the computer workstation is the central component of CAS surgical navigation.
>
> *Display systems.* Current CAS navigation systems utilize a standard computer monitor; other display options, including head-mounted displays or other techniques, are under active development (Figure 1.3).
>
> *Tracking system.* Surgical navigation must include specific hardware for the tracking of surgical instruments. In the late 1980s and early 1990s, instrument tracking via an electromechanical arm was popular; such systems were quite accurate, but they were also cumbersome. More recent systems rely upon optical tracking or electromagnetic tracking. Of course, each particular technology has its own relative advantages and disadvantages. All of these technologies accomplish the same result; that is, they permit the precise localization of instruments in the operative field.
>
> *Specific surgical instrumentation.* Initially, CAS surgical navigation systems provided pointers that could be used for identification of relevant

New Paradigm

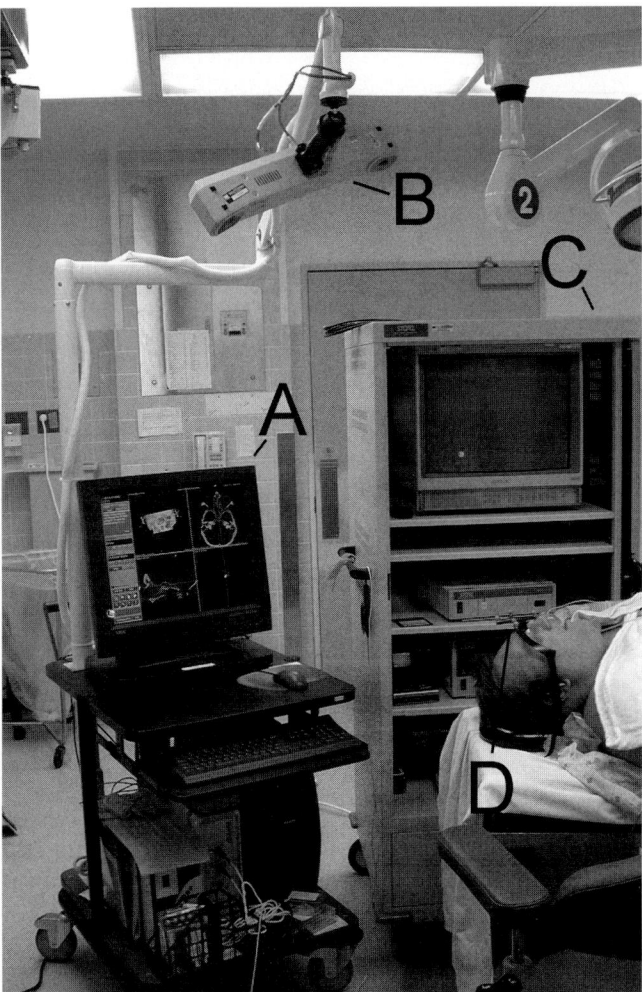

FIGURE 1.2 The basic CAS surgical navigation system includes a computer workstation (A) and tracking system. This representative system (SAVANT .85, CBYON Corporation, Palo Alto, CA) utilizes an optical tracking system. An overhead camera array (B) tracks the relative positions of reflective spheres that are attached to surgical instruments and the surgical field. The SAVANT system is separate from the video tower (C), which is used for endoscopic sinus surgery. The patient wears a special headset to which a dynamic reference frame [also known as a DRF (D)] is mounted; the camera array recognizes and tracks a series of reflective spheres on the DRF.

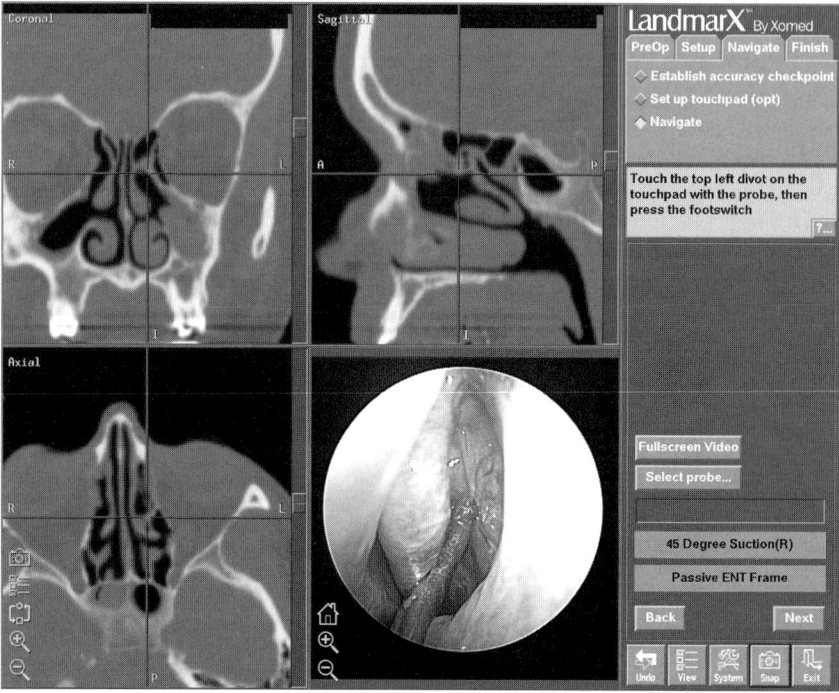

FIGURE 1.3 The CAS surgical navigation system monitor depicts localization data by displaying crosshairs on the preoperative CT images. In this example (LandmarX 3.0, Medtronic Xomed, Jacksonville, FL), the main part of the display is divided into four quadrants, which show the planar CT data (axial, coronal and sagittal planes) in the three orthogonal planes through the calculated location as well as a video input that displays to the location of the pointer tip. The display can be customized for the specific application; surgical planning modes can be shown in the place of the fourth quadrant. The CAS surgical navigation system can be controlled via a variety of menus shown on the right side of the image. Although this display arrangement is probably the most common, other options are also possible.

structures. Today, a variety of standard instruments (such as forceps) have been adapted so that their positions can also be tracked. Even the positions of surgical drills and microdebriders can be monitored through surgical navigation. The use of standard surgical tools has greatly expanded the role of surgical navigation during surgical procedures.

Data transfer hardware. Preoperative imaging data (i.e., the CT or MR) must be transferred to the computer workstation. Such data transfers may

New Paradigm

be accomplished through computer networks that link the scanner and the CAS workstation. Alternatively, the data sets can be transferred on portable digital media, such as DAT tape or CD-ROM.

Software. Finally, software unifies the various hardware components into a functional system. Through software interfaces, surgeons have access to the imaging data and the entire CAS system.

Surgical navigation systems all rely upon two processes that much be successfully executed prior to actual intraoperative use:

Calibration. The desired surgical instrument must be calibrated. Calibration verifies that the anticipate instrument tip position and the actual instrument tip position are identical. Calibration failure will produce significant localization errors.

Registration. All surgical navigation systems require a registration step. Through registration, the software maps points in the preoperative imaging data set volume to the corresponding points in the operative field volume. All further localizations are actually positions that are determined relative to these points. Registration is maintained by keeping a tracking device in the identical position relative to the operative field throughout the entire surgical procedure. In principle, registration is a simple concept; however, in practice registration is challenging, since registration must be accurate, but not intrusive. Multiple registration strategies have been devised. Each of these strategies has been optimized for a specific surgical application.

Although CAS surgical navigation systems are surprisingly simple to use, surgeons must be cognizant of potential errors. Registration errors can produce significant localization inaccuracies. Furthermore, all systems are prone to drift from a variety of causes. For this reason, CAS navigation systems include localization accuracy mechanisms so that the localization accuracy can be monitored (Figure 1.4).

Finally, CAS surgical navigation systems usually include software tools that permit image review, modeling, and surgical planning (Figure 1.5). Because of the importance of surgical navigation, surgeons tend to overlook these other features; however, these tools can be useful in specific circumstances. Using the tools, the surgeon can develop a better understanding of specific three-dimensional anatomical relationships (Figure 1.6). It should be emphasized that the tools can often be adapted for situations for which they were not designed. When surgeons pursue these novel applications, the utility of the CAS system is naturally extended.

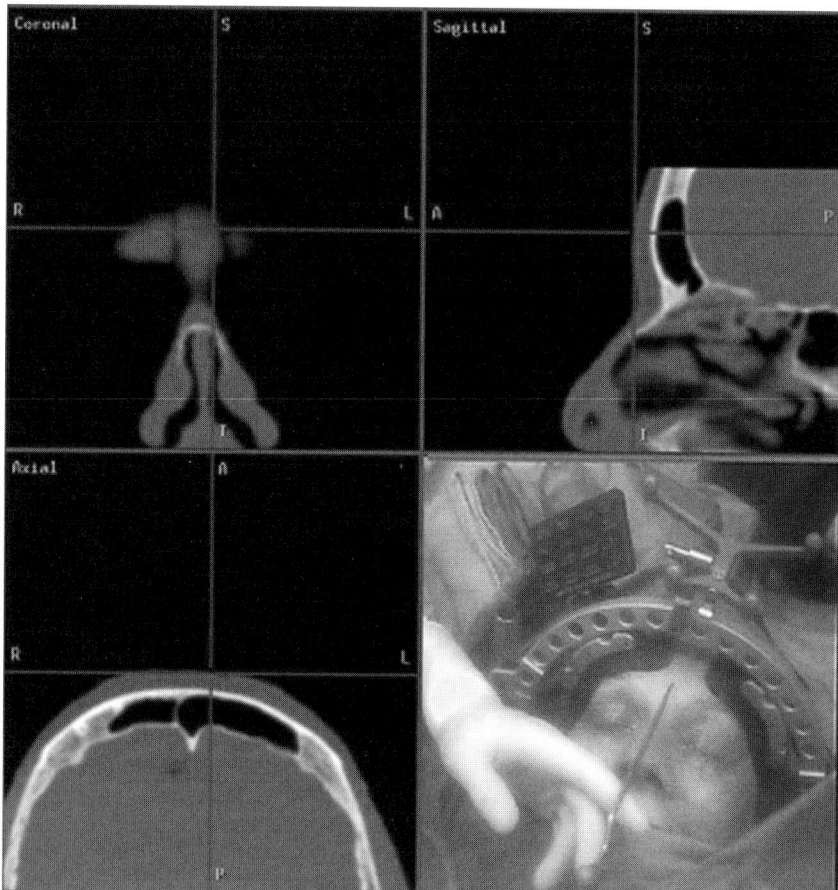

FIGURE 1.4 Registration accuracy must be monitored throughout the entire procedure. Typically localizing to known landmarks can do this; the surgeon then must review the calculated localization and corroborate its accuracy. The surgical navigation platforms typically will provide calculated estimates of registration accuracy. Although such numbers are helpful, they can be misleading. For this reason, the best measure of surgical navigation accuracy is a surgeon's own judgment. It is also important to realize that surgical navigation and registration accuracy can vary at different points in the operating field volume. In this example (LandmarX 3.0, Medtronic Xomed, Jacksonville, FL), acceptable registration accuracy has been achieved.

New Paradigm

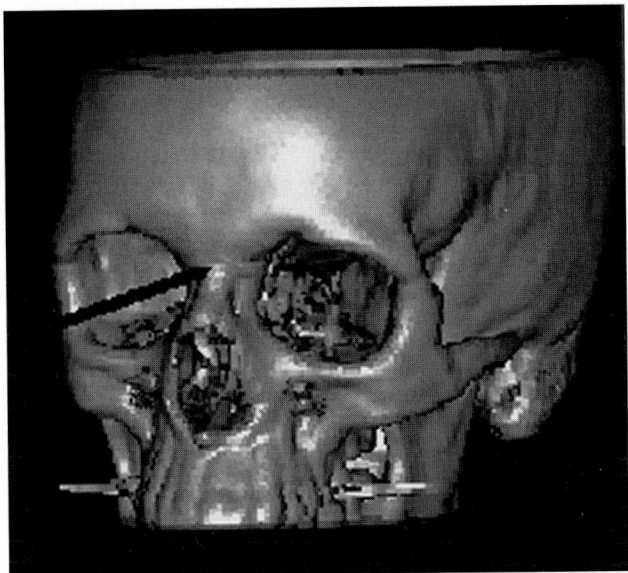

FIGURE 1.5 CAS platforms provide software tools that semi-automatically create accurate three-dimensional models from two-dimensional CT data. This model was made within several minutes on the StealthStation Cranial 3.0 system (Medtronic Surgical Navigation Technologies, Louisville, CO). Before this technology was available, models were not as good, and the process of creating models was time-consuming, expensive, and difficult.

1.5 NEW PARADIGM

The surgical endeavor encompasses distinct but overlapping phases of data collection, diagnosis, planning, and execution. These processes draw upon the collective knowledge base of medicine as well as the surgeon's intuition. CAS in its various manifestations can positively influence each of these various aspects of surgical care.

Since the advent of modern medicine in the late nineteenth century, physicians have sought methods to peer within body spaces. It was accurately believed that visualization would yield more accurate diagnosis and more effective treatment. Eventually, technology began to provide the means for visualization within body spaces—CT and MR provide anatomical information that would have been unimaginable 50 years ago. In addition, minimally invasive surgical techniques, which rely upon telescopes and other optical devices, provide phenomenal surgical access through tiny "portholes." All of this technology still requires a great

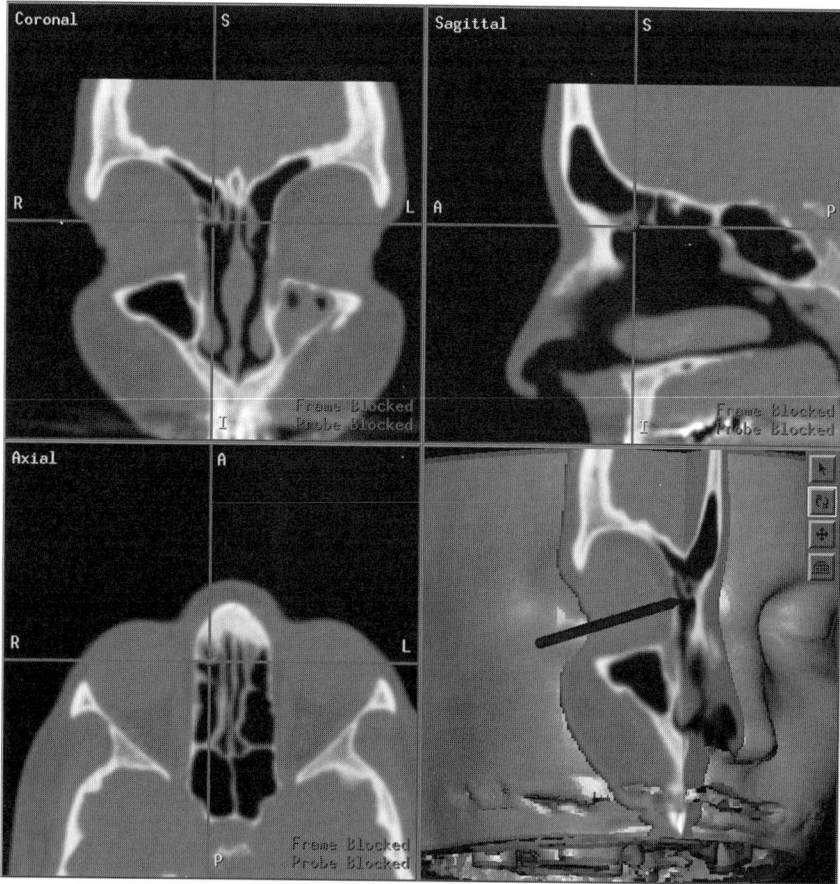

FIGURE 1.6 The software tools that are offered with CAS surgical navigation systems provide unique perspectives that traditional approaches do not. In this instance, LandmarX 3.0 (Medtronic Xomed, Jacksonville, FL) provides a coronal-sagittal "cut" view that highlights the complex frontal recess pneumatization pattern in this patient. Standard coronal CT views do not portray the depth that this "cut" view shows.

deal of mental extrapolation by the surgeon—unless CAS is employed. For instance, the surgeon must mentally reconstruct three-dimensional relationships from two-dimensional planar imaging data, and then this mental model must be applied to the surgical field. Furthermore, minimally invasive surgery relies upon two-dimensional images afforded by surgical endoscopes. Each level of extrapolation introduces potential errors and inaccuracies.

CAS should be considered another tool for the surgeon. CAS provides easy ways to manipulate and view imaging data, and the resultant understanding that the surgeon garners from such manipulations can be directly applied in the operating room through surgical navigation. In these ways, CAS makes the surgical endeavor more precise.

Furthermore, CAS expands the capabilities of surgical care. By providing new vistas on imaging data, CAS can yield previously unrecognized information. CAS also may facilitate delicate surgical procedures. The next generation of CAS platforms will doubtlessly advance surgical care as surgeons recognize the limitations of current technologies, and engineers develop new solutions.

Surgeons can also use computer-based technologies for the more mundane aspects of patient care. The quantity of information is simply immense. Traditional paper records, files and books cannot adequately store this material in a simple way that facilitates retrieval and use. Computers, and more specifically, computer-based communications (such as the Internet), have an obvious role.

The emphasis on the physician-surgeon as an information manager should not dehumanize the delivery of patient care. The amount of information that guides each patient encounter is overwhelming; it is undeniable that even routine medical care now relies upon ever-increasing amounts of medical information. Without specific measures, this avalanche of information will overwhelm the humanistic aspects of the patient-physician relationship.

The mere use of computers does not exacerbate this problem; in fact, computer-based technologies, by offering efficient means for information management, may represent a solution to the information avalanche. CAS applications do not dehumanize the patient-physician relationship; in fact, by increasing available physician time, they may reinject a traditional humanistic element in patient care.

CAS should not be dismissed as a novelty item. CAS applications are diverse and powerful, and they will influence surgical practice for many years. In many ways, the introduction and widespread adoption of CAS will revolutionize how surgeons care for patients.

CAS is an enabling technology. It provides a means for the collection, organization, and manipulation of information and images. CAS will never substitute for the physician in the patient-physician relationship, and it will never replace surgical expertise. In the end, surgeons will rely upon CAS so that they can deliver better patient care.

The technological developments that are powering CAS are leading to new models for diagnosis, disease management, and surgical procedures. Increasingly surgeons are now integrating CAS platforms into their practices. The resultant CAS-driven paradigm represents a critical advance in contemporary surgery, since CAS provides solutions to current challenges and opens new diagnostic and therapeutic vistas for patient care.

REFERENCES

1. Reinhardt H, Meyer H, Amrein E. Computer-aided surgery: Robotik für Hirnoperationen? Polypscope plus 1986; 6:1–6.
2. International Society for Computer-Aided Surgery. Computer-aided surgery: aims and scope. www.iscas.org/aims.html 1999.

2
Historical Perspective

Jack B. Anon, M.D., F.A.C.S.
University of Pittsburgh School of Medicine,
Pittsburgh, Pennsylvania

Ludger Klimek, M.D., Ph.D.
University of Heidelberg, Weisbaden, Germany

Ralph Mösges, M.D., M.S.E.E.
University of Cologne, Cologne, Germany

2.1 FRAMED STEREOTAXY DEVELOPMENT

Stereotactic surgery was first performed to drain abscesses, destroy discrete portions of the cerebrum for the alleviation of pain, perform psychosurgical manipulations, and decrease involuntary tremors. The history of these procedures goes back for many years. Speigel and Wycis were the first to clinically develop and use a stereotactic device in 1947. In the ensuing years, a multitude of instruments were devised. Most of these stereotactic frames were calibrated using plain-film radiographs, anatomical landmarks, and standardized anatomical atlases of the brain. After the computed tomography (CT) scanner was introduced, a number of institutions began applying the new imaging technology to stereotactic surgery and radiotherapy.

In 1976, Bergstrom and Greitz devised a helmet-like plastic fixation device [1]. With this custom-fitted device in place, a metal trajectory ring was placed on the patient's head, and a CT scan was obtained. Limited intracranial instru-

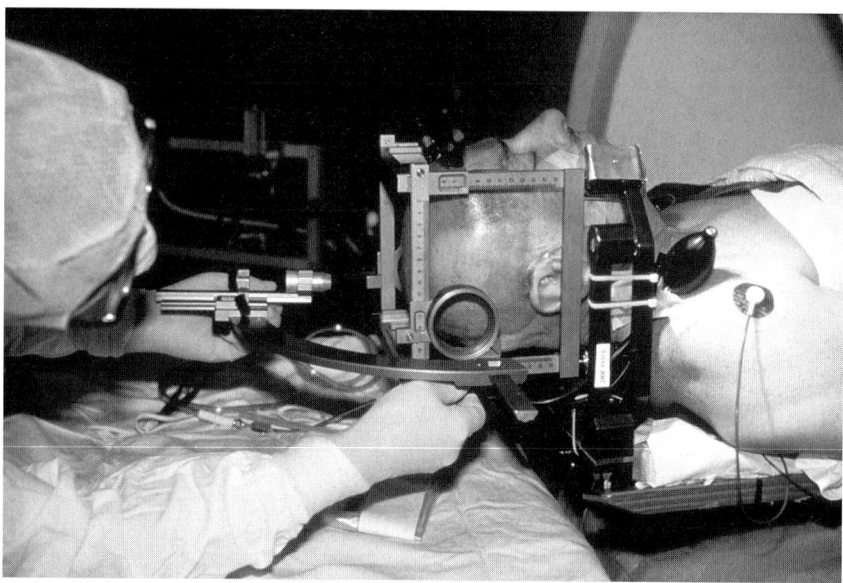

FIGURE 2.1 The rigid stereotactic frame is placed on the patient's head. A CT scan is then performed, and a surgical trajectory can be planned based on coordinate markings.

mentation could then be accomplished. Several years later, Brown developed a system that utilized an acrylic frame and CT data with three-dimensional graphics [2]. In 1980, Perry et al. described a CT-dependent frame with diagonal rods that served as fiducial reference points for the scanner computers. Since stereotaxis was accomplished in the CT scanner itself, repeat scans could be obtained during surgery to confirm the position of the probe tip.

Over the next few years, a variety of framed stereotactic systems were described. Although the equipment was modified, the basic concept of using a rigid frame attached to the patient's head remained constant (Figure 2.1). This strategy carried intrinsic limitations. First, it impeded the approach to the operative site. Furthermore, while an instrument could be positioned along the planned trajectory path, the actual position of the instrument tip was not known.

2.2 FRAMELESS STEREOTACTIC COMPUTER SYSTEMS

Roberts et al. published one of the first reports on a frameless navigational system in 1986 [4]. The patient underwent a preoperative CT scan with three radiopaque glass beads (which served as fiducial markers) taped to his or her head. Then,

Historical Perspective

data from this CT scan were transferred into an IBM PC XT computer located in the operating room. This computer was linked to an operating microscope that had been outfitted with an acoustic localizer. In the operating room, the microscope was fixed on each of the three fiducial markers, and a sonic digitizer recorded their unique positions. The position of the patient relative to the microscope could be calculated through triangulation. The reformatted CT scan was projected through the microscope to the surgeon's eye via a small television monitor. While this frameless device was less cumbersome than framed systems, its accuracy was somewhat lacking (average: 2.0 mm; range: 0.7–6.0 mm).

Watanabe et al. devised the Neuronavigator, a three-dimensional digitizer that had a jointed arm with a surgical probe [5]. The six freely mobile arm joints each contained a potentiometer. Based on the known arm segment lengths and data from the potentiometers, the intraoperative computer (PC-9801E; NEC, Japan) could calculate the relationships of the segments to each other and thus accurately determine the probe tip position. Before surgery, three metal fiducials fiducial markers were placed on the patient's face, and a CT scan was obtained at 10 mm slice thicknesses (2–5 mm thickness for small lesions). Hard copy images were then scanned into the computer. The position sensor arm was used to correlate the patient's intraoperative position to the CT scans. The average error of this system in the operating room was 3 mm.

In 1988, Reinhardt et al. reported on a computerized digitizing arm composed of three aluminum shells containing four potentiometers [6]. Data from the potentiometers were analyzed by an Apple IIE computer (Apple, Cupertino, CA) and then overlaid on a preoperative CT scan imaged by a video camera. The patient's position on the operating table was correlated using plastic fiducial rods attached to a rigid headrest. A clinical accuracy of 2 mm was reported.

The concept of stereotactic surgery was clearly described in 1991 by Guthrie and Adler [7]. They noted that when a digital image of a patient is obtained by CT scanning or magnetic resonance imaging (MRI), any point within the digital image space can be assigned an x, y, or z value, known as a "image coordinate." The correlation requires a minimum of three noncolinear points common to both the image space and the stereotactic (i.e., patient) space.

Guthrie (personal communication) became disenchanted with framed stereotaxis because "the frame dictated the case," rather than acting as an aid to the surgeon. Thus, work was undertaken on the Operating Arm System (Radionics, Boston, MA), an optically encoded multijointed arm coupled to a computer (Silicon Graphics, Mountain View, CA). In this system, skin staples were placed as fiducial markers on the patient's scalp, and then a preoperative CT scan was obtained. In the operating room, registration (namely the mapping of the image space with the patient space) was accomplished by touching the staples in a specific order. The computer matched the CT coordinates of the staples with the coordinates received by the operating arm, and the position of the probe tip was shown as a cursor on the computer screen. The reported accuracy of the system was better than 3 mm.

In 1991, Watanabe et al. reported on the use of a new Neuronavigator system for neurosurgery in 68 patients [8]. The authors believed that their maximum intraoperative error of 2.5 mm was acceptable. The upgraded Neuronavigator Version II (Mizuho Medical Co., Ltd., Tokyo) incorporated the Microsoft Windows 3.2 operating system along with several new features, including a target alarm (Figure 2.2). As the probe approached the target (e.g., tumor), an alarm sounded to indicate close proximity to the target.

Kato et al. described an electromagnetic digitizer for used in computer-assisted neurosurgery in 1991 [9]. Preoperatively, plastic tubes filled with contrast material were placed at four points for a fiducial reference system, and a CT or MRI scan was obtained. Slices of 5 mm thickness were obtained, and a maximum of 24 image slices could be loaded into the computer system. In the operating room, a magnetic field source was attached to the patient, and a sensing probe was used to calibrate the patient's position. Experience with 10 neurosurgical patients demonstrated an accuracy of about 4 mm.

Also in 1991, Leggett et al., who were employees of ISG Technologies, reported their work with the Viewing Wand (ISG Technologies, Mississauga, Ontario, Canada), a localizer that had a six-jointed counterbalanced arm with a sterilizable distal probe (Figure 2.3) [10]. An accuracy of 2–3 mm was reported for skull-base tumor resection, optic nerve decompression, and transphenoidal biopsy. Using a plastic human skull and a custom-designed Plexiglas™ phantom, Zinreich et al. found the Viewing Wand comparable in accuracy to framed stereotactic systems [11].

In a system described by Laborde et al., 50 to 70 2 mm CT slices were reformatted into a three-dimensional (3D) virtual image prior to neurosurgery [12]. For preoperative planning, new software allowed the virtual model to be manipulated so that the surgeon could see the relationship of the pathology to the surrounding tissues. The intraoperative accuracy of 3 mm was enhanced by repeating the registration process.

Barnett et al. published a preliminary report on a frameless, armless system with four components: a probe with two ultrasonic emitters, a receiver microphone array fixed to the operating table, hardware for the timing and control of signal production and reception, and an intraoperative computer [13]. Before surgery, fiducial markers were placed, and a CT or MRI scan was obtained. Microphones arranged in specific positions on the receiver array detected ultrasonic signals generated sequentially by the probe emitters. Localization of the probe tip was calculated based on the time-interval delay of the emitted pulses. An error of 1.5 mm was reported for the initial five patients, whose preoperative scans had been performed at a slice thickness of 1 mm.

In another article, Barnett et al. reported on the use of an ultrasonic localizer

Historical Perspective

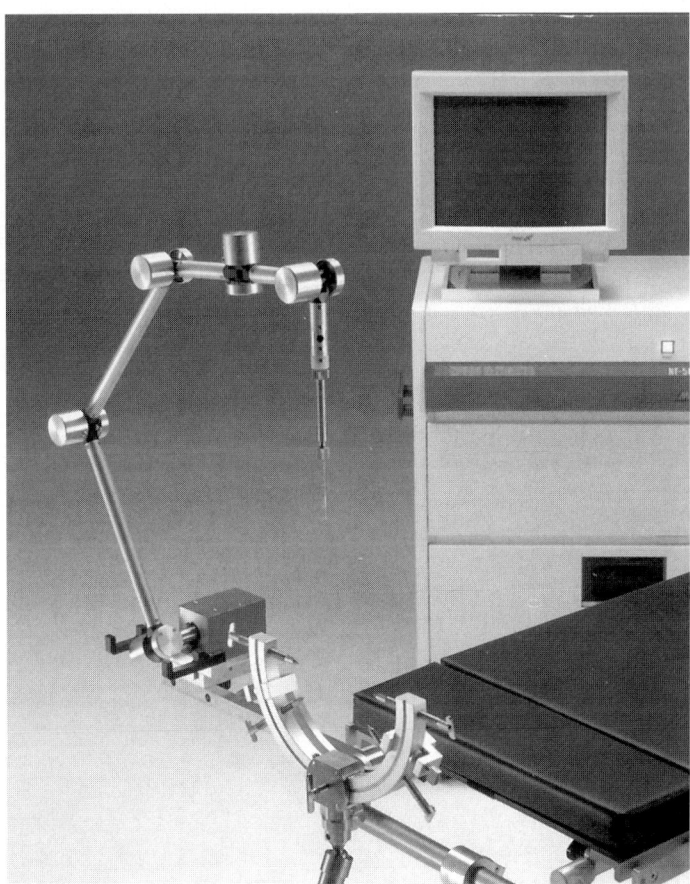

FIGURE 2.2 The Neuronavigator (as developed by Watanabe et al.) incorporated an electromechanical tracking system as well as a computer workstation. The electromechanical arm was rigidly fixated to the operating table, and the patient's head was held rigidly in place.

(COMPASS, Stereotactic Medical Systems, Rochester, MN) in 52 craniotomies [14]. The mean error of the device was 4.8 mm. The authors concluded that although the unit was a reasonable guide for surgery, its imprecision made it unacceptable as a replacement for a framed system.

Klimek et al. in 1993 noted that deep-seated orbital lesions were difficult to access through an endonasal approach and that frameless stereotaxy systems could be advantageous in revision cases or in situations where there was bleeding

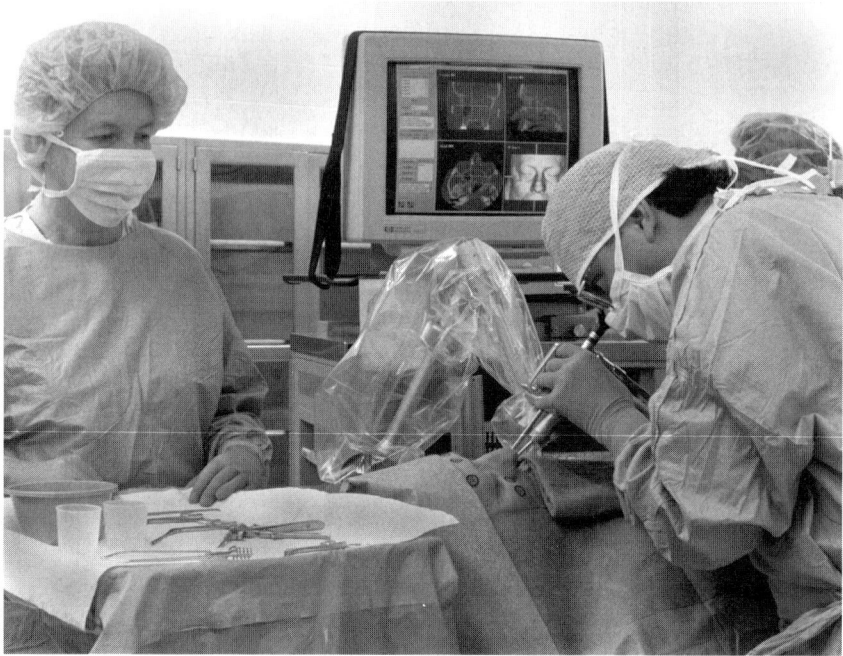

FIGURE 2.3 The ISG Viewing Wand (ISG Technologies, Mississauga, Ontario, Canada) uses an arm-based tracking system. The patient's head must be securely locked into position.

[15]. Using CT scans of 1–2 mm slices, the optical encoder rigid arm had an accuracy of 1 mm in 21 orbital surgeries. The authors felt that the added benefit of orientation outweighed the extra computer registration time and negligible additional operative time.

In 1994 and 1995, other investigators also reported on their experiences with some of the computer-guided systems described above [16–19].

2.3 COMPUTER-AIDED SURGERY IN OTOLARYNGOLOGY

The first experiments using computer-aided surgery (CAS) in the field of otolaryngology were performed at the Aachen University of Technology and the Aachen University Hospital in Germany. In 1986, a group of Aachen investigators described their experience with an industrial passive robot arm (Figure 2.4) [20]. The segments of this arm were connected via five rotary joints. Rotary

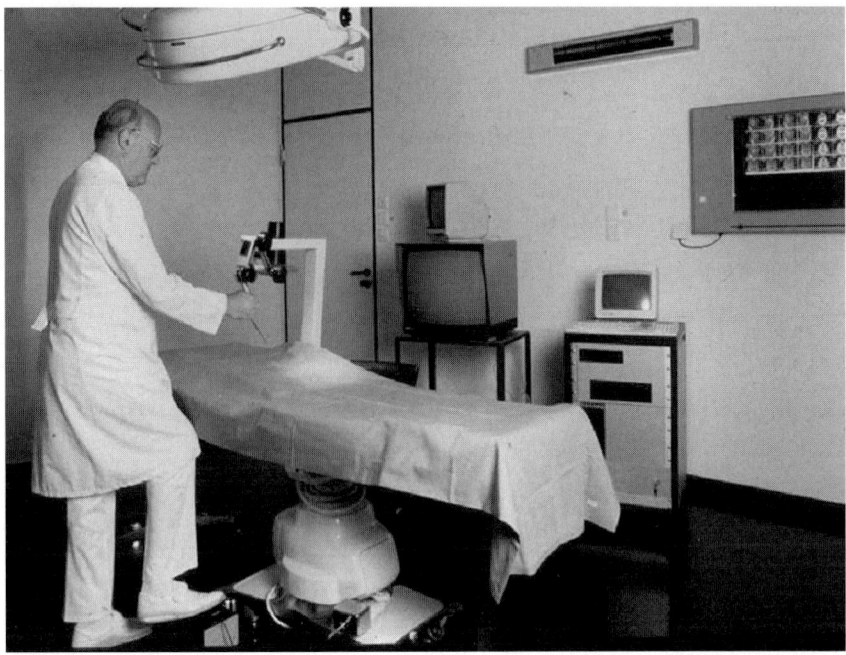

FIGURE 2.4 Professor G. Schlöndorff demonstrates the use of an early Aachen CAS system.

analog potentiometers measured the joint movements and relayed information about the position of the end of the arm to a computer. Hardware and software components were developed to use this robot arm for intraoperative position detection. However, since this device was developed for applications in industry, its handling was cumbersome and its relative inaccuracy (margin of accuracy > 3 mm) was judged insufficient for otolaryngological procedures.

Aachen investigators conducted further research on a counterbalanced six-jointed optical encoder unit linked to a dedicated 68008-microprocessor connected to a main computer. Two-dimensional (2D) data from a preoperative CT scan (2 mm thick slices) were first "merged" to form a 3D cubic "voxel model" with x, y, and z coordinates. This model was displayed on a monitor, along with the original axial (x, y) CT image and the reconstructed coronal (x, z) and sagittal (y, z) views. Four radiopaque reference points were placed on the patient's face before the preoperative CT scan. At surgery, each reference point as visualized on the computer monitor was correlated with the corresponding reference point marked on the patient's face by touching the point with the tip of the digitizer arm. Once all four points were entered, the computer could take any other point on/in the patient (when touched by the tip of the digitizing arm) and match it to the same point on the CT images as displayed on the monitor (shown by a crosshair). This system was used in 64 patients for surgery of the paranasal sinuses, orbit, and skull base, as well as the surgical treatment of central nervous system lesions and lesions within the pterygopalatine fossa. The authors felt that surgery with this CAS platform, which had an accuracy of 1–2 mm, was safer than unaided surgery.

In 1991, the Aachen group updated their experiences in a report on 200 surgical procedures [21]. The indications for CAS were nasal, paranasal sinus, and orbital tumors, skull base procedures, primary and revision paranasal sinus surgery, and acoustic neuromas. The authors also evaluated the risks and benefits of CAS. The risks included extra radiation from the additional CT scan required for the 3D model and the expense of equipment and additional manpower. They noted, however, that the extra radiation dose was minimal and far below the 50% cataract dose. The benefit of CAS was the dramatic increase in surgical information, which led to more efficient surgery and a reduction in operative risks.

Krybus et al. [22], also from Aachen, described the development of an infrared optical localizing probe in 1991. With the infrared free arm, sensors could be attached directly to the operating instruments. Five infrared-emitting diodes were positioned on the handle of an instrument, with three diodes distal to the handle tip and two diodes proximal to it. The distance between these emitters provided for large angles of infrared radiation. Infrared emitters were also attached to the patient. Three sensing cameras were suspended in a circular array 800–1200 mm above the operating table. The position of the instrument tip was located by triangulation calculations based on the known geometry of the infrared diodes on both the instrument and the patient relative to the sensing cameras. The optical localizer took seven measurements per second with a reported accuracy of 1.5 mm. The initial infrared localizing system has since been upgraded.

In 1993, Aachen investigators Mösges and Klimek reported on the application of computer assistance during paranasal sinus surgery [23]. They believed that CAS systems provided helpful intraoperative orientation, especially when there was bleeding or when landmarks were obliterated by tumor or prior surgery. The CT parameters in this report were 1 or 2 mm slice thickness; continuous, nonoverlapping slices; and transverse slices (which avoided dental amalgams). The authors concluded that CAS would reduce the reported 2% complication rate associated with endonasal surgery.

In 1994 Anon et al. published the first report of computer-aided endoscopic sinus surgery in the United States [24]. The ISG Viewing Wand with a 6-inch neuroprobe was utilized in 70 procedures. Using a combination of landmark reg-

Historical Perspective

istration and surface-fitting registration (instead of fiducial marker registration), the authors reported an observed clinical accuracy of 1–2 mm. The indications for CAS included revision cases, massive disease, sphenoid sinus pathology, anomalies such as an Onodi cell, and frontal recess disease.

Carrau et al. also used the Viewing Wand to compare the standard 6-foot Caldwell template with computer guidance for external frontal sinusotomy [25]. The indications for obliteration were frontal sinus fracture (including the frontal recess), severe trauma from a gunshot wound, and chronic frontal sinusitis. The patient's head was secured in a head holder, and registration was performed on landmarks or previously placed fiducial markers. Following exposure of the frontal bone via a bicoronal flap, the 6-foot Caldwell template was placed in position and marked. The Viewing Wand was then used to outline the frontal sinus. The differences between the two techniques ranged from 0 to 1.75 cm (the larger the sinus, the larger the difference). Following the osteotomies, direct visualization into the sinuses showed that the Viewing Wand was more accurate and that penetration into the cranial cavity would have occurred in four of six cases if the template alone had been used.

Gunkel et al. reported on their experiences with the Viewing Wand and the Virtual Patient (ARTMA, Austria), which utilized an electromagnetic digitizer [26]. The transmitter was placed close to the patient's head, and the sensor was attached to various surgical instruments and/or an endoscope. A unique feature of the Virtual Patient system was the ability to decide on the surgical trajectory by marking specific areas on the displayed CT scans along the planned course of surgery. During the operation, colored rectangular frames (representing the trajectory) were superimposed onto the endoscopic view seen on the monitor, thus forming a "highway" for the surgeon to follow. An accuracy of 1.0–2.5 mm was reported for the Viewing Wand. The Virtual Patient system was also quite accurate.

In 1995, Anon et al. updated their experiences with the arm-based Viewing Wand and also introduced the FlashPoint Model 5000 3-D Optical Localizer (Image-Guided Technologies, Boulder, CO) (Figure 2.5) [27]. The latter system used a probe fitted with light-emitting diodes, as well as a dynamic reference frame with three diodes affixed in a triangular arrangement. Unlike the Viewing Arm, which is self-referential and does not tolerate patient motion, the infrared localizer could be used while the patient was under either general or local anesthesia.

In 1996, Tebo et al. repeated their accuracy study on a Plexiglas™ phantom and a plastic skull, using the FlashPoint system (in place of the Viewing Wand) [28]. In this study, 500 measurements were made on the Plexiglas phantom, and 1590 points were evaluated on the plastic skull. The average error was in the range of 2–3 mm, with 95% of the errors ranging from 0 to 5 mm. In three

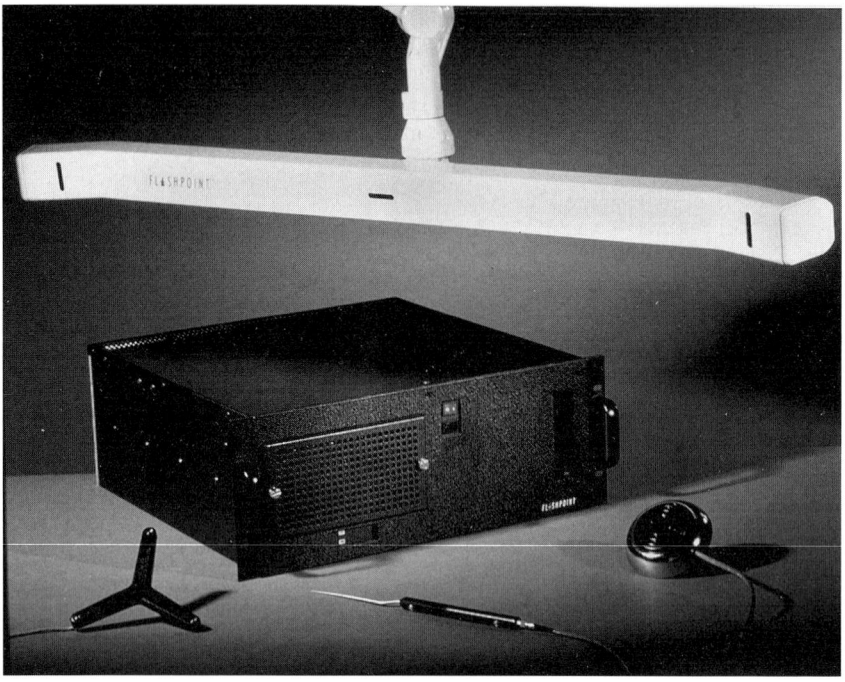

FIGURE 2.5 The Flashpoint 5000 (Image-Guided Technologies, Boulder, CO) uses an active infrared technology.

operations performed by three different surgeons, clinical accuracy ranged from 2 to 5 mm. The authors noted that better hardware, coupled with software improvements, should result in greater accuracy.

Fried et al. [29] published work on an electromagnetic localizer, the InstaTrak system (Visualization Technology Inc., Lawrence, MA) (Figure 2.6). This unit couples electromagnetic tracking to either straight or curved aspirators. With the InstaTrak, no intraoperative complications were encountered in 14 surgical cases. The system was easily integrated into the operating room setting. While complete analysis of the data was deferred until completion of a multisite study, a secondary study using cadaver dissection reported an accuracy of within 2 mm. The authors concluded that the InstaTrak system had overcome many of the limitations of other computer-guided methods.

In 1999, Klimek et al. presented their laboratory and intraoperative findings on a new type of optical computer-aided surgery [30]. The VectorVison (Brain-LAB, Heimstetten, Germany) uses passive reflective optical markers for coordinate determination (Figure 2.7). Laboratory accuracy measurements were ob-

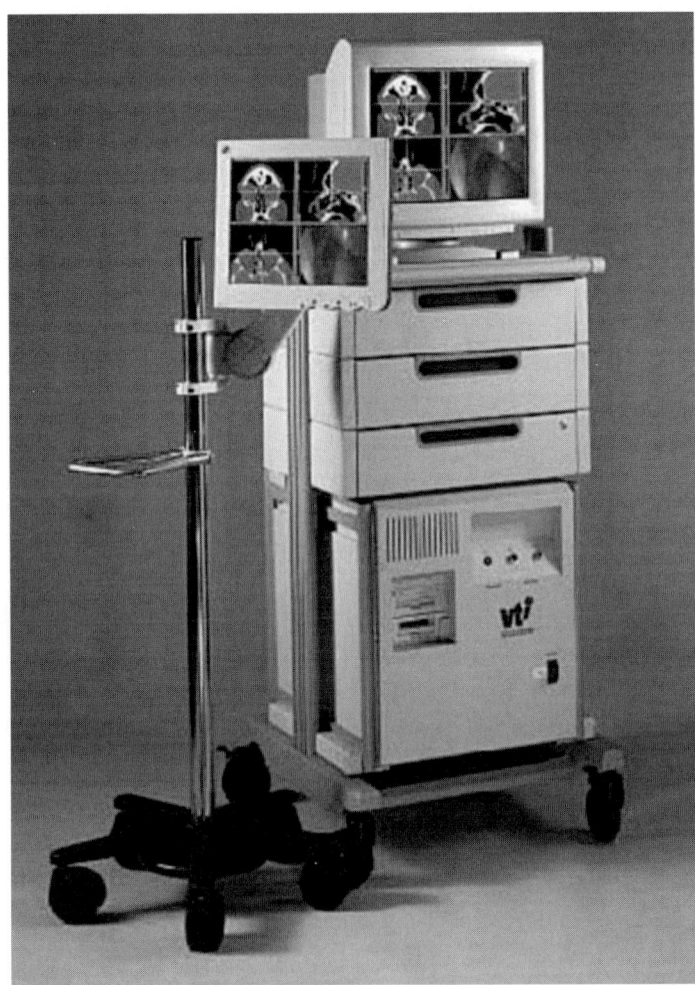

FIGURE 2.6 The InstaTrak (Visualization Technology, Lawrence, MA) was the first commercially available system that used electromagnetic tracking for otolaryngology.

tained on a Plexiglas model with known coordinates. Intraoperative accuracy measurements were recorded from 24 patients undergoing endonasal sinus surgery with two different referencing techniques (fiducial markers and mouthpiece). The system demonstrated laboratory accuracy within 0.86 mm (SD = 0.94 mm). Intraoperative accuracy was within 1.14 mm (SD = 0.57 mm) (fiducial markers) and 2.66 mm (SD = 1.89 mm) (mouthpiece) ($p < 0.05$). One of the main advan-

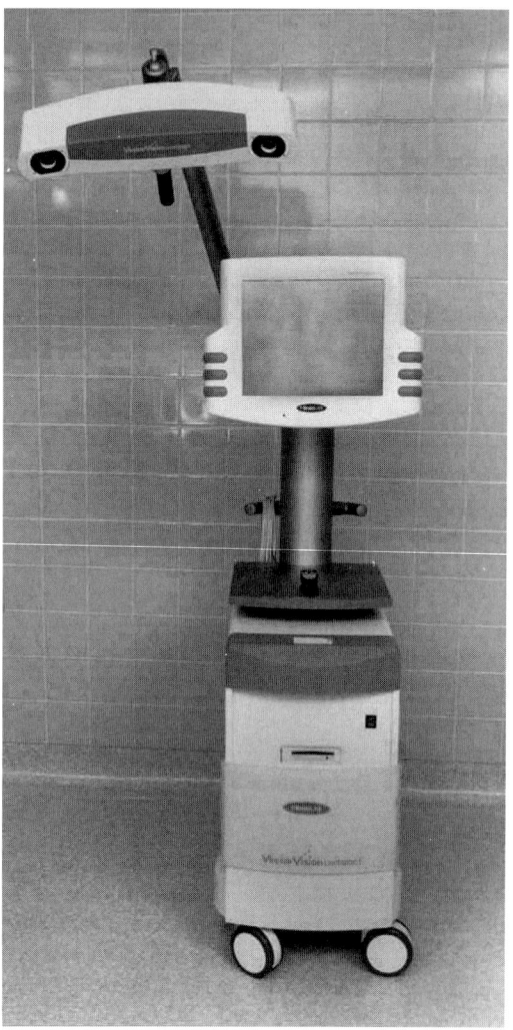

FIGURE 2.7 The VectorVision (BrainLAB, Heimstetten, Germany) utilizes passive infrared tracking technology.

tages of the new technology was the possibility of using any common instrument by attaching the reflective array.

The impact of CAS in the clinical setting was studied by Metson et al. in a combined prospective case study and retrospective analysis of physician surveys [31]. The LandmarX, an active optical-based CAS system (Medtronic

Historical Perspective

Xomed, Jacksonville, FL) was used by 34 physicians to perform 754 sinonasal surgeries over a 2.5-year period at Massachusetts Eye and Ear Infirmary (Figure 2.8). The measured accuracy of anatomical localization at the start of surgery showed a mean value of 1.69 ± 0.38 mm. According to a majority of surgeons questioned, use of the CAS equipment increased operating room time by 15–30 minutes during initial cases and by 5–15 minutes after experience with the equipment had been acquired. More than 90% of their surgeons anticipated the contin-

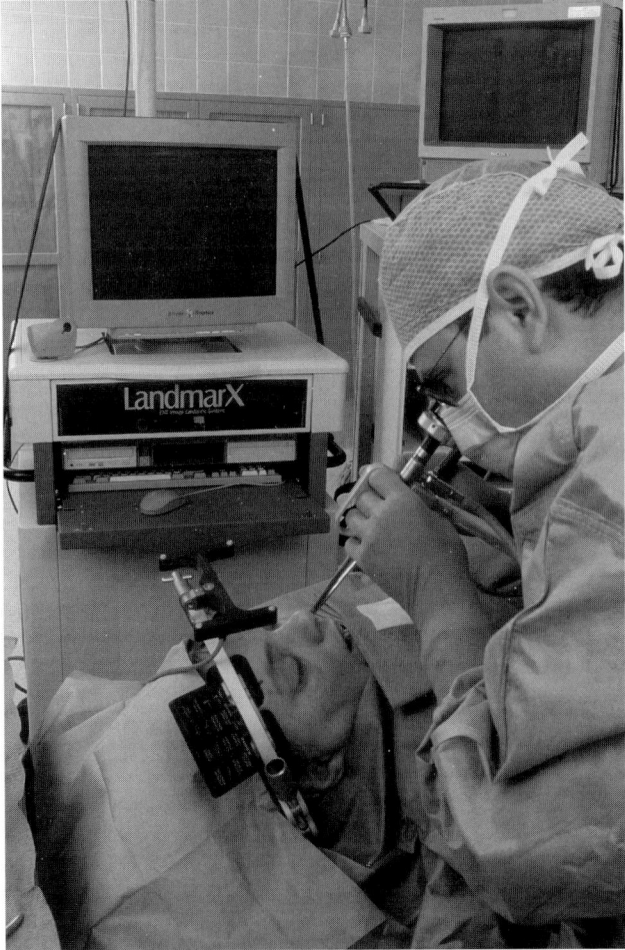

FIGURE 2.8 The LandmarX (Medtronic Xomed, Jacksonville, FL) uses active infrared tracking for surgical navigation.

ued use of CAS equipment for sinus surgery at a similar or greater level in the future.

2.4 TERMINOLOGY

In 1985, Georg Schlöndorff coined the term computer-assisted surgery. At that time, fully automatic robotic systems had been developed for industrial applications and were already in use in areas such as automobile production. Schlöndorff's aim was to give the surgeon a "computerized assistant" that would give additional information during the surgical process, but not replace the human surgeon.

Since 1985, numerous terms—including image-guided surgery (IGS)—have been applied to this discipline. Currently, IGS is commonly used in descriptions of computer-based surgical navigation systems for sinus surgery. In addition, various corporate trademarks are often mentioned.

Today, however, the term computer-aided surgery is the most appropriate term for the entire discipline, which includes surgical navigation, computer-enabled CT/MR review, Internet-based medicine, and surgical robotics. In 1997, an international group of experts chose to incorporate the "computer-aided surgery" terminology (rather than "computer-assisted surgery" or IGS) in the name for a new society dedicated to this area when they formed the International Society for Computer-Aided Surgery (ISCAS).

2.5 CONCLUSION

The history of computer-aided sinus surgery is rewritten every day due to the rapid development of new innovations in hardware and improvements in software. Luxenberger et al. [32] summarized the current status of computer-aided surgery for otolaryngology: CAS "is increasingly acknowledged as useful technology also for endoscopic sinus surgery." They further concluded that CAS is a significant development in sinus surgery. Often CAS is depicted as a replacement for other aspects of the surgical care of patients; however, it should be emphasized that CAS should be considered a helpful surgical tool.

REFERENCES

1. Bergstrom M, Greitz T. Stereotaxic computed tomography. Am J Roentgenol 1976; 127:167–170.
2. Brown R. A computerized tomography-computer graphics approach to sterotaxic localization. J Neurosurg 1979; 50:715–720.
3. Perry JH, Rosenbaum AE, Lunsford LD, et al. Computed tomography-guided stereo-

tactic surgery: conception and development of a new stereotactic methodology. Neurosurgery 1980; 7:376–381.
4. Roberts DW, Strohbehn JW, Hatch JF, et al. A frameless stereotaxic integration of computerized tomographic imaging and the operating microscope. J Neurosurg 1986; 65:545–549.
5. Watanabe E, Watanabe T, Manaka S, et al. Three-dimensional digitizer (Neuronavigator): new equipment for computed tomography-guided sterotaxic surgery. Surg Neurol 1987; 27:543–547.
6. Reinhardt H, Meyer H, Amrein E. A computer-assisted device for the intraoperative CT-correlated localization of brain tumors. Eur Surg Res 1988; 20:51–58.
7. Guthrie BL, Adler JR. Frameless stereotaxy computer interactive neurosurgery. Perspect Neurol Surg 1991; 2:1–15.
8. Watanabe E, Mayanagi Y, Kosugi Y, et al. Open surgery assisted by the Neuronavigator, a stereotactic articulated, sensitive arm. Neurosurgery 1991; 28:792–800.
9. Kato A, Yoshimine T, Hayakawa T, Tomita Y, Ikeda T, Mitomo M, Harada K, Mogami H. A frameless, armless navigational system for computer-assisted neurosurgery [technical note]. J Neurosurg 1991; 74:845–849.
10. Leggett WB, Greenberg MM, Gannon WE, et al. The Viewing Wand: a new system for three-dimensional computed tomography-correlated intraoperative localization. Curr Surg 1991; 48:674–678.
11. Zinreich SJ, Tebo SA, Long DM, et al. Frameless stereotaxic integration of CT imaging data: accuracy and initial applications. Radiology 1993; 188:735–742.
12. Laborde G, Gilsbach J, Harders A, Klimek L, Moesges R, Krybus W. Computer assisted localizer for planning of surgery and intra-operative orientation. Acta Neurochir 1992; 119:166–170.
13. Barnett GH, Kormos DW, Steiner CP, Weisenberger J. Intraoperative localization using an armless, frameless stereotactic wand. Technical note. J Neurosurg 1993; 78:510–514.
14. Barnett GH, Kormos DW, Steiner CP, Weisenberger J. Use of a frameless, armless stereotactic wand for brain tumor localization with two-dimensional and three-dimensional neuroimaging. Neurosurgery 1993; 33:674–678.
15. Klimek L, Wenzel M, Mösges R. Computer-assisted orbital surgery. Ophthalmic Surg 1993; 24:411–417.
16. Murphy MA, Barnett GH, Kormos DW, et al. Astrocytoma resection using an interactive frameless stereotactic wand: an early experience. J Clin Neurosci 1994; 1: 33–37.
17. Kormos DW, Piraino DW. Image-guided surgery attains clinical status. In: Diagnostic Imaging. San Francisco: Miller Freeman Inc., 1994.
18. Pollack IF, Welch W, Jacobs GB, Janecka IP. Frameless stereotactic guidance. An intraoperative adjunct in the transoral approach for ventral cervicomedullary junction decompression. Spine 1995; 20:216–220.
19. Kondziolka D, Lunsford LD. Guided neurosurgery using the ISG Viewing Wand. Contemp Neurosurg 1995; 17:1–6.
20. Schlondorff G, Mosges R, Meyer-Ebrecht D, Krybus W, Adams L. CAS (computer assisted surgery). A new procedure in head and neck surgery. HNO 1989; 37:187–190.

21. Klimek L, Mosges R, Bartsch M. Indications for CAS (computer assisted surgery) systems as navigation aids in ENT surgery. In: Proceedings of the CAR '91. Berlin: Springer Verlag, 1991:358–361.
22. Krybus W, Knepper A, Adams L, et al. Navigation support for surgery by means of optical position detection. In: Proceedings of the CAR '91. Berlin: Springer Verlag, 1991:362–366.
23. Mösges R, Klimek L. Computer-assisted surgery of the paranasal sinuses. J Otolaryngol 1993; 22:69–71.
24. Anon JB, Lipman SP, Oppenheim D, Halt RA. Computer-assisted endoscopic sinus surgery. Laryngoscope 1994; 104:901–905.
25. Carrau RL, Snyderman CH, Curtin HD, Janecka IP, Stechison M, Weissman JL. Computer-assisted intraoperative navigation during skull base surgery. Am J Otolaryngol 1996; 17:95–101.
26. Gunkel AR, Freysinger W, Thumfart WF, Pototschnig C. Complete sphenoethmoidectomy and computer-assisted surgery. Acta Otorhinolaryngol Belg 1995; 49: 257–261.
27. Anon JB, Rontal M, Zinreich SJ. Computer-assisted endoscopic sinus surgery—current experience and future developments. Op Techn Otolaryngol Head Neck Surg 1995; 6:163–170.
28. Tebo SA, Leopold DA, Long DM, et al. An optical 3D digitizer for frameless stereotactic surgery. IEEE Comput Graph Applic 1996; 16:55–64.
29. Fried MP, Kleefield J, Gopal H, Reardon E, Ho BT, Kuhn FA. Image-guided endoscopic surgery: results of accuracy and performance in a multicenter clinical study using an electromagnetic tracking system. Laryngoscope 1997; 107:594–601.
30. Klimek L, Ecke U, Lubben B, Witte J, Mann W. A passive-marker-based optical system for computer-aided surgery in otorhinolaryngology: development and first clinical experiences. Laryngoscope 1999; 109:1509–1515.
31. Metson RB, Cosenza MJ, Cunningham MJ, Randolph GW. Physician experience with an optical image guidance system for sinus surgery. Laryngoscope 2000; 110: 972–976.
32. Luxenberger W, Kole W, Stammberger H, Reittner P. [Computer assisted localization in endoscopic sinus surgery—state of the art? The Insta Trak system]. Laryngorhinootologie 1999; 78:318–325.

3

Surgical Navigation Technology: Optical and Electromagnetic Tracking

Ralph B. Metson, M.D.
Harvard Medical School and Massachusetts Eye and Ear Infirmary, Boston, Massachusetts

3.1 INTRODUCTION

The performance of surgery in the head and neck demands a high degree of precision and allows little room for misjudgments regarding anatomical relationships. These demands can be particularly challenging when operating on a patient with poor anatomical landmarks, as is often the case from extensive disease or previous surgery. In an attempt to enhance surgical safety and efficacy of otolaryngologic procedures, navigational systems have been developed that can track the movement of a surgical instrument in the operative field. This information is used to provide the surgeon with real-time localization of the instrument on a three-dimensional (3D) video display of the patient's preoperative computed tomography (CT) or magnetic resonance (MR) scan.

The earliest intraoperative guidance systems were developed in the 1980s for neurosurgical procedures. They utilized a stereotactic frame that required fixation of the patient's head during surgery with cranial screws [1]. An articulated mechanical arm or "wand" held a probe, which could be localized in the surgical field by means of electromechanical sensors. A frameless system was eventually developed [2], which was used for a variety of sinonasal procedures [3–5]. However, many surgeons found this system to be awkward to use and time-consuming [6,7]. In addition, the patient's head still had to be immobilized during surgery. The introduction of wandless and frameless systems in the mid-1990s greatly facilitated the utility of image-guided technology for otolaryngologic surgery [8–14]. These devices required neither articulated arms nor head immobilization and could be readily adapted for use during commonly performed endoscopic sinus procedures.

Commercially available systems are currently based upon two different tracking technologies—optical and electromagnetic. The optically based systems utilize an infrared camera array to track light-emitting diodes (LEDs), which are attached to the surgical instrument and a headset worn by the patient. Some optical tracking systems are "passive," i.e., the infrared camera array tracks the positions of highly reflective spheres, which are substituted for the standard LEDs. In this approach, the camera array also houses an infrared emitter, which illuminates the reflective spheres so that the camera array can recognize their positions. Obviously, the passive systems eliminate the need for wires for the tracking system in the operative field. The electromagnetically based systems track the position of the surgical instrument relative to the patient by means of a radiofrequency transmitter mounted to the headset and a radiofrequency receiver incorporated in the surgical handpiece. These two different navigational systems have both demonstrated their ability to provide the surgeon with accurate information regarding anatomical localization during surgery [10]. However, the different technologies utilized by these systems result in distinct differences in design and function, which can be used to formulate individual surgeon's preferences for equipment selection.

3.2 EQUIPMENT OPERATION

Certain operational features—calibration, registration, and accuracy verification—are common to all navigational systems. These steps are necessary to ensure the integrity of the equipment at the start of surgery and the accuracy of localization throughout the procedure. For the purposes of this discussion, the mechanics of surgical navigation for endoscopic sinus surgery will be emphasized, since this specific application of surgical navigation is the most well-developed application of this technology within the domain of otorhinolaryngology–head and neck surgery.

3.2.1 Calibration

Prior to utilization of the navigational system, the surgeon must perform calibration. It is typically done after the patient is draped and the cables from the headset

Surgical Navigation Technology

and handpiece have been attached to the computer. This step usually requires the surgeon to hold the tip of the surgical instrument (usually a straight probe or suction) in a divot on the patient headset while stepping on a pedal. The system verifies the proper geometric relationships between the handpiece and headset to ensure that the equipment is in proper working order and that the surgical instrument has not been bent or damaged.

3.2.2 Registration

Registration is the process whereby the patient's digitized preoperative CT or MR scan is aligned with the patient's actual anatomy in the operating room. The reference points used to perform this function are known as fiducial points. Most surgical navigation systems that use optical tracking generally rely upon anatomical fiducial points, which are selected by the surgeon prior to surgery from surface landmarks on the 3D video model. Registration is completed when the surgeon touches these same points on the patient while activating the footpedal.

The electromagnetic system uses fiducial points, which have been embedded into the patient headset. Since the patient wears this headset during both the preoperative CT scan and surgery, the computer can align the CT scan with the patient's anatomy. The surgeon performs the registration process by holding the tip of the suction handpiece in a divot in the center of the headset and rotating the instrument around the tip at 90° increments.

It should be noted that registration protocols do not reflect the limitations of either optical or electromagnetic tracking. In theory, both electromagnetic and optical tracking systems can support anatomical fiducial point registration and automatic headset-based registration. The engineers of each system have developed approaches to registration independently of the design for tracking technology.

3.2.3 Sustained Accuracy

Slippage of the patient headset or equipment malfunction can result in a loss of system accuracy during surgery. In order to assure that anatomical drift has not occurred, navigational systems incorporate timed reminders for the surgeon to verify system accuracy. This process requires the surgeon to select a precise anatomical point at the start of surgery, usually at the nasion. This point can be identified with an ink spot or adhesive strip with a central divot. The tip of the probe or suction is touched to this point at the start of surgery and at regular intervals throughout the procedure. If anatomical drift of more than 2 mm has occurred, the system should be reregistered prior to continuing its use.

It is strongly recommended that the surgeon develop a habit of checking the image-guidance system against known anatomical landmarks prior to its use for surgical navigation. For example, before using the probe to identify the level of the ethmoid roof, it should be touched to the tip of the middle turbinate or the posterior wall of the opened maxillary sinus to verify that the information the system is providing is accurate and correct.

3.3 OPTICAL TRACKING SYSTEMS

Optical image-guidance systems (Figure 3.1) for otolaryngologic surgery include the LandmarX (Medtronic Xomed, Jacksonville, FL), StealthStation (Medtronic

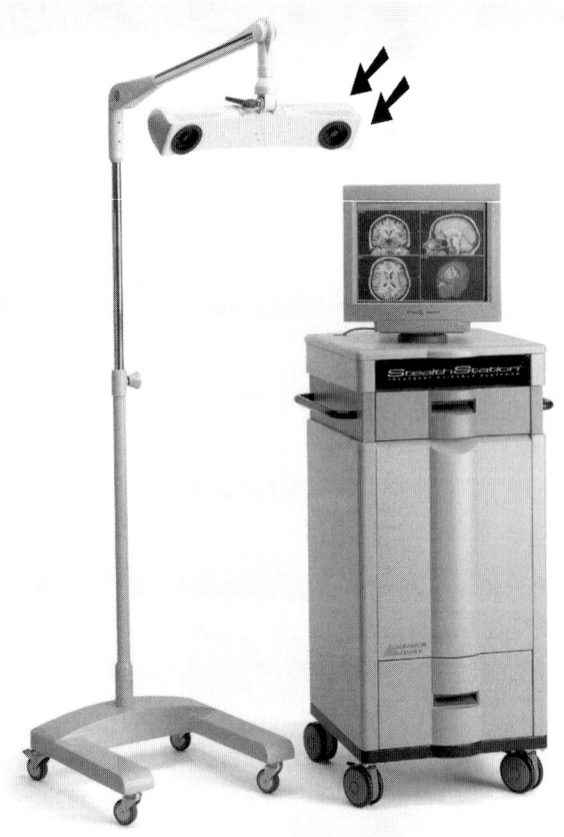

FIGURE 3.1 The LandmarX surgical navigation system (Medtronic Xomed, Jacksonville, FL) utilizes optical tracking technology incorporates an infrared camera array (arrows) to monitor the position of light emitting diodes (LEDs) mounted to the surgical instrument and patient headset.

Surgical Navigation Technology

Surgical Navigation Technologies, Louisville, CO), Surgical Navigator (Zeiss, Montauk, NY), Optical Tracking System (Radionics, Burlington, MA), SAVANT (CBYON, Palo Alto, CA) and VectorVision (BrainLab, Tuttlingen, Germany). Most of these systems have software and hardware packages available that upgrade existing neurosurgical and orthopedic systems for use during otolaryngologic surgery. Most manufacturers also offer dedicated, less expensive systems, which are equipped only for ENT procedures.

These optical systems employ an infrared tracking system to locate the real-time position of surgical instruments on the patient's preoperative CT scan. The tip of the instrument is depicted by crosshairs on a video display of a reformatted 3D image, as well as axial, coronal, and sagittal CT views (Figure 3.2). The optical sensor is an array of two or three infrared cameras mounted in a mobile, horizontal bar. Positioning of the cameras approximately at their focal length (typically 6 feet) from the head of the operating table provides optimal

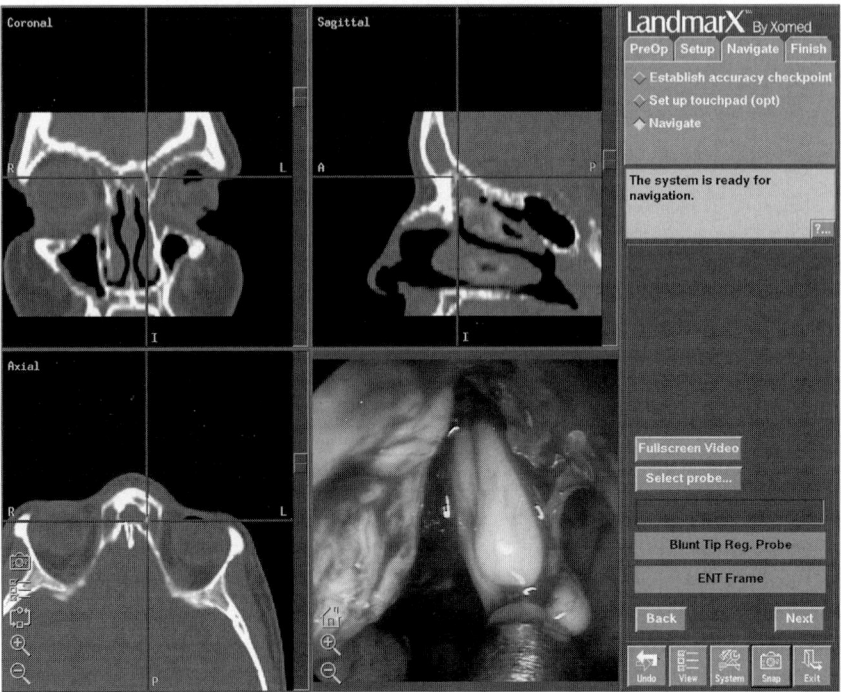

FIGURE 3.2 During surgical navigation, the instrument tip localization is depicted relative to the preoperative CT scan. A representative screen capture from the LandmarX system (Medtronic Xomed, Jacksonville, FL) is shown.

resolution. The cameras monitor the coordinate position of LEDs that are attached to standard sinus instruments or a straight probe (Figure 3.3). A separate set of LEDs is mounted in a dynamic reference frame (DRF), which is connected to the headset worn by the patient during surgery to monitor head movement (Figures 3.4 and 3.5). (In passive optical systems, reflective spheres serve the same functions as the LEDs, as described above.) This information is processed by an optical digitizer and computer workstation.

In most optical systems, patients do not wear a headset during the preoperative CT scan. Since the SAVANT and VectorVision support automatic headset-based registration as well as anatomical fiducial registration, the patient may wear the SAVANT or VectorVision headset at the time of the scan, if the surgeon wishes to use the headset-based registration protocol. Scanning protocols vary among manufacturers but generally utilize standard spiral CT scan techniques. Nonoverlapping axial slices of 1–3 mm thickness can also be used. Images are transferred to the guidance system through the hospital's computer network or by means of optical disk or storage tape.

The surgical handpiece is calibrated by placing the tip of the instrument in a divot on the headset DRF array while the foot pedal is depressed. The registration process involves correlating points in the operative field with the corre-

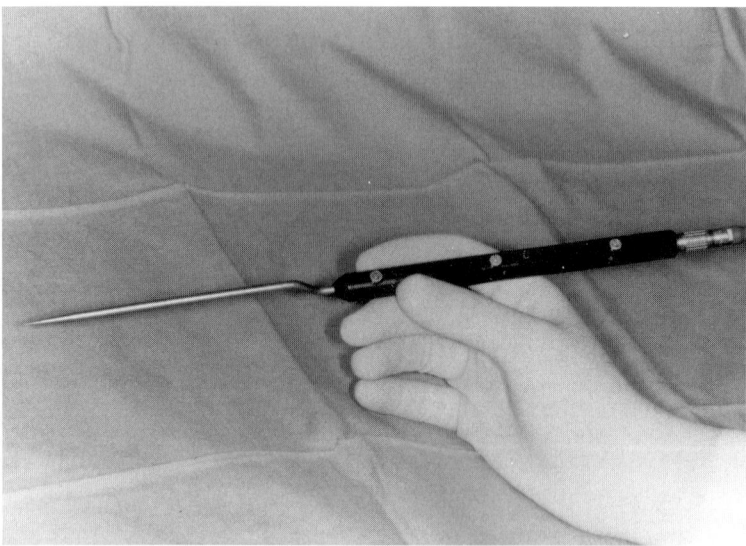

FIGURE 3.3 A standard surgical pointer for surgical navigation incorporates a LED array, which can be tracked by the overhead camera array. (LandmarX, Medtronic Xomed, Jacksonville, FL).

Surgical Navigation Technology

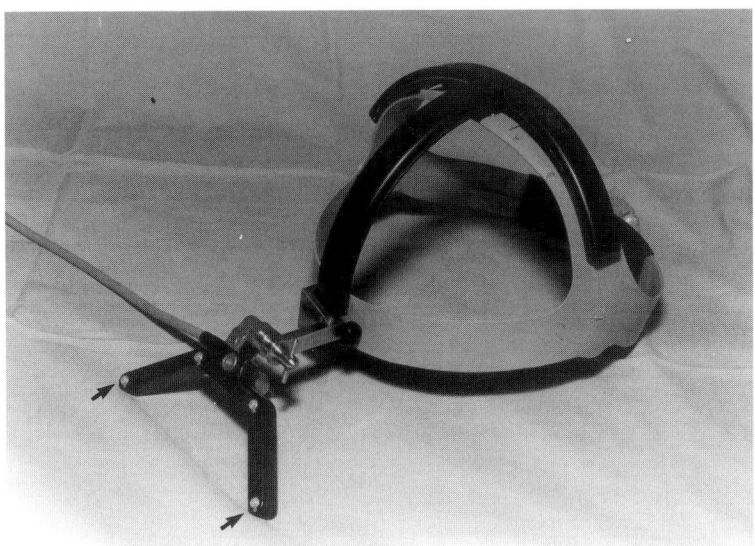

FIGURE 3.4 This headset from the StealthStation ENT module (Medtronic Surgical Navigation Technologies, Louisville, CO) supports anatomical fiducial point registration. The headset contains LEDs (arrows) that are tracked by an infrared camera. This headset compensates for any intraoperative head movement and/or repositioning.

sponding points on the CT images. If an anatomical fiducial point registration protocol is used, the surgeon, resident, or nurse selects five to seven anatomical fiducial points on the 3D reconstructed model at the computer workstation with a standard computer mouse. This selection process can be done anytime prior to surgery, but it is often convenient to perform this step just prior to the patient's arrival in the operating room. The most commonly used anatomical fiducial points are the nasal dorsum at the level of the medial canthi, the tip of the nose (at the point of greatest anterior projection), the base of the nose (where the columella meets the upper lip), the right and left lateral orbital rims at the level of the lateral canthi (the bony rims can be palpated), and the right and left ear tragus (at the points of greatest lateral projection). Although any anatomical sites on the head can be used for fiducial points, it is preferable for the points to surround the surgical field (i.e., the paranasal sinuses) in order to optimize navigational accuracy. Sites at which skin is in close proximity to underlying bone have been found to provide the most reliable reproducibility and result in the least amount of distortion during surgery.

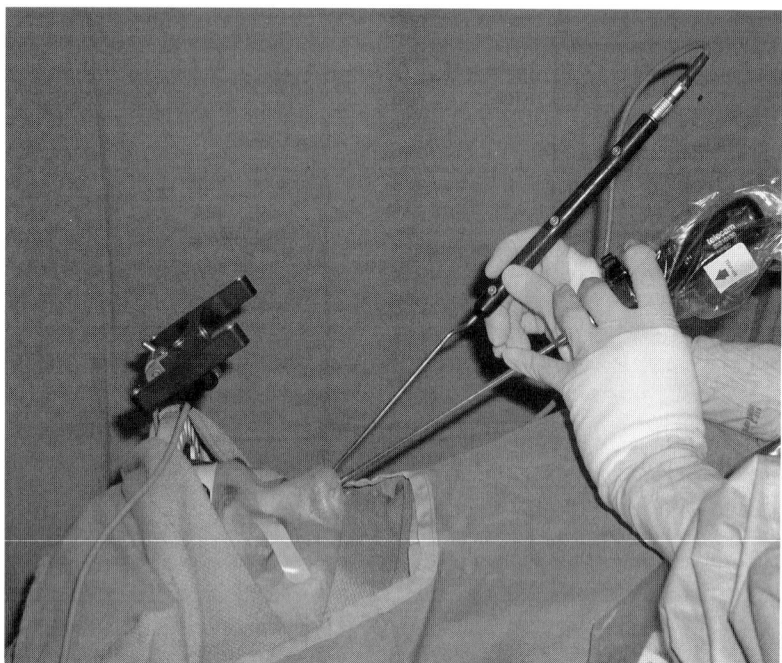

FIGURE 3.5 This intraoperative photograph shows the relative positions of the headset and instruments during surgical navigation with an optically based system using anatomic fiducial point registration.

The location of the selected surface fiducials on the patient's face are then touched with the tip of a calibrated probe or surgical instrument while depressing the foot pedal. For the remainder of the surgery, the location of the instrument tip is displayed on the CT images whenever the foot pedal is depressed. When the foot pedal is released, the current location of the instrument is frozen on the computer display. The system can also be set with the foot pedal in a "locked on" position, so that localization of the surgical instrument remains activated throughout the surgery, even when the foot pedal is not depressed.

For automatic headset-based registration for the SAVANT, the patient wears a special headset, which houses fiducial points, at the time of the preoperative CT scan. The patient wears the same headset at the time of surgery. Since the headset can fit each patient in only one way, the spatial relationships between the headset's fiducial points and the patient's anatomy are maintained. Furthermore, the relationship between the headset DRF and the fiducial points is fixed. During registration, the SAVANT computer automatically recognizes the fiducial

Surgical Navigation Technology

points on the preoperative CT scan and calculates the registration. Surgical navigation may then proceed. The VectorVision automatic registration protocol is similar.

At approximately 15-minute intervals, many systems display a screen icon, which notifies the surgeon that navigational accuracy needs to be verified. For this step, the surgeon places the tip of a calibrated instrument on the previously selected point (typically a point on the nasal dorsum), while depressing the foot pedal. This step ensures that anatomical drift, which could result in a significant decrement in system accuracy, has not occurred. Such drift is usually the result of inadvertent movement of the headset during surgery. If the system demonstrated a decrement in accuracy of more than 2 mm, the registration process should be repeated before continuing with surgery.

3.4 ELECTOMAGNETIC TRACKING SYSTEMS

The first navigational system (Figure 3.6) introduced for sinus surgery was the InstaTrak (Visualization Technology, Inc., Lawrence, MA), which utilizes electromagnetic tracking technology. This system employs a radiofrequency transmitter mounted to a specialized headset that is worn by the patient during the operative procedure (Figure 3.7). A radiofrequency receiver is incorporated into the handpiece of a nonmagnetic suction (Figure 3.8). Cables connect both the transmitter and receiver to the computer workstation. The tip of the suction cannula is depicted by crosshairs on axial, coronal, sagittal images of the patient's preoperative CT displayed on a video monitor (Figure 3.9).

The InstaTrak imaging protocol requires the patient to wear the exact same headset during both the preoperative CT scan and the operative procedure. When placing the headset, care must be taken not to allow objects that can cause distortion to push against the headset during the scan. Using helical mode, the scans are obtained with 3 mm slice thickness by 3 mm table movement and reconstructed to 1 mm table increments in the bone algorithm. If direct coronals are needed, the headset must be removed before scanning. The patient is scanned from the bottom of the maxilla to approximately 2.5 cm above the most superior of the seven metal spheres incorporated in the headset. Multiplanar CT views are obtained by reformatting the axial images. The digitized CT data is loaded into the InstaTrak directly by transporting the unit to the radiology department, via the hospital's computer network, or from an optical storage disk.

The patient must bring the same headset worn during the CT scan to the hospital to wear during the surgery. The headsets are neither interchangeable nor reusable. The headset serves two functions—it compensates for head movement during the procedure and it serves as a method for automating registration. Registration is the means by which digitized CT data in the computer workstation is correlated with the patient's actual anatomy. This system uses an automatic

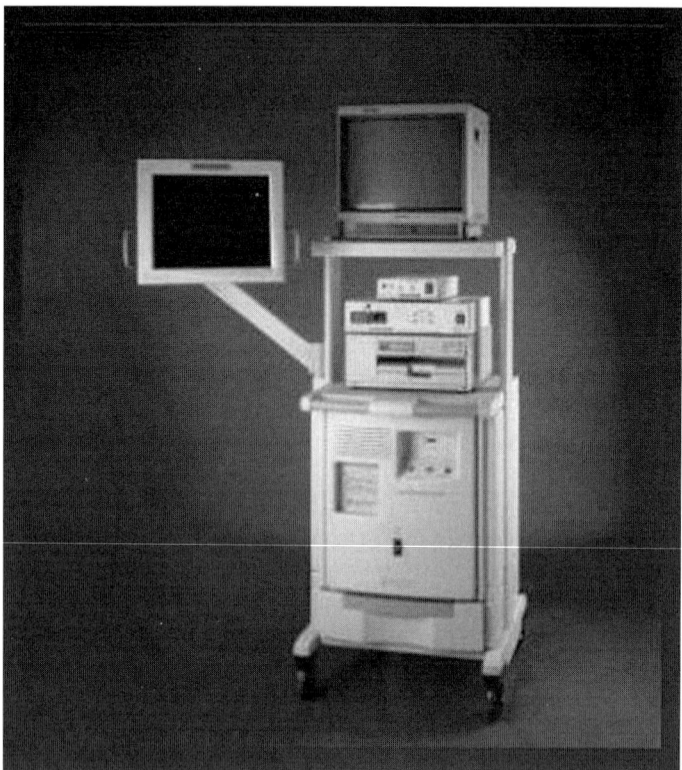

FIGURE 3.6 The InstaTrak system (Visualization Technology, Lawrence, MA) uses electromagnetic tracking technology with a radiofrequency transmitter mounted to the patient headset and a receiver attached to the surgical handpiece.

registration process where fiducials embedded in the patient's headset, rather than anatomical landmarks, are used to align the CT data and patient anatomy.

The suction instrument is calibrated by holding its tip in a divot in the center of the headset, while the shaft is rotated 360° around the tip at 90° increments. Next, a verification point is established to ensure the system's accuracy throughout surgery. This verification point is an adhesive strip with a central divot placed on the skin of the nasal dorsum. The tip of the suction is placed in the divot at 15-minute intervals to verify the sustained accuracy of the system. If the measurement is found to be greater than 2 mm (indicating drift), the registration process can be repeated.

Because the electromagnetic system uses radiofrequency transmission, metallic objects in the field will disrupt the operational signal. Distortion of the

Surgical Navigation Technology

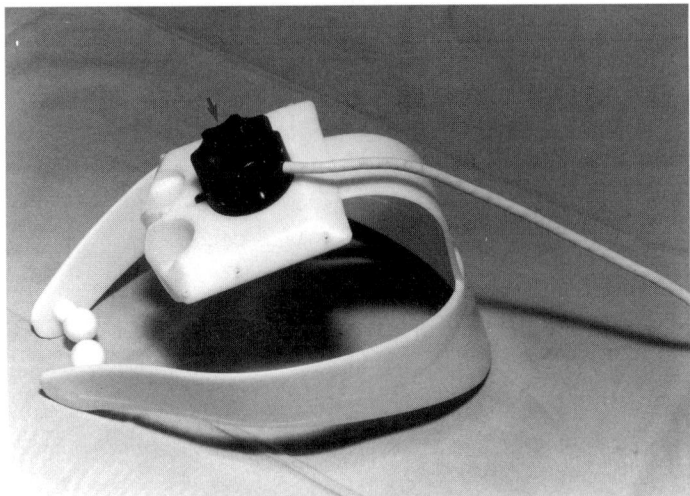

FIGURE 3.7 The headset for the InstaTrak system (Visualization Technology, Lawrence, MA) must also be worn by the patient during the preoperative CT scan. An electromagnetic transmitter (arrow) is attached to the headset at the start of surgery.

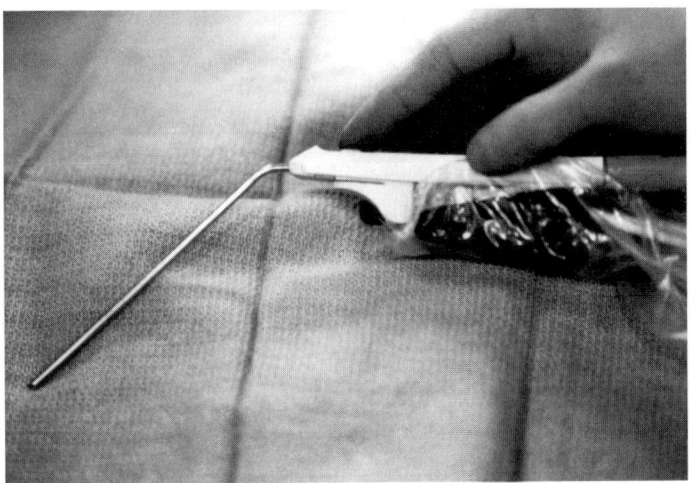

FIGURE 3.8 A suction aspirator also may prove useful in specific circumstances. The suction apparatus from the InstaTrak system (Visualization Technology, Lawrence, MA) is made from nonferrous (i.e., nonmagnetic) metal, since the InstaTrak uses an electromagnetic tracking system.

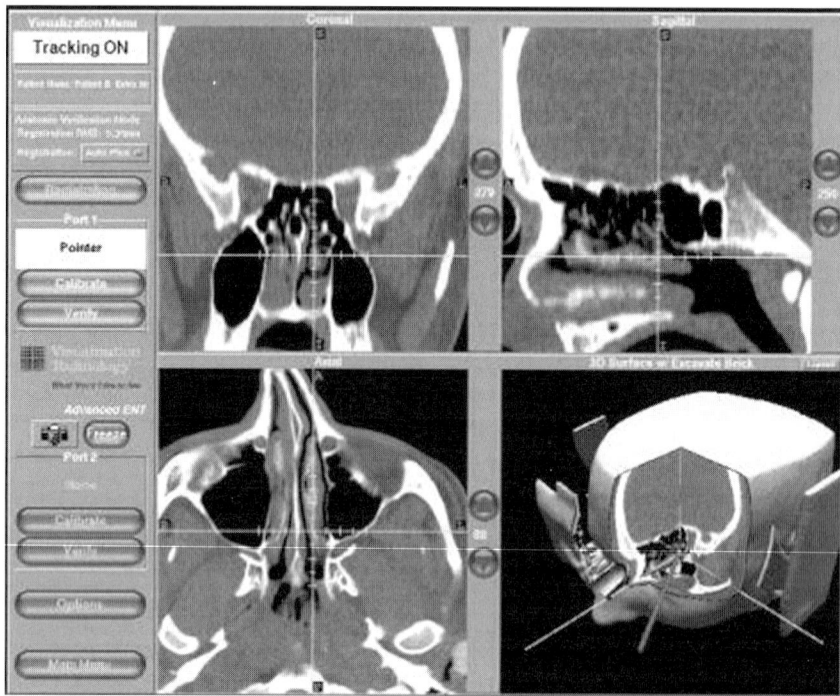

FIGURE 3.9 During surgical navigation, the instrument tip localization is depicted relative to the preoperative CT scan. A representative screen capture from the InstaTrak system (Visualization Technology, Lawrence, MA) is shown.

electromagnetic field, which is necessary for surgical navigation, will interrupt the system's operation. A window on the computer monitor will notify the surgeon when such a disruption occurs. It may be necessary to place two mattress pads between the patient and the metal operating table in order to minimize potential metal artifact. In addition, instrument tables, anesthesia equipment, and other sizable metallic devices generally have to be positioned an appropriate distance from the surgical field.

3.5 SYSTEM COMPARISONS

Both the optical and electromagnetic navigational systems have demonstrated ease of use and reliability for otolaryngologic surgery, particularly for those procedures involving the paranasal sinuses [8,10,14]. Nevertheless, they possess sev-

Surgical Navigation Technology

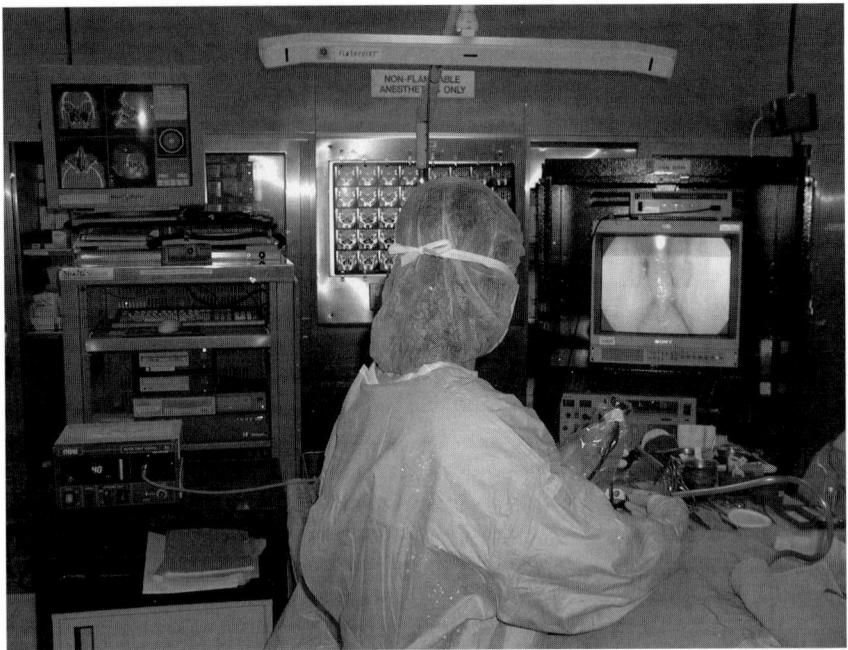

FIGURE 3.10 This intraoperative photograph shows the relative positions of the headset and instruments during surgical navigation with an optically based system using infrared tracking.

eral practical differences in terms of clinical utility based upon differences in their hardware and software design.

3.5.1 Signal Distortion/Blocking

Because the optical-based system relies upon an infrared signal for correct operation, it is necessary to maintain a clear line of sight between the infrared camera and the DRFs mounted on the surgical instruments and patient headset. Therefore, the surgeon must hold the instrument with the DRF uncovered and pointed in the direction of the infrared camera whenever the system is activated. Furthermore, operating room personnel and equipment cannot be placed between the patient's head and the camera array lenses, which are positioned at their focal length (generally 6 feet) above the head of the table (Figure 3.10).

Since the electromagnetic system utilizes a radiofrequency signal for localization, metallic objects in the surgical field cause signal distortion. To ensure proper operation of the electromagnetic system, patients have to be placed on two surgical table mattress pads to increase the distance between the metal operating table and the electromagnetic emitter and sensor. This step may not be necessary in operating rooms where thicker mattresses are used. In addition, instrument tables, anesthesia equipment, and other sizable metallic devices must be positioned at an appropriate distance from the immediate surgical field.

3.5.2 Patient Headset

Automatic headset-based registration protocols require patients to wear a headset during the preoperative CT scan. Although patients occasionally report discomfort when wearing the headset, this issue rarely prevents completion of the scan. Use of the headset may contribute to patient and physician inconvenience, particularly if the patient forgets to bring the headset on the day of surgery.

Unlike the headset for manual registration, which is held in place by a band or rubber pads that encircle the head at the level of the brow, the headsets for automatic registration are secured at the ear canals and nasal bridge. This configuration necessitates intraoperative coverage of a portion of the medial orbit and frontal regions. For most sinus surgery, this design is not of clinical importance; however, it does preclude use of headsets with this design for procedures, which involve external incisions or manipulations in the frontal, medial canthal, or auricular regions.

All registration protocols for sinus surgery require a headset to be worn in the operating room. Because these devices must be secured in a fashion to minimize slippage during surgery, they may cause patient discomfort when surgery is performed under local anesthesia. In addition, temporary skin erythema at the headset contact points is commonly observed. In rare instances of prolonged surgery performed under general anesthesia, superficial skin necrosis has been observed at these contact points. The regular use of foam tape between the headset and skin appears to add to skin protection without increasing headset slippage.

3.5.3 Operating Room Time

The use of image-guided technology requires additional time for equipment setup and operation. Surgeons have reported 15–30 minutes per case of increased operating room time when first learning how to use the image guidance system [14]. Once the surgeon and nursing staff became familiar with the equipment, this time is reduced to 5–15 minutes. An automated registration process would actually be expected to save time as compared to a manual registration process, which requires the surgeon to preselect anatomic landmarks for fiducial points. In a study that compared the use of an optical system with manual registration and electromagnetic system with automatic registration at a single institution, total operating room time averaged 17 minutes longer for the electromagnetic system. However, this difference was thought to reflect the fact that the electromagnetic system was the first image-guidance system used at the institution [10].

3.5.4 Expense

The use of image-guidance technology increases operating room expense. In one study, hospital charges were increased by approximately $500 per case when a surgical navigation system was used [12]. In addition to the capital outlay for equipment purchase, one must consider the cost of nonreusable supplies. If the system requires the use of disposable headsets and suction handpieces, greater operating costs may be anticipated.

3.5.5 Surgical Instrumentation

The electromagnetic system uses a specialized, nonmetallic suction, which was found to be helpful when brisk bleeding was present. However, difficulty may be encountered when trying to reach into the frontal sinus with the curved version of this suction because of its diameter and unusual tip configuration. The optical systems often use standard endoscopic sinus surgery instruments, which are mated to DRFs for localization. This feature may be especially advantageous when working in the region of the frontal recess. The narrow, curved, olive-tip suction can be readily inserted into the frontal sinus and can even verify the localization of different compartments within a large sinus.

Since the introduction of image-guidance technology, the number and variety of surgical instruments, which can be used with surgical navigation systems, has greatly increased. Many of the optical systems now offer universal instrument registration. With this process almost any standard surgical instrument can be digitized during surgery and used for anatomical localization.

Optical systems are also available that offer passive infrared technology. The camera array emits an infrared signal that is reflected by specialized spherical surfaces on the surgical handpiece. This technology allows for the use of wireless instrumentation and eliminates the problem of multiple cables, which may become tangled entwined.

3.5.6 Accuracy of Localization

Anatomical localization has been shown to be accurate to within 2 mm for both the electromagnetic and optical systems [10,12]. Although this degree of accuracy can be very reassuring to the surgeon, navigational systems have been found to be most useful to confirm the identity of large compartments within the sinus cavities, rather than to distinguish between millimeter increments. For example, the straight probe or suction is commonly used to confirm the identity of the exposed ethmoid roof or to verify that the sphenoid sinus had been entered, rather than a large posterior ethmoid cell. The curved suction cannula is most useful to demonstrate that an ostium that has been opened in the frontal recess leads to the true frontal sinus, rather than an adjacent supraorbital ethmoid cell.

The positions of fiducial points may influence the accuracy of localization. For instance, the arrangement of fiducial markers in a planar surface may compromise accuracy at points distant from that plane. The selection of fiducial points in an array that surrounds the surgical site should theoretically increase system accuracy deep at points throughout the operative field. It is for this reason that the left and right tragus are typically used as fiducials during anatomical fiducial point registration. Similarly, the SAVANT headset for automatic registration incorporates fiducial markers that are separated in depth (i.e., out of plane).

3.5.7 Patient Selection

Intraoperative image-guidance systems have been found to be most useful for cases which present the surgeon with the greatest technical challenge due to abnormal anatomy or distorted landmarks [14]. Both types of systems have been widely utilized to facilitate sinus surgery in patients who have extensive disease or require revision surgery. Because the headsets used for automatic registration preclude access to the medial orbital and frontal regions, they cannot be used for surgeries, which require external access to these regions (e.g., frontal trephination, external ethmoidectomy, frontal sinus obliteration, or endoscopic dacryocystorhinostomy).

3.6 CONCLUSION

Navigational systems have demonstrated their clinical utility and relative ease of use for surgical procedures of the head and neck. Their greatest benefit appears to be for patients who have poor surgical landmarks from extensive disease or previous surgery. Both the optical and electromagnetic tracking systems provide the surgeon with accurate information regarding anatomical localization during sinus surgery. The different technologies utilized by these systems result in distinct differences in their design and function that can be used to formulate individual preferences for equipment selection.

REFERENCES

1. Goerss SJ, Kelly PJ, Kall BA, Alker GJ Jr. A computed tomographic stereotactic adaptation system. Neurosurgery 1982; 10:375–379.
2. Zinreich SJ, Tebo S, Long DL, et al. Frameless stereotaxic integration of CT imaging data accuracy and initial applications. Radiology 1993; 188:735–742.

3. Anon JB, Rontal R, Zinreich SJ. Computer-assisted endoscopic sinus surgery-current experience and future developments. Operative techniques. Otolaryngol Head Neck Surg 1995; 6:163–170.
4. Carrau RL, Snyderman CH, Curtin HB, Weissman JL. Computer-assisted frontal sinusotomy. Otolaryngol Head Neck Surg 1994; 111:727–732.
5. Gunkel AR, Freysinger W, Martin A, et al. Three-dimensional image-guided endonasal surgery with a microdebrider. Laryngoscope 1997; 107:834–838.
6. Freysinger W, Gunkel AR, Martin A, et al. Advancing ear, nose, and throat computer-assisted surgery with the arm-based ISG Viewing Wand: the stereotactic suction tube. Laryngoscope 1997; 107:690–693.
7. Roth M, Lanza DC, Zinreich J, et al. Advantages and disadvantages of three-dimensional computed tomography intraoperative localization for functional endoscopic sinus surgery. Laryngoscope 1995; 105:1279–1286.
8. Fried MP, Kleefield J, Gopal H, et al. Image-guided endoscopic surgery: results of accuracy and performance in a multicenter clinical study using an electromagnetic tracking system. Laryngoscope 1997; 107:594–601.
9. Anon JB, Lipman SP, Oppenheim D, et al. Computer-assisted endoscopic sinus surgery. Laryngoscope 1994; 104:901–905.
10. Metson R, Gliklich RE, Cosenza MJ. A comparison of image guidance systems for sinus surgery. Laryngoscope 1998; 108:1164–1170.
11. Klimek L, Ecke U, Lubben B, Witte J, Mann W. A passive-marker-based optical system for computer-aided surgery in otorhinolaryngology: development and first clinical experiences. Laryngoscope 1999; 109:1509–1515.
12. Metson R, Cosenza MJ, Gliklich RE, Montgomery WW. The role of image-guidance systems for head and neck surgery. Arch Otolaryngol Head Neck Surg 1999; 125:1100–1104.
13. Neumann AM, Pasquale-Niebles K, Bhuta T, Sillers MJ. Image-guided transnasal endoscopic surgery of the paranasal sinuses and anterior skull base. Am J Rhinol 1999; 13:449–454.
14. Metson RB, Cosenza MJ, Cunningham MJ, Randolph GW. Physician experience with an optical image guidance system for sinus surgery. Laryngoscope 2000; 110:972–976.

4
Principles of Registration

Martin J. Citardi, M.D., F.A.C.S.
Cleveland Clinic Foundation, Cleveland, Ohio

4.1 INTRODUCTION

Although computer-aided surgery (CAS) systems offer a wide variety of features, including preoperative planning, intraoperative surgical navigation has attracted the most interest among practicing otorhinolaryngologists. Discussions of CAS surgical navigation tend to focus upon the impact that surgical navigation has on surgical procedures. Unfortunately, that emphasis tends to minimize the importance of registration, which is a critical step for all surgical navigation. Since clinically useful surgical navigation requires accurate registration, it is at least inappropriate and probably dangerous to overlook the registration process that underlies the intraoperative applications of CAS.

This chapter will describe the concept of registration as well as various approaches for registration in the surgical setting. Rather than present information about mathematical estimates of tracking accuracy, this chapter will discuss strategies for registration; the approach is to provide clinically relevant information that clinicians can employ when they use CAS-based surgical navigation in the operating room.

4.2 REGISTRATION BASICS

The elements of a simple CAS platform for surgical navigation include a computer workstation and a tracking system as well as software that integrates the hardware components, provides a user interface, and displays image data. The tracking system can monitor the relative position of instruments in three-dimensional (3D) space.

Tracking technology has improved dramatically over the past 15 years. Early systems relied upon electromechanical arms. A series of acoustic emitters and receivers also can also serve as a mechanism for tracking. Most CAS surgical navigation platforms rely upon an optically based technology, that incorporates light-emitting diodes (LEDs) or highly reflective spheres into arrays (known as intraoperative localization devices, or ILDs) that are integrated into surgical instruments (Figure 4.1). Finally, an electromagnetic emitter and receiver can also provide localization data. Each of these specific technologies has its relative advantages and disadvantages, but it is important to realize that the principles of registration apply to all tracking systems and are not specific to any one tracking technology. Regardless of the specific hardware, the CAS surgical navigation system must have the capability to "learn" the location of the operative field.

Conceptually, all points in the operating field volume may be assigned a unique x, y, z coordinate value that defines the position of the point in relation to all other points in the operating field volume. Similarly, all points in the volume depicted by the preoperative imaging may be assigned a unique x, y, z coordinate value that defines the position of the point in relation to all other points in the preoperative imaging data set volume. During registration, the CAS system simply maps selected points (known as fiducial points) in the operating field volume with their corresponding points in the preoperative imaging data set volume. In this way, there is a one-to-one relationship between corresponding points in the real world and imaging data set.

The data generated by the registration process then serve as the basis for all surgical navigation. All further localizations are relative to the registration data. If the registration data are inaccurate or if the registration data become corrupted, then surgical navigation will suffer accordingly. Surgical navigation depends upon registration.

Inaccuracies in surgical navigation may be traced to a variety of problems, but often the biggest problem is poor registration. An active, optically based tracking system under laboratory conditions (not in the operating room) theoretically has submillimetric precision, while other tracking technologies are only slightly less precise. Clinically, the best surgical navigation accuracy is perhaps 1–2 mm and often 2–3 mm. This dramatic difference in accuracy illustrates the challenge of registration. The challenge is not tracking instrument position in a precise manner; the challenge lies in calculating instrument tip positions relative to the preoperative imaging. Registration protocols are answers to this challenge.

Principles of Registration

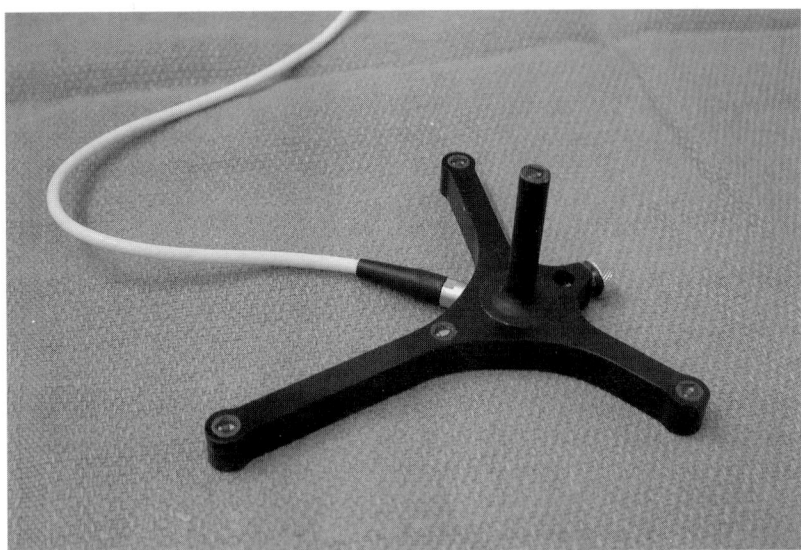

(a)

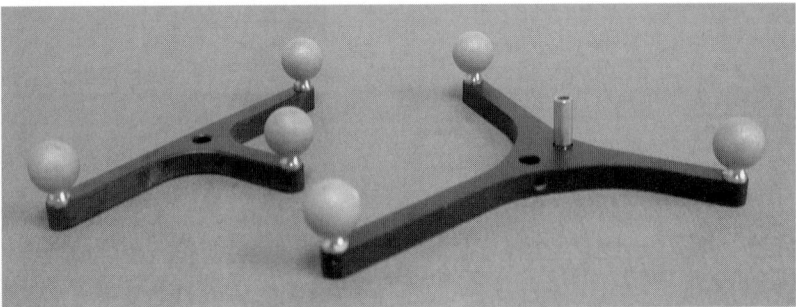

(B)

FIGURE 4.1 (A) An array of light emitting diodes (LEDs) can provide information about the relative positions of instruments in the operating field volume; an overhead camera array senses the light emitted by the LEDs and triangulates their position. This example shows the typical characteristics of an optical ILD. (B) Optical tracking can also occur passively; i.e., the ILD does not emit an active signal. Instead, an array of highly reflective spheres is used. The overhead camera array emits an infrared signal that is reflected by the spheres. Two representative passive ILDs are shown.

The ideal registration protocol would yield a precise correlation between corresponding points in the operating field volume and the image space. For practical reasons, it is also desirable that surgeons can easily and simply implement the registration without significant disruption of the typical operating room activities. Unfortunately, combining the features of precision and simplicity is not a simple task; in fact, skeptics would propose that precision and simplicity in registration are inversely related to each other. As a practical matter, the easiest registration protocols tend to offer greater potential for inaccuracies, and the most precise registration protocols are the most cumbersome. The registration protocols that are commercially available are compromise solutions that seek to balance the need for precision and the need for usability.

Almost all registration protocols support dynamic registration, which compensates for patient movement during surgical navigation. Dynamic registration can be achieved by simply attaching an ILD to the volume of interest patient. This ILD, which may be more precisely termed a dynamic reference frame (DRF), then functions as a frame of reference for the coordinate system of the operating field volume, since all localizations are relative to the DRF (Figure 4.2). (Colloquially, ILD and DRF are used interchangeably, since for all practical purposes they serve the same function, i.e., they permit tracking by CAS tracking systems.)

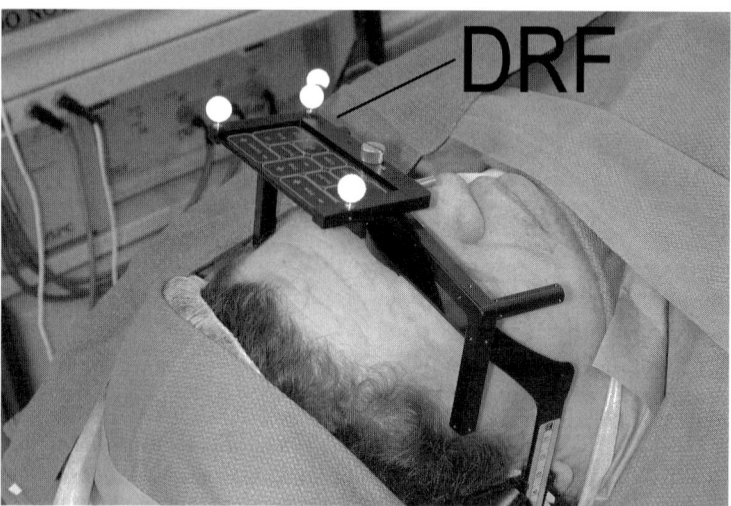

FIGURE 4.2 An ILD that is attached to the patient monitors the position of the operating field volume. This ILD, known as a DRF, may be a standard ILD, or a special ILD may be adapted for this purpose. The CBYON ENT headset (CBYON, Palo Alto, CA) with its DRF is shown.

Principles of Registration

Of course, maintaining a constant 3D relationship between the DRF and the operating field volume is critical. In this arrangement the CAS tracking system is tracking the position of the patient. After dynamic registration is achieved, the CAS system must track both the DRF and a second ILD, which is attached to a surgical instrument. This arrangement involves tracking two ILDs (the instrument ILD and the DRF, which is the ILD attached to the patient). Tracking two ILDs is inherently less precise than tracking a single ILD; however, this tradeoff in accuracy is small and not clinically significant. Since dynamic registration greatly enhances the usability of CAS in the real work, it is felt that dynamic registration is an essential feature for almost all registration protocols.

Obviously it is critically important that the DRF maintain a constant geometric relationship to the target area of interest in the operative field volume if dynamic registration is used. For this reason, dynamic registration works best for most sinus surgery and neurosurgery procedures. In these cases the DRF can be attached directly to the patient's head or skull through a variety of means. In contrast, dynamic registration is not feasible for any surgery involving soft tissues of the neck, since the tissue will inevitably deform before, during, and after registration. Similarly, registration for the bony spine is also problematic, since the vertebra to which the DRF is attached may move in relation to adjacent vertebrae. Consequently, robust registration strategies for spinal surgery is a very active area of technological development.

At the conclusion of the registration protocol, the CAS software calculates an error value, which summarizes the average calculated error of each fiducial point relative to all of the fiducial points. This calculation, known as the root mean square (RMS), expresses the standard deviation of each fiducial point of the registration data set compared to the entire set. Clinical experiences indicate that lower RMS values are associated with better surgical navigation accuracy, but this is not necessarily true in every case.

RMS data may be presented graphically as regions in which the mathematical calculations indicate the greatest statistical likelihood of precise registration (Figure 4.3). Although a graphical representation portrays more information than a single value, it should not be considered a substitute for direct estimation of surgical navigation accuracy.

Of course, smaller RMS error values are desirable; however, a registration with a small error value does not guarantee that the surgical navigation will provide accurate localizations. For this reason, it is critically important that surgeons verify the accuracy of surgical navigation by localizing against known landmarks so that practical limitations of the system for each case are fully known. Surgeons should also recheck accuracy by localizing against known landmarks throughout the entire case so that inadvertent drift caused by shifting ILDs can be recognized early. Similarly, surgeons should monitor surgical navigation accuracy at multiple landmarks widely separated in 3D space in the operating field volume. It is con-

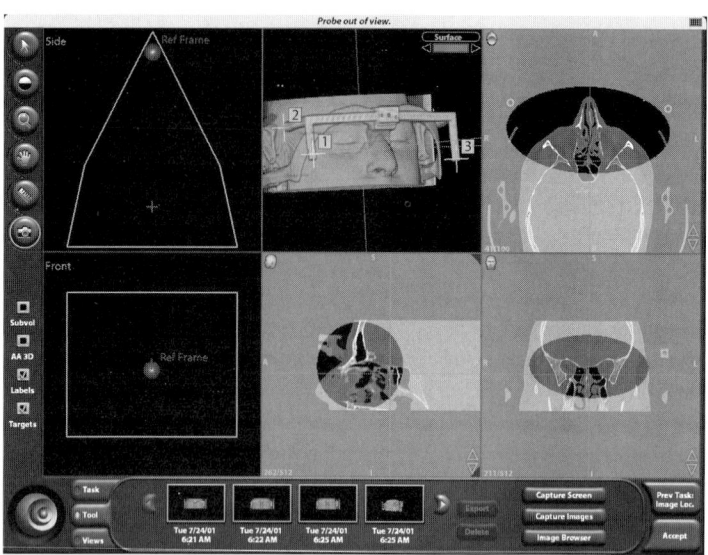

FIGURE 4.3 Registration error may be calculated mathematically; this information can then be presented in a graphical format. The CBYON Suite (CBYON, Palo Alto) displays zones of anticipated accuracy by displaying yellow or red masks on the preoperative axial, coronal, and sagittal CTs; the central zone—where the unaltered imaging is shown—shows the area of maximum anticipated accuracy. In this screen capture, the two left images convey information about the relative positions of the CAS pointer and DRF, and the central image on the upper row shows the current set of fiducial points.

ceivable that registration may yield good surgical navigation accuracy in one part of the operating field volume while the surgical navigation accuracy is quite poor in an adjacent region.

After registration is complete, CAS surgical navigation systems provide a means for monitoring the continued performance of the system; i.e., the systems will permit calculations of so-called sustained accuracy or verification points. (CAS vendors have applied multiple names to this function; in general, they all serve the same purpose.) In order to use this feature, the surgeon must localize to an arbitrary point, whose coordinates are stored by the CAS software. Throughout the case, the surgeon may localize the same target, and the system will indicate the drift (distance between the initial point and subsequent localizations). Any drift can be ascribed to DRF movement, CAS pointer damage, tracking failure, and other factors.

It should be emphasized that registration and calibration are not synonymous. Calibration confirms the geometry between the instrument tip and the

Principles of Registration

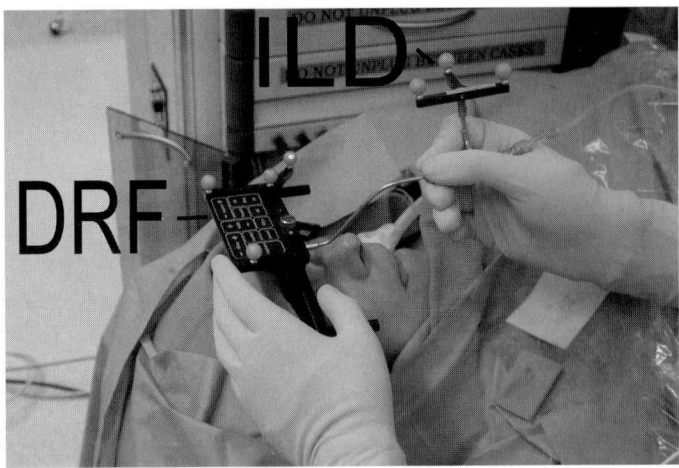

FIGURE 4.4 For instrument calibration, the desired CAS pointer (in this case, a modified suction with an attached DRF) is placed in a calibration divot/tube that is incorporated into the DRF. Both the CAS pointer and calibration point must have attached ILDs. (From CBYON, Palo Alto, CA)

attached ILD (Figure 4.4). In some systems, this geometry is predefined, and calibration only verifies the programed parameters that describe the relative positions of the ILD and instrument tip. If the instrument cannot be calibrated, then it is probably bent damaged. Obviously, this damaged pointer cannot be used. In other systems, an ILD can be clamped to any instrument at the discretion of the surgeon. Since CAS computer does not have a profile that describes the relationship between the instrument tip and this ILD, manual calibration must be performed. For manual calibration, the surgical instrument with the ILD must be touched to a predefined point while the surgeon clicks a specific button that initiates the calibration routine. Of course, if the position of the ILD is altered, the calibration step must be repeated. It also should be noted that some systems require periodic recalibration or at least verification of calibration so the usage of a damaged pointer can be minimized.

4.3 MANUAL REGISTRATION PARADIGMS

As described above, all registration paradigms deliver a system for aligning corresponding fiducial points in the operating field volume and the preoperative imaging data set volume. In manual registration, the surgeon must select points the fiducial points in the preoperative imaging data set and then localize with the surgical navigation pointer to the corresponding points in the operating field volume (Figure 4.5).

The steps for manual registration are as follows:

1. The surgeon reviews the preoperative images on the computer workstation and selects the desired fiducial data points. This step can be performed at almost any time after the preoperative images have been transferred to the computer workstation.
2. At the beginning of surgery, the CAS equipment must be set up as necessary. This step includes DRF placement. For sinus surgery, the DRF is typically attached to the patient's head with a band or vise-type device (Figure 4.6). For neurosurgery, the patient's head is placed in a Mayfield head holder, and the DRF is bolted to the Mayfield head holder.
3. Next, the CAS pointer (namely the operative instrument with an attached ILD) must be calibrated by localizing to a fixed point on the DRF.
4. Subsequently, the surgeon then localizes against the selected fiducial points.
5. The CAS software calculates the registration by mapping the coordinates of the points from the operating field volume with the corresponding coordinates from the preoperative imaging data set volume.
6. If the registration error is below a critical value, the system may automatically accept it, or the surgeon may need indicate that the registration is acceptable.
7. Of course, the surgeon must confirm accuracy of surgical navigation by localizing against known anatomical landmarks.

A variety of fiducial markers may be used. Bone-anchored fiducial markers are rigidly fixed to bone, while external fiducial markers are merely taped to the patient's skin (Figure 4.7). Sometimes, simple skin staples can serve as fiducial markers. Of course, all of these fiducial markers must be placed before the preoperative imaging study.

Bone-anchored fiducial markers are cumbersome, but they are clearly the gold standard since they provide excellent data for registration. The obvious practical issues limit their widespread use. External fiducial markers are often acceptable, but there are limitations. The external soft tissues exhibit a surprising amount of varying deformation so that the positions of the taped-on fiducial markers demonstrated a surprising amount of movement between the preoperative imaging and the actual surgery. The taped-on markers also cannot be moved until the manual registration is complete; therefore, the preoperative imaging must be done shortly before the planned surgical procedure.

Principles of Registration

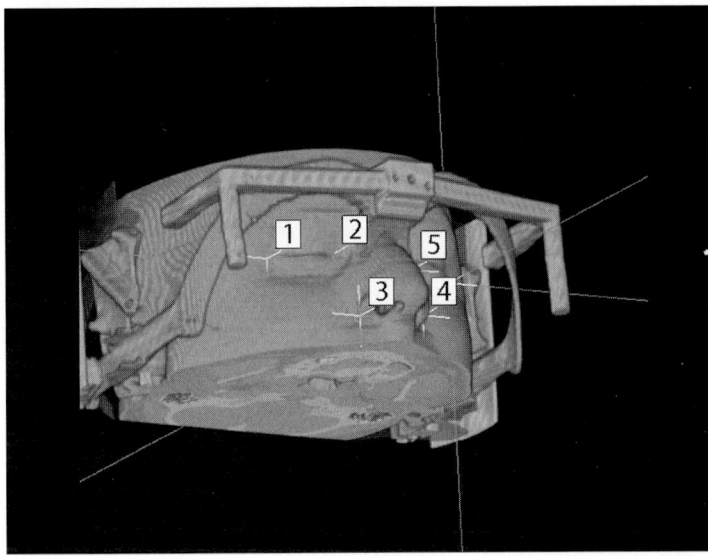

(A)

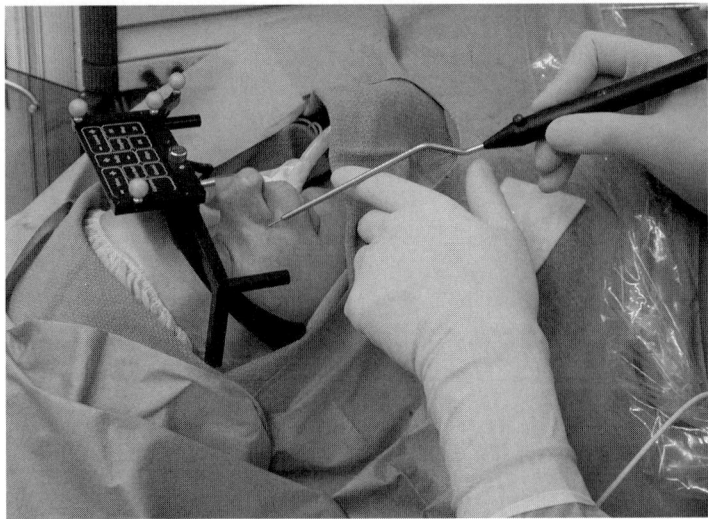

(B)

FIGURE 4.5 (A) In manual registration, fiducial points must be selected. In this example, five anatomical points were chosen. (B) For manual point mapping, the user must localize to the corresponding fiducial points in the operating field volume. In this example, the indicated fiducial point corresponds to point 3 in (A). (From CBYON, Palo Alto, CA)

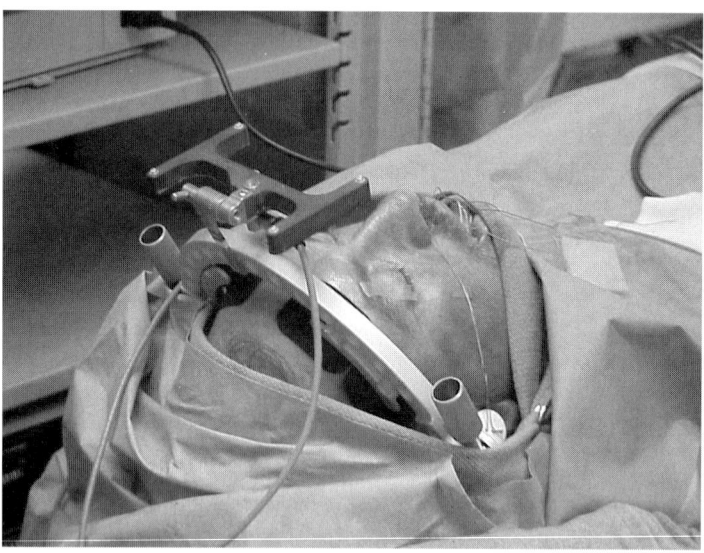

FIGURE 4.6 In manual registration, the ILD must be attached to the patient securely. This example shows the ENT headset for LandmarX (Medtronic Xomed, Jacksonville, FL).

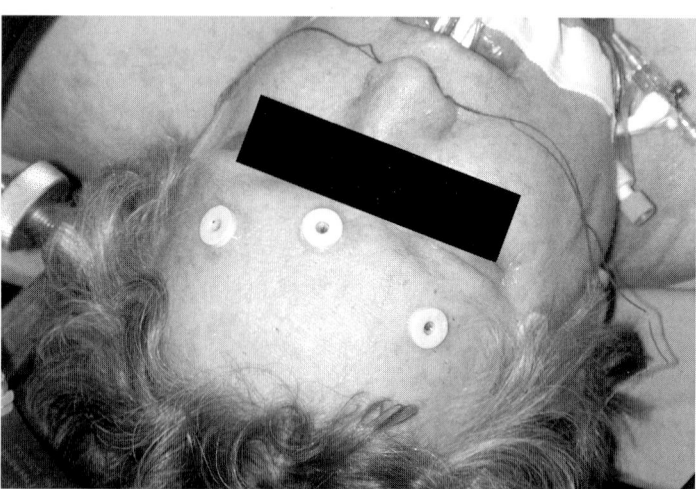

FIGURE 4.7 External fiducial markers may be simply taped to the patient's skin. In this instance, seven other markers were attached to other areas of the patient's head; these other markers are not seen in this image.

Principles of Registration

Anatomical fiducial landmarks can also support registration. Other limitations apply here. In some patients, the landmarks may be difficult to reproducibly identify. For instance, identification of facial landmarks on very round faces of obese patients can be problematic. Also, surgeons must learn to select these points reliably, and there are no rigid rules to guide this anatomical fiducial landmark selection.

4.4 AUTOMATIC REGISTRATION PARADIGMS

All automatic registration paradigms share similar features; i.e., they require the use of a relocatable frame that may be reproducibly placed on a patient in a noninvasive fashion. The frame contains a series of fiducial points that the computer software can automatically recognize. Intraoperatively, a DRF is attached to the relocatable frame so that the relationship between the DRF and the fiducial points in the relocatable frame is fixed. Intraoperative surgical navigation occurs by CAS computer projection of the tip of the CAS instrument onto the preoperative imaging study relative to the fiducial points in the relocatable frame. Since the relocatable frame fits the patient in only one way, this serves to show localization information relative to the patient's unique anatomy.

Automatic registration is uniquely suited to sinus surgery procedures. The CBYON ENT headset (CBYON, Palo Alto, CA) and the InstaTrak headset (Visualization Technology, Laurence, MA) both achieve automatic registration for most sinus surgery procedures (Figure 4.8). The fiducial system in the CBYON ENT headset is contained in a series of bars that are arranged in a cage-like shape. The InstaTrak headset houses a series of small, metallic spheres that act as fiducial points.

The steps for automatic registration are as follows:

1. The preoperative imaging is performed with the patient wearing the relocatable frame.
2. After the preoperative imaging data set is loaded into the computer, the CAS software must process the data so that the fiducial points are recognized. This step may occur automatically after loading the data, or the software may require an input from the user to proceed (Figure 4.9).
3. If the calculated error is within acceptable limits, the registration is complete. The registration process does not truly require that the relocatable frame be on the patient, although the user interface for the software may suggest that this is necessary.
4. The relocatable headset is placed on the patient (Figure 4.10), and function of the tracking system is confirmed.
5. The CAS probe is calibrated.
6. The surgeon must confirm the accuracy of surgical navigation by localizing against known anatomical landmarks.

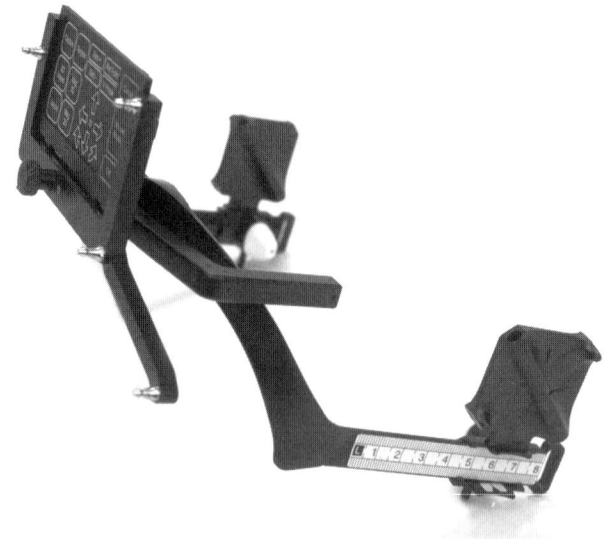

(A)

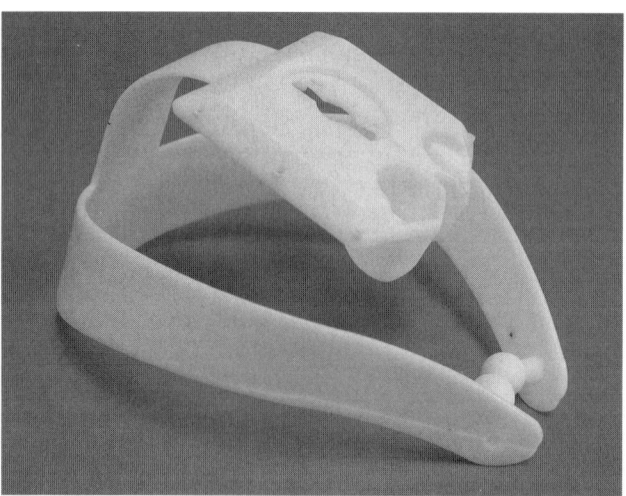

(B)

FIGURE 4.8 (A) The CBYON ENT headset (CBYON, Palo Alto, CA) incorporates the standard features of relocatable headsets for registration. The headset is designed so that it may be reproducibly placed on the patient's nose and ears. Built-in fiducial bars support registration. (B) The InstaTrak headset (Visualization Technology, Laurence, MA) is similar to the CBYON headset (shown in (A)). Built-in metallic spheres support registration.

Principles of Registration

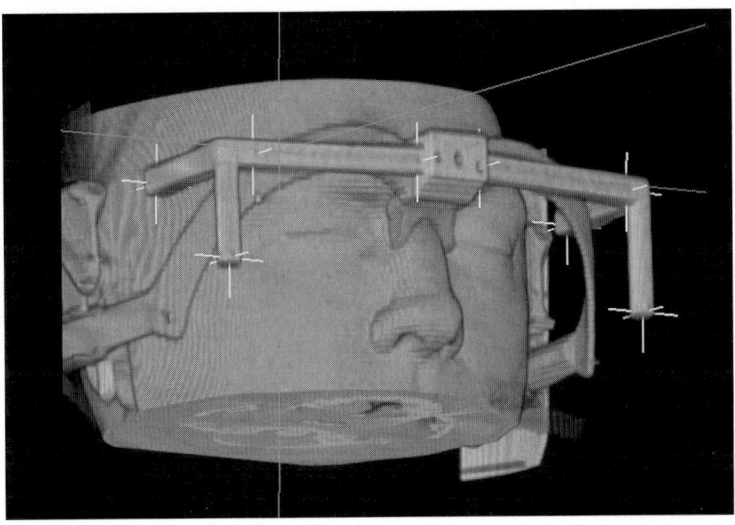

FIGURE 4.9 During automatic registration, the CAS software finds the position of the fiducial markers directly. In this screen capture (CBYON, Palo Alto, CA), the positions of the fiducial points are indicated by crosses.

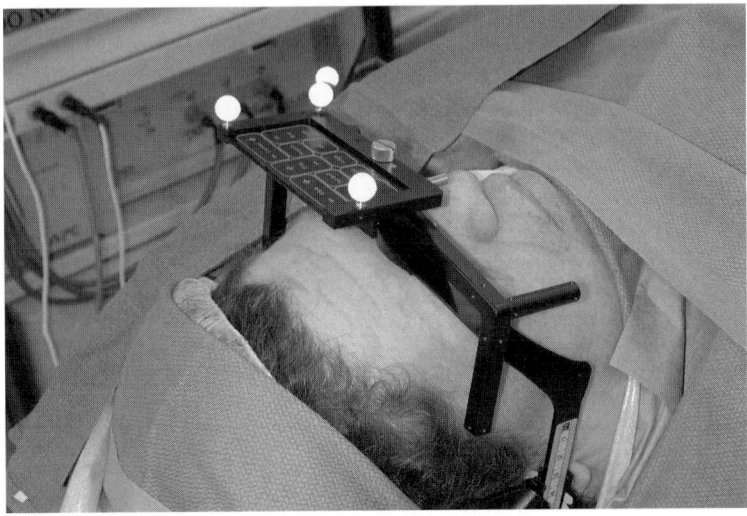

FIGURE 4.10 After automatic registration is complete, the special relocatable headset must be place on the patient as shown here. (From CBYON, Palo Alto, CA)

In automatic registration protocols, registration is complete after the software recognizes the location of fiducial points and calculates the relationship between these points and the defined position of the DRF. The relocatable frame does not need to be on the patient. As a result, registration accuracy in an automatic registration approach reflects the quality of the preoperative imaging data set, and surgical navigation accuracy depends upon a variety of factors, including repositioning of the relocatable frame and the registration accuracy, among other factors.

In automatic registration paradigms, RMS calculations only summarize the overall quality of the preoperative imaging study and the software's ability to locate the fiducial points of the headset. In this approach, the geometric relationship of the fiducial points is fixed—there is no significant variation between the anticipated and real positions of the points, since the points are all fixed in an array that does not change. As a result, the concept of RMS does not apply to automatic registration in the same way as it applies to manual registration, where the deviations between the anticipated and the actual positions of fiducial points are routinely encountered. In manual registration, the array of fiducial points (analogous to the fixed fiducial system in automatic registration) is defined for each case by the selection of fiducial points on the preoperative images; as a result, the geometric relationships among these points is unique for each case. As corresponding points from the surgical field are manually mapped to these points, deviations between their actual and anticipated positions are inevitable. RMS summarizes the degree of deviation between the actual and anticipated position for each point.

The design of the system for automatic registration is important for the success of automatic registration. Because the software performs the registration with almost no opportunity for user input, the software must accurately reconstruct models based on the preoperative image data, and the software must precisely identify the location of the fiducial markers in the preoperative imaging data set. To the extent that these processes introduce errors due to miscalculation, incorrect assumptions, etc., the overall robustness of automatic registration suffers. In addition, the arrangement of the fiducial markers in the relocatable frame is also very important. Ideally, these markers should be set so that they surround the anticipated area of interest. For this reason, the fiducial system for the CBYON ENT headset (CBYON, Palo Alto, CA) is configured like a box that surrounds the region of the paranasal sinuses.

The relocatable frames can also be adapted to support a semi-automated registration paradigm (Figure 4.11). In this approach, the surgeon performs manual point mapping to points on the relocatable frame. The steps are as follows:

1. The surgeon manually selects the fiducial points on the relocatable frame in the preoperative imaging data set.

Principles of Registration

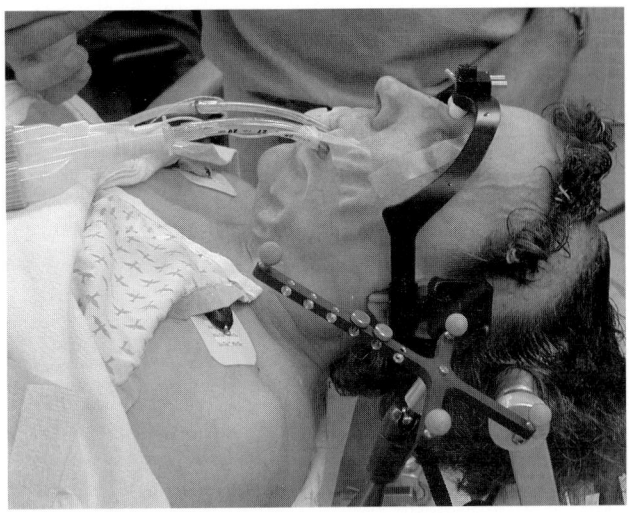

(A)

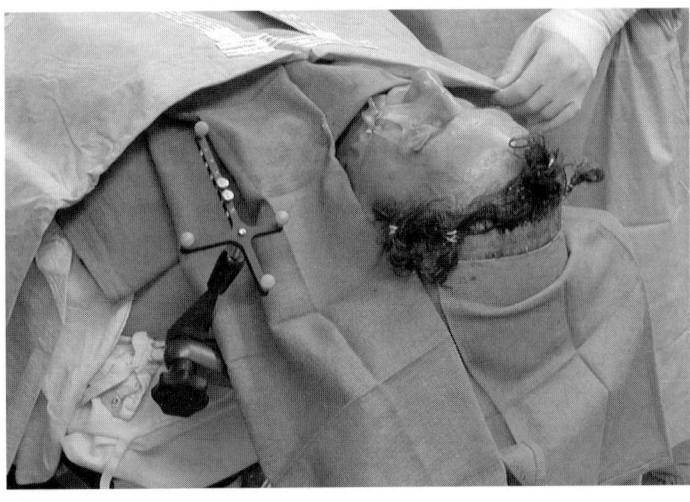

(B)

FIGURE 4.11 (A) In semi-automatic registration, the ILD (which is more accurately described as a DRF in this situation) must be directly attached to the patient. Fiducial markers on the headset in the preoperative imaging must be manually selected in the preoperative CT scan. Subsequently, the headset must be removed. Because the DRF is attached directly to the patient, the headset is no longer needed when point mapping is complete. (From CBYON, Palo Alto, CA). (B) In this photo, the CBYON headframe has been removed, since is use is redundant after semi-automatic registration has been achieved.

2. The DRF is secured directly to the patient, typically through a neurosurgical Mayfield head holder or a similar device.
3. The relocatable frame is placed on the patient.
4. The tracking system is prepared, and its function is confirmed.
5. The surgeon then localizes to the fiducial points on the relocatable frame.
6. The computer software calculates the registration.
7. The relocatable head frame is removed.
8. The surgeon must confirm the accuracy of surgical navigation.

Although semiautomatic registration has many features associated with manual registration paradigms, semiautomatic registration tends to be much faster. In semiautomatic registration, the initial selection of fiducial points in the preoperative imaging data set is very rapid, since small markers on the headset are easier to locate than standard fiducial markers and anatomical landmarks. Similarly, intraoperative localization to the fiducial points is faster for semiautomatic registration, since the points are easier to recognize than traditional fiducial points.

4.5 CONTOUR MAPPING REGISTRATION PARADIGMS

Registration may also be achieved by mapping surface contours from models derived from the preoperative imaging and the corresponding areas of the operating field (Figure 4.12). In theory this approach provides a large number of fiducial points; the resultant registration should be very high quality.

The basic steps for registration that is based upon contour maps are as follows:

1. The computer builds three-dimensional models from the two-dimensional preoperative imaging data through a process known as segmentation. Early segmentation routines were manual and required a great deal of user input; contemporary segmentation routines are mostly automated, although some user input may be necessary.
2. The tracking system, including DRF, is set up in the standard fashion.
3. The surgeon then localizes to a large number of points on various curvilinear surfaces.
4. The computer then calculates a registration that fits the contour defined by the intraoperative localization data to the contour defined by the segmentation models.
5. The surgeon must confirm surgical navigation accuracy by localizing against known landmarks.

Principles of Registration

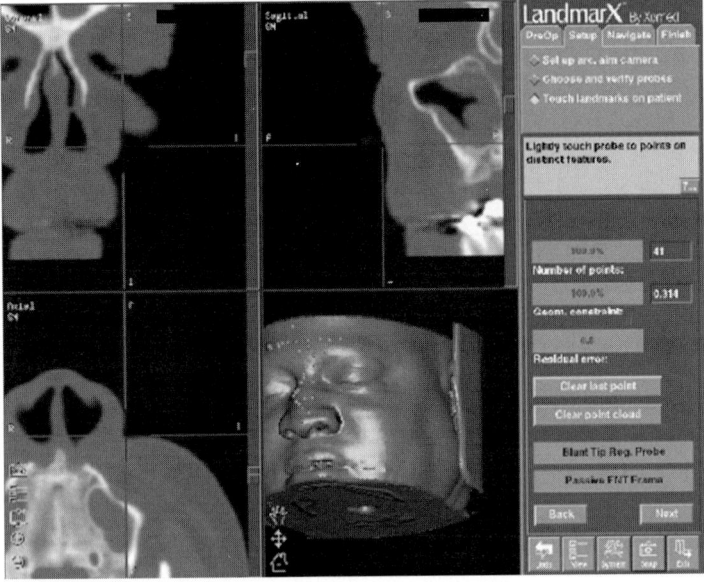

(A)

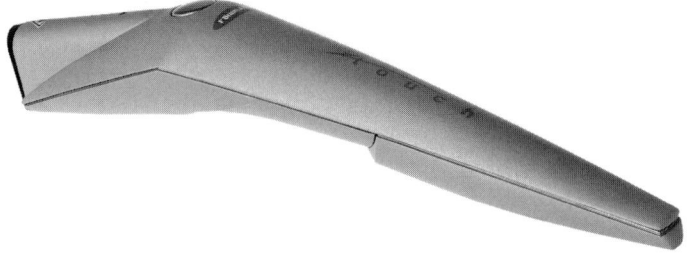

(B)

FIGURE 4.12 (A) The SurfaceMerge registration protocol for the LandmarX system (Medtronic Xomed, Jacksonville, FL) serves as an enhancement of the system's standard manual registration. After initial manual registration, the surgeon can choose an additional 40 random points along curvilinear surface contours by simply localizing at these points. The computer then calculates a contour from these points and fits it to the surface contour generated by segmentation modeling of the preoperative imaging data set. This screen capture shows the distribution of points along the patient's forehead, glabella, and external nose. Points at each tragus are not shown. (B) The VectorVision z-Touch registration system (BrainLab, Heimstetten, Germany) uses a laser light, whose reflection from the surface contour serves to define that contour. The z-Touch laser handpiece is shown here. In this approach, standard manual point mapping is not necessary, and a relocatable headset does not need to be used.

Initial contour mapping routines required multiple manual localizations (typically 30–40 or more, depending on the specific area of interest). Contour mapping has also been used as a refinement step that can be performed after simple point-mapping registration. Newer approaches utilize a laser, whose reflected light provides localization data about the intraoperative surface contour.

Contour-based registration is an attractive alternative. It seems simple, and the large number of fiducial points suggests good registration accuracy. Unfortunately, early reports have suggested that contour-based registration is less than precise than comparable routines based upon standard manual point mapping.

Contour-based registration has not been widely adopted for a number of reasons. First, the protocols for contour-based registration are newer, and surgeon familiarity with them is limited. Furthermore, these early protocols likely require additional refinement that will take additional time.

Additional technical improvements can be anticipated in the segmentation routines that drive the development of contours. This type of registration is dependent upon segmentation routines for the reconstruction of precise three-dimensional models, from which the contours are derived. If the segmentation routines are compromised by concerns imposed by limited computer memory and microprocessor speed, by poor preoperative imaging quality and/or by poor software design, then contour-based registration will always be suboptimal. Admittedly, faster, more affordable computer hardware is becoming available, but the software that is currently available or will be available in the foreseeable future is often designed to run on hardware with poorer performance. (It is less expensive to use older hardware, operating systems, and software drivers, and the various flaws in older computer equipment have mostly been discovered and corrected.) The quality of the preoperative imaging also must be considered. The best segmentation models require fine-cut computed tomography (CT) data (1 mm slice thickness or better); many scanners cannot provide the large number of slices of that thickness without overheating. Newer and better scanners will solve this problem. Since the high-resolution scanners are more expensive to purchase and operate, the availability of the appropriate CT scans cannot be assured.

Certain limitations are inherent to all contour-based registration protocols. It is doubtful that any amount of development will overcome these intrinsic features. The distribution of the fiducial points as well as their number influences the quality of the registration. A large number of points that are coplanar or nearly coplanar will provide a poor registration, and surgical navigation error will grow as one localizes to points further from the plane of fiducial points. In fact, the three-dimensional geometry of the fiducial points may be more important than the number of points. Contour-based registration typically relies upon a large number of points from areas such as the forehead and cheeks, which are relatively flat and coplanar; this is simply not an optimal arrangement. Furthermore, the

Principles of Registration 67

involved contours are not fixed; changes in facial expression, overall body weight, and skin turgor will all influence the contours.

4.6 IMAGE FUSION

Image fusion refers to a software technique that blends corresponding images from two different imaging data sets. In this way, two different CT scans or two different magnetic resonance imaging (MRI) scans can be merged. Alternatively, a CT scan and an MRI scan can be merged. In this way it is possible to morph between two different sets of images.

The process of aligning the corresponding images is a type of registration, since it involves mapping corresponding points. Registration for image fusion is relatively straightforward. It requires that the user identify corresponding fiducial points in each data set. The computer then maps the corresponding points to each other and thereby aligns the images. The fiducial points may be standard external fiducial markers, bone-anchored fiducial markers, anatomical landmarks, and/or markers built into relocatable frames. The CAS software may contain specific software tools that facilitate this process. Such tools are helpful, but not mandatory for successful registration for image fusion.

4.7 IMAGE-ENHANCED ENDOSCOPY

In image-enhanced endoscopy (IEE), a new feature in the CBYON Suite (CBYON, Palo Alto, CA), the CAS computer calculates the perspective view from the tip of the surgical telescope and projects both the virtual endoscopic view of the preoperative imaging data and the real world endoscopic view in real time (Figure 4.13). Both the perspective view generated by the software and the endoscopic view through the telescope must be tightly aligned for useful IEEE. This requires a specific registration protocol. The system must also reconstruct a high-quality perspective three-dimensional model with movement, and the tracking system must monitor instrument position. Of course, the analog video single from the endoscopic camera must be sent to the CAS computer's video card for digital conversion.

During IEE registration, the telescope is focused on a grid pattern; the software can recognize this pattern and align a perspective model of a similar grid (Figure 4.14). In this way, the real view and virtual view are aligned.

IEE must be especially robust, since even a small amount of error renders IEE useless. Obviously, the major factor in the IEE registration process is its software, since so much of the entire process is software-derived segmentation and modeling. Powerful computers with sophisticated graphics cards are necessary to run this graphics-intensive software.

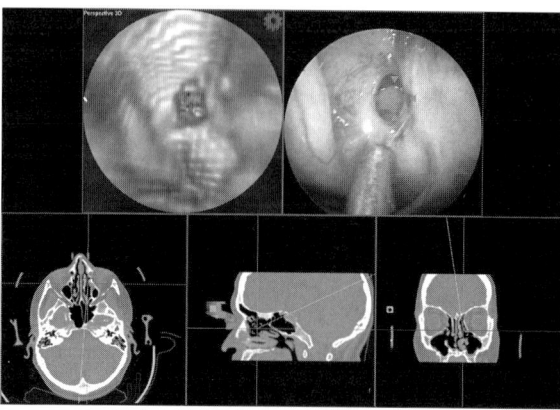

FIGURE 4.13 This still image capture from CBYON Suite Image-Enhanced Endoscopy (CBYON, Palo Alto, CA) depicts the view provided by the telescope (upper right panel) and the corresponding view of the virtual model (upper left panel). The virtual model shows the optic nerve in green, but the optic nerve cannot be seen in the standard telescopic view. In this way, IEE provided anatomical information that was supplementary to the view afforded by the nasal telescope. The lower panels depict the relative position of the tip of the suction (seen in the real endoscopic image).

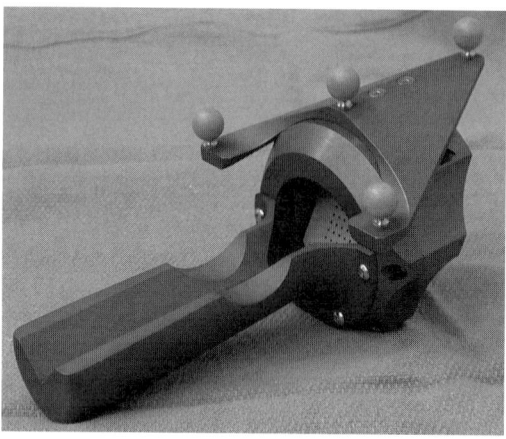

FIGURE 4.14 IEE registration of the perspective virtual model and the real endoscopic view is performed with this device, which houses a special grid pattern that serves to register the endoscopic view. The attached passive ILD indicates the location and orientation of the device during IEE registration. The user simply orients the telescope in the long axis of the device and the software processes the endoscopic image of the registration grid pattern. This data then permits co-registration of both the standard endoscopic view and the virtual endoscopic view.

Principles of Registration

4.8 REGISTRATION FAILURES

It is important to distinguish between problems with surgical navigation and problems with registration. Since registration maps corresponding fiducial points in the preoperative imaging data set volume and the operating field volume, registration failures reflect misalignment of these points. Surgical navigation fails when the estimated accuracy of the system against known landmarks is suboptimal. In fact, surgical navigation errors may arise, and the registration may still be in tact. (Admittedly, surgical navigation and registration errors can overlap, and from a clinical perspective the implications can be very similar. However, users of CAS must be able to understand the fundamental issues so that they can troubleshoot the technology effectively.)

Probably the most important factor in the fidelity of registration is the quality of the fiducial points as well as their arrangement in 3D space around the area of surgical interest. The best fiducial points can be easily recognized on the preoperative images and in the operating field. Even in automatic registration paradigms, the software routines must be able to locate the fiducial markers in the preoperative imaging. During manual registration using anatomical fiducial landmarks, it is critical that the surgeon precisely identify the selected points in the operative field during registration and that these points precisely match the fiducial points selected on the preoperative images.

All registration approaches require a theoretical minimum of three fiducial points. In practice, a greater number of fiducial points are used, since the greater number tends to enhance the precision of the resultant registration; however, above a certain number (approximately 6–12 points, depending on the application), the impact of each additional fiducial point on the overall registration is progressively less critical. For this reason, large numbers of fiducial points are not used unless contour mapping is the basis of the registration. (In registration based on contour mapping, corresponding contours are aligned; these contours are defined by large numbers of individual points, but the individual points themselves are not mapped to their corresponding points.) In fact, a large number of fiducial points may degrade the net registration accuracy, since an aberrant fiducial point, which becomes more likely as all of the preferred fiducial points have been used, will have a profound impact on the registration process.

The spatial distribution of the fiducial points influences registration fidelity. Ideally, the fiducial points are distributed in 3D space around the entire surgical area. If some or all of the fiducial points are coplanar (i.e., in the same plane) or the fiducial points are located far from the operative field, then the registration in the area of interest will be poor. For instance, if all fiducial points are located on the skin surface overlying the frontal bone, then the registration may be acceptable in the immediate frontal area; however, the registration will deteriorate as one moves from the area of fiducial points to other regions of the paranasal sinuses. On the other hand, arranging the fiducial points so that they surround the sinuses will yield a much higher registration throughout the paranasal sinuses. In this example, the placement of fiducial points at the tragus or temple areas as well as the anterior frontal area provides very good registration.

The quality of the preoperative imaging data set greatly influences the results of all types of registration. Higher resolution scans provide better data for the localization of fiducial markers preoperatively. This is true both in automatic systems, where software locates the markers automatically, and in manual systems, where the user must choose the fiducial points. Simply stated, a thin 1 mm axial CT is always preferable to a similar CT scan performed at a greater slice thickness. In a sense, the thickness of the slice determines the functional limit of registration accuracy (and surgical navigation). The system cannot be more precise than the slice thickness in the preoperative imaging data. As a result, recommendations for the use of 2 mm (or 3 mm) slices effectively sets the lower limit of accuracy at 2 mm (or 3 mm) under the best possible circumstances. When these thicker slices are used, it may be unreasonable to anticipate accuracy of better than 2 mm.

Since registration procotols are driven by the software that runs them, the precision of the software processes influences registration. In early CAS systems, limited hardware resources for manipulation of large amounts of image data led programmers and designers to approximate some image manipulations so that the software would run efficiently. Obviously, these choices compromised the ultimate fidelity of calculations for the sake of speed. In addition, inadvertent software code error (poor programming) also can degrade registration. For many applications (especially early applications), these issues were not significant; however, as the surgical applications have grown more sophisticated and as the resultant demands on the CAS systems have increased accordingly, these limitations may be more problematic, especially when older CAS systems are used for more complicated applications.

In manual registration, the tracking system also must function well so that the surgeon can perform point mapping. Failure of the tracking apparatus and damaged (i.e., bent) instruments can compromise intraoperative tracking.

User error can also cause poor manual registration. To the extent that the actual location of the CAS probe tip differs from the position intended by user during point mapping, the calculated RMS value for the registration will rise and the resultant registration will suffer. In other words, if the user intends to place the CAS probe tip at one location, but the tracking system localizes the probe tip to another location, then that difference is a mapping error. Each mapping error contributes to the total error of the registration. Contemporary tracking systems can track instruments with a precision of 1 mm (or even better) in laboratory settings; when a registration error occurs due to misalignment of corresponding points, failure of the tracking system rarely causes this problem. The real issue

Principles of Registration

is usually incorrect selection of the point in the preoperative imaging data set and/or in the operating field volume. Both of these are user errors.

User errors rarely influence the accuracy of automatic registration, since the registration process simply localizes the fiducial markers on the relocatable headset in the preoperative imaging data set. As a practical matter, user error can compromise the next step in these systems. If the relocatable headset is not correctly placed on the patient, then differences between the intraoperative placement and the placement used at the time of preoperative imaging leads to obvious errors. For this reason, radiology personnel and operating room personnel (including the surgeon) must be familiar with the relocatable headset.

Registration protocols are designed to support surgical navigation. If registration fails, then surgical navigation will be impossible. In some cases, registration may seem successful, but the surgical navigation accuracy will be poor. For this reason, surgeons must continually check the fidelity of surgical navigation by localizing against known anatomical landmarks in the operating field volume throughout the case. When surgical navigation accuracy is compromised, the cause usually can be tracked to one of the following problems:

1. The initial registration was not as robust as it initially appeared.
2. The DRF has shifted relative to the operating field volume.
3. The CAS pointer is damaged, or the CAS pointer is no longer calibrated due to even a slight shift in the alignment of the tip relative to the ILD.
4. The tracking system has failed. The actual hardware can fail. Transient errors are more common. If the line of sight between the ILDs and the camera array is not maintained for optical systems, then the system cannot track. Similarly, distortions of the electromagnetic field can disrupt tracking based on electromagnetic sensors.
5. The CAS software can freeze/crash. These bugs can be obvious, but they can be more subtle. If the latter is true, then detection of this error can be much more difficult.

4.7 CONCLUSION

Registration refers to the process through which corresponding fiducial points in the preoperative imaging data set volume and the intraoperative operating field volume are aligned. As a result, registration serves as the foundation for surgical navigation. Paradigms for registration may be divided into the categories of manual point mapping, automatic registration (with a relocatable headset), and contour mapping. Each of these approaches offers specific advantages and disadvantages. Because of the complexity of registration and its impact on clinical applications, surgeons should be familiar with registration principles. This will serve to enhance the overall clinical effectiveness of CAS.

5

Intraoperative Magnetic Resonance Imaging

Neil Bhattacharyya, M.D., F.A.C.S., and Liangge Hsu, M.D.
Brigham and Women's Hospital, Harvard Medical School, Boston, Massachusetts

Marvin P. Fried, M.D.
Albert Einstein College of Medicine and Montefiore Medical Center, Bronx, New York

5.1 INTRODUCTION

The surgical anatomy of the head and neck is replete with a higher density of vascular, nervous, and specialized soft tissue structures than virtually any other portion of the human body. Surgery within the head and neck therefore confronts the otolaryngologist with a complex array of interrelated three-dimensional structures that govern the approach, safety, and efficacy for operative procedures within the head and neck. The otolaryngologist is often faced with balancing complete extirpation of the lesion, preservation of complex functions, avoidance of vitally important surrounding structures, and cosmesis when considering surgery within the head and neck.

The advent of multiplanar imaging technology has had a profound impact on the diagnosis and surgical treatment of otolaryngologic disease. Computed tomography (CT) has virtually supplanted plain film radiography in the diagnosis of chronic rhinosinusitis, chronic otitis media, and upper airway anatomy [1]. It is now widely employed in the staging of head and neck tumors, both at the primary site and as a screening tool for nodal metastases to the neck. CT is also extremely valuable in the preoperative anatomical planning for endoscopic sinus surgery and extirpative procedures for head and neck neoplasia [2]. CT derives its utility mainly from its highly accurate delineation of bony and soft tissue detail, separating the morphology of pathological processes from normal anatomy. More recently, magnetic resonance imaging (MRI) has seen wider utilization in the diagnosis of otolaryngologic disease. It is now considered the gold standard test for the diagnosis of acoustic neuroma and neoplastic conditions of the skull base. While both of these modalities provide excellent spatial resolution, MRI has the advantages of imaging in multiple planes and better delineation of soft tissue detail [3].

Until recently, both CT and MRI have been primarily employed in the preoperative diagnosis and surgical planning for lesions within the head and neck; real-time or intraoperative use of these modalities has been quite limited. Several groups have explored CT for localization and needle biopsy of head and neck tumors [4]. CT has shown promise in adding to the accuracy of fine needle biopsy for nodal staging of head and neck tumors [5]. Even more recently, intraoperative MRI has been explored as a surgical adjunct for biopsy and operative treatment of head and neck lesions [3,6]. The advent of new technology has largely been responsible for these contemporary advances.

Intraoperative multiplanar imaging may present several advantages for surgery within the head and neck. First, as a navigational tool, it may assist the surgeon in avoiding important surrounding structures while performing the surgical procedure within the intended anatomy. In addition, it may provide real-time confirmation that the intended lesion has been biopsied, removed, or appropriately modified by the procedure [7]. These potential advantages have driven current investigators to pursue intraoperative or interventional magnetic resonance imaging (I-MRI) and to develop additional technologies to provide such information intraoperatively.

5.2 DESCRIPTION OF THE TECHNOLOGY
5.2.1 Description of the Open MRI Unit

While several interventional MRI units are under construction or in early use, only a few have been employed with published data for head and neck purposes. We describe here in the prototype open MR interventional suite currently in use

Intraoperative Magnetic Resonance Imaging

at the Brigham and Women's Hospital and Harvard Medical School [8]. This magnet has been operational since January 1994.

The prototype open MRI magnet is housed in a 3500 square foot suite within a 25 × 25 feet procedure room (Figure 5.1). The design was implemented by General Electric in 1987 in collaboration with the Brigham and Women's Hospital, Boston, and installed in January 1994. The magnet itself is a 0.5 Tesla superconducting magnet constructed for the sole purpose of providing image guidance for minimally invasive surgical procedures. The unit itself has an "open" configuration, with six superconducting coils arranged to accommodate a split cryostat, allowing a 56 cm wide vertical gap. This vertical gap allows the surgeon "bedside" access to the patient, similar to that provided in the conventional operating suite configuration. This essential vertical gap for access to the patient is achieved by modifying the two-coil Helmholtz design, and altering the superconducting material by using niobium-tin with the slightly higher transition temperature of 18.1 K (versus niobium-titanium with a transition temperature of 10.1 K). This small difference in temperature permits the coils to operate at a higher temperature for which a two-stage cryocooler assembly is adequate, thus obviating the need for the liquid helium bath. The absence of this liquid helium bath permits an increase space between the superconducting coils, thus allowing for the vertical gap [9]. Three pairs of superconducting coils are housed in a

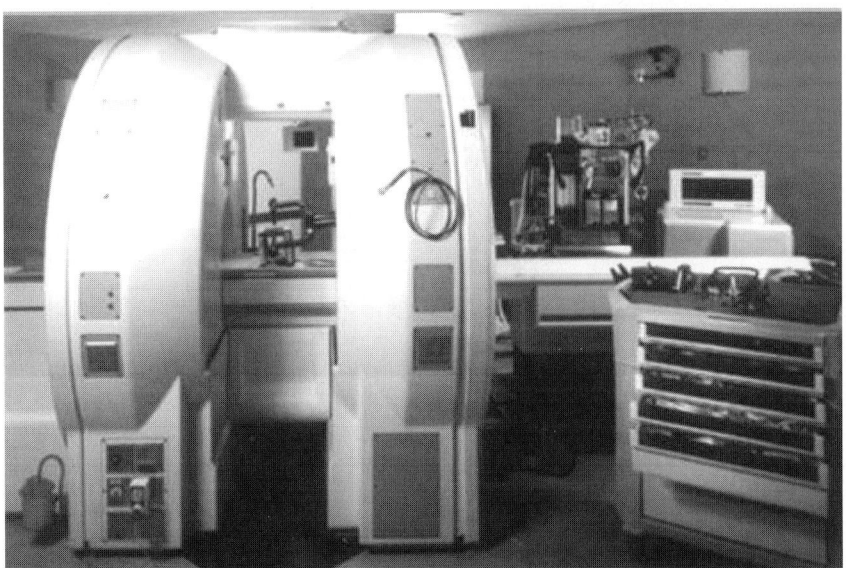

FIGURE 5.1 Open magnet interventional magnetic resonance imaging unit.

separate but communicating cryostat, which provides a homogeneous spherical imaging volume approximately 30 cm in diameter. Surface flexible transmission and receiving radio frequency coils are placed over the area of interest for image acquisition. The system is also designed to allow differing patient positions, including the sitting position, as well as allowing the operate surgeon to be positioned sitting or standing at either the patient's head or side (Figure 5.2). A high-quality two-way audio system provides communication between the operating surgeon and radiology personnel during the procedure (Figure 5.3).

In addition to the magnet, the operating suite is specially designed to merge features of a radiology suite with the essential features of a traditional operating room. In order to do so, multiple special innovations were conceived to allow the introduction of many of the basic instrumentation, anesthesia, and monitoring devices into and around the magnetic field. The relevant concerns include safety of both the patient and health-care personnel and the compatibility of instruments, monitoring devices, and anesthesia delivery, as well as proper functioning of various image display and integration systems.

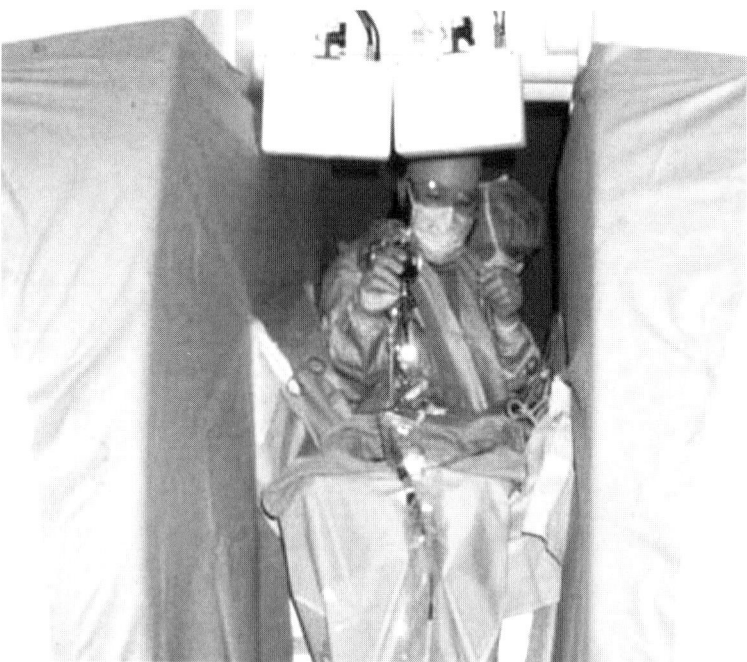

FIGURE 5.2 Open magnet interventional magnetic resonance imaging unit. The surgeon's access to the operative field is demonstrated.

Intraoperative Magnetic Resonance Imaging

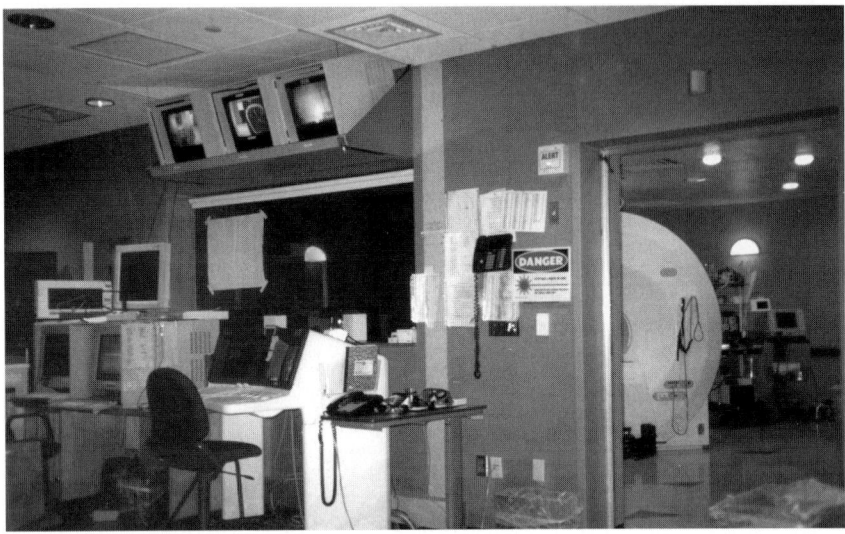

FIGURE 5.3 Interventional MR console. The radiologists and MR technicians control the I-MRI unit through this interface. Direct interaction with the surgical team influences the progress of the surgical procedure.

5.2.2 Anesthesia Considerations

All of the anesthesia equipment employed in the I-MRI suite must be magnetic resonance (MR) compatible. The anesthesia workstation (XL10 MRI Compatible Anesthesia Station: Ohmeda, Madison, WI), ventilator (Omnivent, Topeka, KS), and monitoring equipment systems, including pulse oximetry, electrocardiogram, automated noninvasive blood pressure and invasive pressure transducer, were specially designed to be MRI compatible. Most of the other anesthesia equipment such as intravenous lines, needles, and syringes are standard, and no modifications were required. Other items meeting modification included aluminum oxygen tanks and IV poles as well as nonmagnetic lithium batteries. Unfortunately, MRI-compatible infusion pumps and intubating devices are not currently available. This requires that patients be intubated outside the operating enclosure, followed by subsequent transfer into the I-MRI procedure room [8].

One of the major concerns for patient safety involves the inability to perform a standard 12-lead EKG within the procedure room because of the ST wave distortion caused by the magnetic field. A limited monitoring EKG system was developed with EKG leads composed of carbon-fiber or fiber optics to provide intraoperative cardiac monitoring. In the event of a potential intraoperative cardiopulmonary event, the patient would be brought outside the procedure room immediately. The magnetic field may then be "quenched" within 70 seconds and cardiac defibrillation performed; cardiac defibrillation itself is not MRI compatible.

5.2.3 Surgical Instrumentation

As most standard surgical instrumentation is made of stainless steel or other ferromagnetic products, special equipment must be designed that is MR compatible. This is especially important in otolaryngology, where multiple sets of specialized instruments are required for various procedures. Special equipment has been designed in conjunction with surgical instrument manufacturers to be used in the I-MRI suite [8]. Most are made from material such as low iron content stainless steel, copper, or titanium. Surgical instruments made from brass, ceramic, and carbon fiber have an additional advantage in that they demonstrate the least imaging artifact on intraoperative MRI scans. For procedures such as endoscopic sinus surgery (ESS), additional special instrumentation was required including endoscopes, forceps, and probes (Storz Surgical Instruments, St. Louis, MO) [10]. High-speed pneumatic drills (Midas Rex, Fort Worth, TX) are similar to conventional drills except that the drill bearings are made of ceramic materials.

5.2.4 Image-Guidance Methodologies
5.2.4.1 Optical Tracking System

Image guidance during the surgical procedure is provided by near real-time MR imaging via a three-dimensional optical tracking system that utilizes two infrared light-emitting diodes (LED) mounted on a handpiece or incorporated into various surgical instruments. Three high-resolution digital cameras mounted overhead within the magnet track the position of the handpiece, in an arrangement that is similar to other optical tracking devices. Spatial position and three-dimensional coordinates are then calculated and MR images in three orthogonal planes are generated on the MR images, providing image localization. A 5-inch square liquid crystal display monitor, which is mounted within the vertical gap, displays a crosshair on any one of three orthogonal MR images, thus providing the surgeon with image localization of the surgical instrument [11]. Other investigators have also developed nonoptical image tracking techniques that can be localized via real-time MR scanning [12]. Such systems have the advantage of not being subject to optical signal loss, which can occur in a confined imaging volume due to spatial limitations.

5.2.4.2 Real-Time MRI During Surgery

In addition to the optical tracking system, the I-MRI unit is capable of real-time MRI scans of the operative field during the surgical procedure. A methodology

Intraoperative Magnetic Resonance Imaging 79

known as "interactive scan plane control" has been developed to allow interactive scanning with the plane to be scanned determined by the operating surgeon. The scan plane is determined by the surgeon at discrete times during the procedure by using a single-purpose pointer brought into the surgical field [8]. The position of this pointer is recognized by a detection system utilizing infrared LED that are mounted above the vertical operating gap within the magnet. The position of the LED is then calculated by computer algorithm providing coordinates in the sagittal, axial, and coronal planes. The pointing device is then visualized by the surgeon as a small crosshair on the MRI console and the liquid crystal display, and the position of the pointing device is verified. The main purpose of the pointing device is to dictate the three-dimensional planes to be imaged by the real-time scan. Once the desired position has been confirmed, a real-time MR scan may be obtained, and multiplanar MR images centered on the desired position in the surgical field can be visualized. This allows active verification of surgical position within the operating field and shows changes in anatomy produced by the procedure itself [8].

Static pointing devices have also been developed for use in surgical localization. Such pointers can be constructed of gadolinium-filled or labeled tubes and instruments. When real-time scans are conducted with these instruments in the surgical field, these pointers appear as high-intensity objects on T_1-weighted MR images. This type of pointing device is non interactive and does not dictate the plane to be imaged, but rather serves to verify surgical position, even when anatomy has changed due to the surgical procedure.

5.2.4.3 Acquisition Times

With the current technology, images may be acquired at discrete intervals during surgery with a mean acquisition time of 14 seconds using a "fast spin echo" sequence, with a relaxation time (TR) of 400 msec and an excitation time (TE) 26 msec. This acquisition time compares quite favorably to conventional spin echo sequences, which require minutes for acquisition. Even faster acquisition times of images during the procedure can be achieved with "fast gradient sequences." However, though these images only require 1–2 sec to compose, these sequences provide less signal-to-noise quality, and thus provide significantly less anatomical resolution. They have been found to afford good intraoperative instrument localization.

5.2.5 Training of Personnel

Accompanying the development of any innovative technology is a learning curve required to employ the technology effectively. This is even truer in the I-MRI suite because of the complex interactions between the operating surgeon, radiology personnel, and anesthesia personnel. Prior to utilizing the I-MRI suite in clinical trials, extensive training was conducted with cadavers [8]. Such training was conducted not only to familiarize operating surgeons with the spatial limitations of the open magnet system, but also to verify the MR compatibility of the surgical instrumentation. In addition, studies were conducted to verify the accuracy and precision of the optical tracking system and the intraoperative MR images. The three-dimensional optical tracking system has been found to be linear to within 1% through the 30 cm imaging volume. The tracking accuracy of the instrument within the imaging volume exhibits a 1 mm tolerance. During training, it was evident that one problem with the optical tracking system is that it is extremely sensitive to changes in instrumentation angle, which may obscure optical tracking of the LED. Such considerations must be carried over into clinical preparations and planning.

In addition to the surgeon's operative training, extensive training for support staff and personnel is required to orient them to the unique safety and efficiency considerations required by the open magnet system. A special team of anesthesia personnel familiar with the I-MRI and its limitations was assembled and trained. Similar considerations were employed in assembling the nursing staff for head and neck I-MRI procedures. Patients and operating room personnel with cardiac pacemakers or aneurysm clips that have not been verified as MR compatible must be excluded from the operating suite. Special protocols for emergencies, equipment failure, and unforeseen circumstances must be constructed and implemented in order to ensure proper patient safety [8].

5.3 APPLICATIONS
5.3.1 MRI-Guided Biopsy of Head and Neck Lesions

Fine needle aspiration biopsy (FNAB) is now commonplace in the diagnosis of head and neck lesions. It may be used to provide an initial cytological diagnosis for primary lesions arising in major salivary glands, submucosal lesions in the upper aerodigestive tract, and cervical lymphadenopathy. It has been shown to be highly sensitive, specific, and reliable [13,14].

Extensive work has been done with coupling FNAB to various imaging modalities. Such a linkage offers the attractive benefit of ensuring that the desired tissue is actually sampled. Increasing accuracy for FNAB has been demonstrated when ultrasound or CT guidance is used to direct and confirm the biopsy [15,16]. Sensitivity and specificity may be increased to up to 95% with these adjunctive techniques. Image-guided biopsy techniques are essential when the lesion is not palpable, situated within the deeper structures of the head and neck, or when vital structures lie between the scan and the lesion of interest [16].

MR-guided FNAB may provide distinct advantages over other image-

Intraoperative Magnetic Resonance Imaging

guided biopsy techniques. First, with the capacity to image in multiple planes, three-dimensional confirmation that the target tissue has been sampled may be realized. Second, of the major imaging techniques, MRI provides the best resolution and distinctions of the various soft tissues within the head and neck [17]. Since in many cases it is desirable to follow the biopsy needle from its entry point continuously until it reaches the target tissue, multiple scans are often required. In this situation, iterative CT scans will result in additional radiation exposure to the patient (and health-care personnel), and such CT scans may require administration of intravenous contrast with potential attendant side effects. Although ultrasound imparts no radiation to the patient, it is less efficient at delineating soft tissue/soft tissue interfaces than MRI. Because of its favorable imaging characteristics (Table 5.1) and the lack of radiation exposure, MR-guided biopsy in the head and neck has recently been explored [3,6].

Fried and associates [3] reported on their initial patient experience with MR-guided needle biopsies within the head and neck. In their series of seven patients, none of the lesions requiring biopsy could be palpated or visualized on routine examination. Target lesions included four parotid gland lesions, two tumors of the parapharyngeal space, and one lesion of the second cervical vertebra. Using intraoperative fast-gradient echo pulse sequences, with 2–4 sec acquisition times, interactive MR-guided biopsies were performed. The authors were able to successfully localize the desired tissue for biopsy using both the previously described optical tracking system as well as sequential intraoperative scanning. Notably, the authors found that the needle trajectory required alteration several times based on the intraoperative images. In five of seven cases the MR-guided

TABLE 5.1 Summary of Important Distinctions Between Potential Intraoperative Imaging Modalities

	Intraoperative imaging modality		
	Ultrasound	Computed tomography	Magnetic resonance imaging
Portability	Yes	No	No
Imparts radiation exposure	No	Yes	No
Multiplanar imaging	Single plane	Multiplanar (2 planes)[a]	Multiplanar (3 planes)
Strength of imaging	Cystic lesions	Bone/soft tissue interface	Soft tissue interfaces

[a] The third (sagittal) imaging plane may be viewed from reconstructed images, but this consumes additional time and is not yet widely employed intraoperatively.

needle biopsies were diagnostic and accurate. This is especially notable because none of these lesions were palpable or located in easily accessible regions. No complications were encountered.

An example of an interactive MR-guided needle biopsy is shown in Figure 5.4. A 57-year-old male noted left upper neck swelling for 1 month without a palpable mass. Further evaluation disclosed the lesion on MRI, and an MR-guided FNA was performed as demonstrated. The cytological findings were consistent with a pleomorphic adenoma, which was subsequently excised.

In a recent study by Davis and associates [6], a series of 21 patients were submitted for MR-guided biopsies of head and neck lesions. Of these, 9 were nonpalpable lesions, and 8 lesions involved deeps tissue spaces within the head and neck not conventionally accessible by standard FNAB techniques. Two patients had previously unsuccessful needle biopsies of their lesion. The authors found a concurrence rate of 92% between the MR-guided needle biopsy technique and subsequent open biopsy or surgical therapy. No complications were encountered within this patient series. The authors concluded that the use of MR-guided needle biopsy added to the accuracy and safety of the needle biopsy procedure. Furthermore, several patients were able to avoid potentially morbid and disfiguring surgeries based on the MR-guided needle biopsy results. Similar findings were noted in a series of 24 patients reported by Wang and associates [18].

Further work needs to the established to verify the accuracy and safety of MR-guided needle biopsy in the head and neck. The intuitive advantages of MR imaging coupled with the ability to perform scans track the biopsy needle trajectory may potentially offer the most reliable integrated needle biopsy technique in the head and neck. Further work is currently being conducted to develop active real-time tracking systems for the needle biopsy instrument and to develop alternative trajectory approaches for difficult to reach lesions [12].

5.3.2 MRI-Guided Endoscopic Sinus Surgery

Image guidance during endoscopic sinus surgery (ESS) has been a major focus in otolaryngology-head and neck surgery [2,19,20]. The impetus for image guidance during ESS comes from the "key hole" nature of the surgery and the two-dimensional view provided by the nasal endoscope, as well as the complex surrounding anatomy. ESS can be technically challenging because of the proximity of the central nervous system and orbital structures and because of the anatomical variations that may be encountered [2]. Furthermore, extensive disease, such as sinonasal polyposis, as well as the relatively frequent need to perform revision surgery in a field that has been previously altered may add to the surgical complexity and risk of the procedure.

Although ESS is an ideal situation for the application of intraoperative MR-guided surgery, it has not been yet studied extensively. Fried and associates [10]

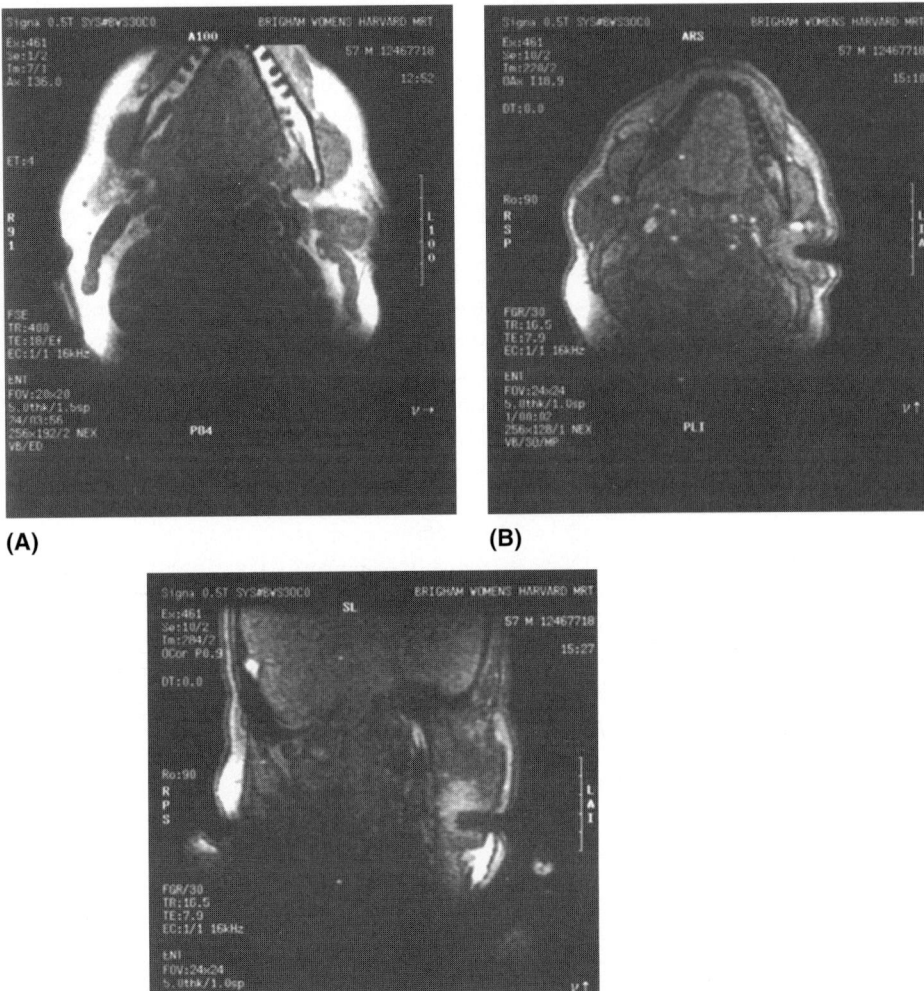

FIGURE 5.4 (A) Axial MR image demonstrating a left upper neck lesion just posterior to parotid gland. This lesion was not palpable on physical exam. (B) Similar axial MR view with fast image sequence for image-guided biopsy. The needle is seen as the dark linear artifact entering the lesion from the patient's left. (C) Coronal MR image showing the needle in the tumor, confirming that the center of the lesion is being sampled.

reported on an initial patient experience in the open magnet system with MR-guided ESS. In this series, 12 patients underwent MR-guided surgery: 11 for chronic rhinosinusitis and one for an inflammatory tumor. Four of these cases were revision procedures. The authors reported no complications for the procedures performed in the MRI operating suite. Image acquisition time approximated 14 sec per image and was found to be helpful during the procedure to delineate changes within the soft tissues. Although these procedures took longer than standard surgical times, subsequent cases have been able to be performed in a streamlined fashion after clinical familiarity with the MR-guided surgery unit has been acquired. The major limitation encountered with MR-guided ESS was found to be the relative unavailability of specialized ESS instrumentation compatible with the MR unit. Specifically, MR-compatible light cables, endoscopes, and sinus instruments were available, but the lack of an MR-compatible microdebrider and drill did influence the completeness of the surgical procedures in certain cases. A representative image sequence from interactive MR-guided ESS is presented (Figure 5.5). As indicated, the ability to image in real time in three orthogonal planes is ideal for image-guided sinus surgery.

Although this study and other accruing patient series have demonstrated the safety of MR-guided ESS, its efficacy and advantages are yet to be determined. Significant advances are yet to be realized in terms of ESS instrumentation compatibility and availability. In addition, although image quality is satisfactory for ESS purposes, further refinements in image quality will be necessary to fully apply MR-guided ESS to the expected patient population. Those patients requiring revision procedures and patients with anatomical variations that make standard surgical approaches more risky could prove to be the patient population in whom MR-guided ESS has greatest applicability and efficacy. Furthermore, patients with sinonasal tumors that can be approached endoscopically would also be ideal candidates for MR-guided ESS, since the amount of tumor resected could be followed with real-time imaging. Similar advantages of real-time intraoperative imaging would be helpful in cases of extensive sinonasal polyposis. As further patient experience is gathered with MR-guided ESS, it will likely have a role in selected cases.

5.3.3 Additional Surgical Horizons

Image-guided surgery with MRI has been espoused by other surgical disciplines including neurosurgery [21]. With the recent advances in MR-guided surgical technology and the already present experience in the neurosurgical literature, it is logical that MR-guided surgery for skull base lesions will be an area of increasing interest. MRI has the ability to distinguish several tissue types within the skull base region, offering the surgeon valuable anatomical localization for the procedure, as well as information regarding the extent of resection for a given tumor

Intraoperative Magnetic Resonance Imaging

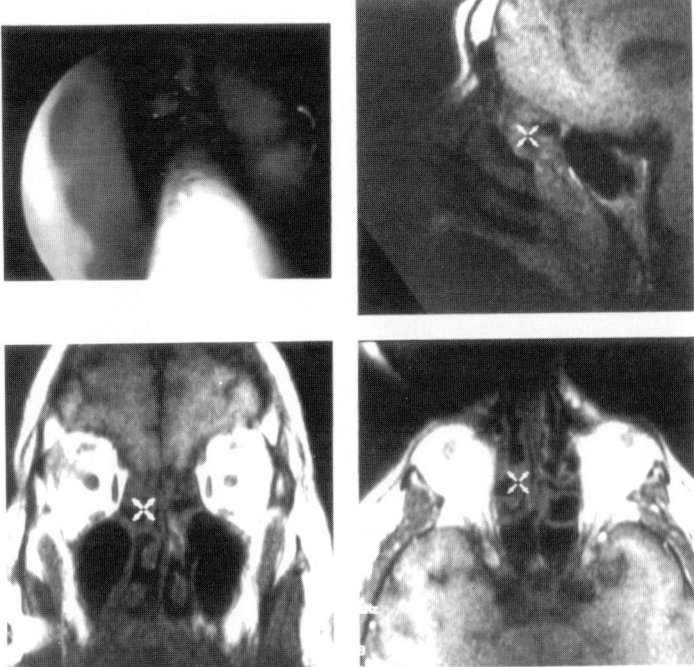

FIGURE 5.5 Images from MR-guided endoscopic sinus surgery. Upper left view demonstrates the interactive pointer approaching the right ethmoid sinus from the bottom of the screen. The pointer position (crosshair) is confirmed within the right ethmoid sinus complex on intraoperative MR images in the sagittal, coronal, and axial planes. (From Ref. 10.)

[22]. Similarly, MR-guided pituitary surgery may prove to be advantageous. Often the extent of the pituitary resection is determined by both visualization and intraoperative imaging confirmation. Intraoperative MR-guided surgery may significantly facilitate these procedures.

5.4 ADVANTAGES OF MRI-GUIDED SURGERY

As with any novel technology, acceptance in the surgical arena proceeds relatively slowly and cautiously. However, from the initial patient studies accumulated thus far, MR-guided surgery will offer significant advantages over current tracking techniques. These advantages can be related to the MRI as an imaging modality. In addition, specially designed MRI units have the ability to perform near real-time images during surgery.

Because MR is more sensitive to soft tissue morphology, it will likely have an increasing role in the diagnosis and treatment of head and neck lesions. As otolaryngologists become more familiar with MR as an imaging tool, they are more likely to consider it as an adjunctive tool in surgery. The MR image has the ability to demonstrate anatomy in true three-dimensional planes rather than a reconstructed sagittal plane. This will prove to be a significant advantage in the complex three-dimensional anatomy of the head and neck. Because MRI does not involve radiation exposure, it is better suited for intraoperative image guidance than intraoperative CT.

Although intraoperative real-time imaging would be the most advantageous system for image-guided surgery within the head and neck, this has yet to be realized. The image scan times currently available for MR-guided surgery in otolaryngology are acceptable and provide a surgeon with discrete information about the progress of the surgical procedure. This is not possible with the currently available electromagnetic or optical tracking systems. With such systems, judgments on instrument localization and extent of surgery need to be based on the real-time endoscopic image that guides the surgeon and the static preoperative CT image. Intraoperative real-time MR imaging may present a distinct advantage in this regard. Such intraoperative imaging will allow the surgeon to follow the procedure and determine what anatomical changes have been rendered by the surgery. For example, as the surgeon proceeds with the intranasal polypectomy in ESS, use of intraoperative imaging may assist in determining how much of the polypoid disease has been resected and how much remains. Because MR can also document heat-related tissue changes, intraoperative MR guided laser or thermal ablation of tumors has recently been explored [23]. This ability to track the progress of the surgical procedure as it is being undertaken also may have applicability in surgery for tumors of the head and neck, when the lesion cannot be removed from surrounding attached surfaces.

5.5 DISADVANTAGES OF MR-GUIDED SURGERY

Although intraoperative MR-guided surgery has several intuitive but yet realized advantages, it is not without attendant disadvantages. Probably the most important disadvantage of MR-guided surgery is the initial start-up expense and capitalization costs encountered in developing an I-MRI surgical suite. Such development takes an extraordinary amount of planning and economic resources for given institution. Presently, we are aware of only three actively employed MR-guided surgery suites used for head and neck surgical procedures. In addition to the tremendous capitalization costs, additional economic resources need to be devoted to the purchase and development of MR-compatible instrumentation [8]. In a specialty field such as otolaryngology–head and neck surgery, with the multiple types of instrumentation required, these secondary costs can be prohibitive as well.

MR-guided surgery within the head and neck may also suffer from other problems, including imaging artifact from instruments that are only partially compatible with the MR suite and a relatively low signal-to-noise ratio based on current technology. There is an inherent trade-off in the time required to produce a real-time scan (both image acquisition time and image processing time) and the quality of the image. In addition, if the surgeon desires imaging with several sequences (i.e., both T_1- and T_2-weighted images), significant additional scanning time will be required, which will in turn slow the operative procedure. As MR technology improves, these time factor issues should have a diminishing impact.

5.6 FUTURE DIRECTION

Although the experience with MR-guided surgery within otolaryngology/head and neck surgery has been somewhat limited, its exploration has been sparked by an increasing interest in image-guided surgery among otolaryngologists. The current technology is somewhat limited, since it is bounded by expense as well as imaging and technical constraints. As further technological developments are incorporated into the I-MRI suite, we anticipate that this technology will become more widely available. This will subsequently lead to more experience with the unit and adaptation for certain clinical applications, which will in turn lead to greater efficacy. Planning for future work continues in several areas. Aside from the continuing accrual of clinical experience with the current unit, further work on the adaptation of specialized otolaryngology surgical instruments is being undertaken. Newer generations of scanners that require less space and may provide more vertical access to the patient undergoing an MR-guided procedure. Further study is being conducted on mobile MR-guided units. With such anticipated advantages, MR-guided surgery within the head and neck is an entirely realizable possibility.

REFERENCES

1. Witte RJ, Heurter JV, Orton DF, Hahn FJ. Limited axial CT of the paranasal sinuses in screening for sinusitis. Am J Roentgenol 1996; 167(5):1313–1315.
2. Fried MP, Morrison PR. Computer-augmented endoscopic sinus surgery. Otolaryngol Clin North Am 1998; 31:331–340.
3. Fried MP, Hsu L, Jolesz FA. Interactive magnetic resonance imaging-guided biopsy in the head and neck: initial patient experience. Laryngoscope 1998; 108(4 Pt 1): 488–493.
4. DelGaudio JM, Dillard DG, Albritton FD, Hudgins P, Wallace VC, Lewis MM. Computed tomography—guided needle biopsy of head and neck lesions. Arch Otolaryngol Head Neck Surg 2000; 126(3):366–370.
5. Takes RP, Righi P, Meeuwis CA, Manni JJ, Knegt P, Marres HA, Spoelstra HA,

de Boer MF, van der Mey AG, Bruaset I, Ball V, Weisberger E, Radpour S, Kruyt RH, Joosten FB, Lameris JS, van Oostayen JA, Kopecky K, Caldemeyer K, Henzen-Logmans SC, Wiersma-van Tilburg JM, Bosman FT, van Krieken JH, Hermans J, Baatenburg de Jong RJ. The value of ultrasound with ultrasound-guided fine-needle aspiration biopsy compared to computed tomography in the detection of regional metastases in the clinically negative neck. Int J Radiation Oncol Biol Physics 1998; 40(5):1027–1032.
6. Davis SP, Anand VK, Dhillon G. Magnetic resonance navigation for head and neck lesions. Laryngoscope 1999; 109(6):862–867.
7. Lamb GM, Gedroyc WM. Interventional magnetic resonance imaging. Br J Radiol 1997; 70:S81–88.
8. Fried MP, Hsu L, Topulos GP, Jolesz FA. Image-guided surgery in a new magnetic resonance suite: preclinical considerations. Laryngoscope 1996; 106(4):411–417.
9. Silverman SG, Jolesz FA, Newman RW, Morrison PR, Kanan AR, Kikinis R, Schwartz RB, Hsu L, Koran SJ, Topulos GP. Design and implementation of an interventional MR imaging suite. Am J Radiol 1997; 168:1465–1471.
10. Fried MP, Topulos G, Hsu L, Jalahej H, Gopal H, Lauretano A, Morrison PR, Jolesz FA. Endoscopic sinus surgery with magnetic resonance imaging guidance: initial patient experience. Otolaryngol Head Neck Surg 1998; 119(4):374–380.
11. Hsu L, Fried MP, Jolesz FA. MR-guided endoscopic sinus surgery. Am J Neuroradiol 1998; 19(7):1235–1240.
12. Leung DA, Debatin JF, Wildermuth S, Heske N, Dumoulin CL, Darrow RD, Hauser M, Davis CP, von Schulthess GK. Real-time biplanar needle tracking for interventional MR imaging procedures. Radiology 1995; 197(2):485–488.
13. Fulciniti F, Califano L, Zupi A, Vetrani A. Accuracy of fine needle aspiration biopsy in head and neck tumors. J Oral Maxillofac Surg 1997; 55(10):1094–1097.
14. Shaha A, Webber C, Marti J. Fine-needle aspiration in the diagnosis of cervical lymphadenopathy. Am J Surg 1986; 152(4):420–423.
15. Elvin A, Sundstrom C, Larsson SG, Lindgren PG. Ultrasound-guided 1.2-mm cutting-needle biopsies of head and neck tumours. Acta Radiol 1997; 38(3):376–380.
16. Robbins KT, vanSonnenberg E, Casola G, Varney RR. Image-guided needle biopsy of inaccessible head and neck lesions. Arch Otolaryngol Head Neck Surg 1990; 116(8):957–961.
17. Trapp T, Lufkin R, Abemayor E, Layfield L, Hanafee W, Ward P. A new needle and technique for MRI-guided aspiration cytology of the head and neck. Laryngoscope 1989; 99(1):105–108.
18. Wang SJ, Sercarz JA, Lufkin RB, Borges A, Wang MB. MRI Guided needle localization in the head and neck using contemporaneous imaging in an open configuration system. Head Neck 2000; 22:355–59.
19. Anon JB, Klimek L, Mosges R, Zinreich SJ. Computer-assisted endoscopic sinus surgery: an international review. Otolaryngol Clin North Am 1997; 30:389.
20. Fried MP, Kleefield J, Taylor, R. New armless image-guidance system for endoscopic sinus surgery. Otolaryngol Head Neck Surg 1998; 119:528–532.
21. Hall WA, Martin AJ, Liu H, Nussbaum ES, Maxwell RE, Truwit CL. Brain biopsy

using high-field strength interventional magnetic resonance imaging. Neurosurgery 1999; 44(4):807–814.
22. Kruckels G, Korves B, Klimerk L, et al. Endoscopic surgery of the rhinobasis with a computer-assisted localizer. Surg Endosc 1996; 10:453.
23. Vogl T, Mack M, Muller P, et al. Recurrent nasal pharyngeal tumors: preliminary clinical results with interventional MR imaging-controlled laser induced chemotherapy. Radiology 1995; 196:725–733.

6
Internet-Enabled Surgery

Ronald B. Kuppersmith, M.D.
Virginia Mason Medical Center, Seattle, Washington

6.1 INTRODUCTION

The application of Internet technology to the practice of surgery is currently in its infancy. The conversion of atoms to digital information (bits) and the unique properties of bits allow information technology to provide many advantages over traditional atom-based technologies. The potential applications are widespread and could potentially affect all aspects of the evaluation and management of surgical patients. The digital transformation also will have a broad impact on surgical training methods. Predicting how surgical practice will be transformed by information technology and networked computers is difficult at best. This chapter discusses the potential impact that the Internet will have on surgical practice and education.

The practice of surgery is increasingly information intensive, and the volume of information required to make fully informed decisions will eventually exceed the ability of any individual to store, manage, and retrieve all relevant information. The net result is that it will become increasingly difficult to provide optimal care without the aid of information technology. This information may include, but is not limited to, concepts of pathophysiology, therapeutics and their interactions, anatomy and its variations, surgical approaches to conditions that are infrequently encountered, radiographic information, genetic information, demographics, and social data as well as administrative and legal requirements imposed on the physician. Some information has a life shorter than the time required to disseminate it through traditional methods of professional communication (medical charts, textbooks, print journals, continuing medical education, and face-to-face conversation). Additionally, many traditional forms of clinical information (radiographs, endoscopic examinations) are rapidly being converted into digital information (bits) that can easily be stored, manipulated, duplicated, and disseminated.

Fortunately, decreasing costs per computational unit and advances in information technology will make this information more manageable and more accessible. Several technological trends are going to affect this transformation significantly:

Widespread broadband access. Broadband access will allow physicians to have instant access to information-intensive resources, such as large databases, radiographs, intraoperative video, video from patient encounters, and video conferencing from remote locations. Broadband will also facilitate information sharing and consultation with colleagues regardless of location.

The emergence of application service providers. Through subscription fees, application service providers will give practitioners access to computational capabilities over the Internet, without the need to maintain expensive hardware or develop or purchase expensive software.

The proliferation of wireless Internet technologies. The wireless Internet will allow physicians to access and manage information from any location using handheld devices, freeing them from traditional computers. These wireless devices will allow physicians to refill medications with the touch of a button, answer queries from the office without having to call on the phone and wait on hold, and provide access to patient information and other medical databases.

The increasing complexity of health care delivery. Socioeconomic factors and regulatory issues, as well as the greater sophistication of even routine diagnostic modalities and therapeutics, are driving a greater complexity in almost all healthcare delivery settings.

Expansion of the medical knowledge base. Medical research has greatly expanded the entire medical knowledge base. This expansion will likely accelerate, as the pace of the acquisition of additional information about human genomics accelerates. The technological revolution that facilitates the field of genomics and its related disciplines will ultimately impact healthcare.

As the Internet and information technology will transform the practice of surgery, it also creates several new responsibilities for physicians. Prior to the Internet, physicians were the main source of medical information because access

Internet-Enabled Surgery

to information from medical journals and textbook was difficult and expensive for non–healthcare providers. Widespread access to medical information on the Internet has the benefit of allowing patients to be more educated about their ailments, but this occurs at the risk of exposure to inaccurate and potentially harmful information. Physicians now must guide patients to sources of accurate information and provide context and interpretation of information that may be found on the Internet but that ultimately proves to be of questionable accuracy.

Additionally, surgeons must take responsibility to protect the confidentiality and privacy of their patients, since the Internet and other new information technologies potentially represent a serious threat to these important aspects of the physician-patient relationship and represent major medicolegal risks for the physician.

6.2 TECHNOLOGIES THAT MAY AFFECT THE EVALUATION AND MANAGEMENT OF SURGICAL PATIENTS

The patient's initial contact with the surgeon's office will likely take place online. After being referred to a surgeon, the patient will access the surgeon's Internet presence from home and/or from the referring physician's office. In addition, other access methods, including wireless Internet devices, are feasible. The patient will be able to review information about the surgeon and other background information on the website. Using a secure form, the patient will then be able to request an appointment on the site in an arrangement that will be similar to booking an airline ticket. When the patient requests an appointment, he or she will be able to specify a preference for time and date. An algorithm within the system will automatically determine when an appointment will be available based upon the patient's preferences, the surgeon's existing schedule, and criteria set by the surgeon. For instance, if the surgeon only wants to see one vertigo patient per clinic day, once that appointment is taken a second patient with a similar complaint cannot be scheduled on that particular day without an override from the surgeon or his office staff. Insurance preauthorization will automatically be obtained and documented before confirmation of the appointment. Copayments and other fees will be collected through an online secure credit card transaction during appointment scheduling.

Internet-based appointment scheduling can also support other advanced functions. Patients will enter their demographic information, insurance information, chief complaint, medical history, and all other required preregistration information. This may potentially be transferred from the primary care physician's records or from an online medical record repository that the patient maintains. Based on their chief complaint, the patient will be automatically queried about previous studies (e.g., x-rays, diagnostic tests) and consultations. Appropriate release forms will be generated for the patient to acquire all appropriate studies and records, and the patient will be advised to obtain and bring these materials to the scheduled consultation.

When patients arrive at the surgeon's office, they will be able to log in and update any of their information. In the waiting room, they will have access to online educational materials via the Internet. The surgeon may select these materials so that patients may review information relevant to their symptoms, conditions, and possible therapeutic interventions. Before seeing the patient, the surgeon will have access to all of the information given by the patient on a handheld device or desktop system.

While the surgeon sees the patient, they will have instant access to decision support software. Based on information mined from a database of the physician's past experiences, data aggregated in large outcome's databases and patient-specific criteria, the physician will be able to provide estimates of treatment success and long-term outcome.

The physician will be able to view diagnostic studies, including images, and show these to the patient. Algorithms will compare new diagnostic images to previous imaging studies, and differences will automatically be calculated. Images will also be compared to image libraries that are stored on the Internet for additional diagnostic information.

Educational materials and videos will be designated for the patient to review at a later time when they log on to the surgeon's Internet site. Any diagnostic tests ordered will be routed to the appropriate lab through secure Internet connections. After completion of these tests, the physician will automatically be notified and the patient will be able to review the results with interpretation provided by the physician. This feedback can be automated based on the results of the test and annotated with specific information by the physician when warranted.

Prescriptions will be routed to the appropriate pharmacy and automatically delivered to the patient at a convenient time and place. When attempting to prescribe a particular medication, it will be checked against the formulary supported by the patient's insurance company, the specific cost of the pharmaceutical, the potential interactions with existing prescriptions, the efficacy with respect to the current diagnosis, and the side effect profile. If better alternatives exist, they will be suggested by the system.

Of course, the physician will enter information into the patient's medical record, but this record keeping will be much easier and less burdensome. Dictation, voice recognition software, handwriting recognition, keyboard, or even another interface may provide a means of record keeping that is comfortable for the surgeon, since it fits the work flow. Clinical images obtained in the clinic will be integrated into the record. Documentation will be consistent and encoded so that specific data will be able to be measured and compared between encounters or between patients. Diagnostic and evaluation and management coding will be done automatically and will appropriately reflect the level of documentation. Data collection required for participation in multisite or multi-institution research studies will be facilitated by the system and automatically captured.

The patient's entire record, including diagnostic tests, images, and video, will be able to be transported over the Internet for consultation with experts anywhere in the world. These consultations can be done in real time with video teleconferencing or in a store-and-forward manner, whereby the expert will review the material at his or her convenience and then render an opinion. General discussions about patient care among groups of physicians on the Internet already take place, and the addition of the ability to easily and quickly share images, video, and other data will greatly enhance the utility of these services.

Prior to entering the operating room, the surgeon may load radiographic and other information into a surgical planning system and determine the best surgical approach. The system may suggest alternatives correlating outcomes with experiences. Over the Internet and using a shared environment, the surgeon may walk through the surgical plan with other surgeons who will be involved in the case or with consulting experts. This may be done in real time or may be done asynchronously, depending on the availability of the individuals.

In the operating room, the surgeon will have access to the entire record, including imaging studies. They will be able to add intraoperative findings, images, and video to the record. Additionally, the surgeon will be able to access archived cases that may be similar in nature in order to determine the best approach to the current problem. Consulting surgeons can be available for remote tele-mentoring (to provide support and teaching during difficult cases), and tele-proctoring (to provide training). Both tele-mentoring and tele-proctoring may also support surgeons undergoing remediation.

When patients return home they will be able to review their medical records via a secure connection. All of the technical medical language within the records will automatically be translated into lay terms. Appropriate internal and external links to reference materials, support groups, and other resources will be provided for patient education purposes. This may include videos and interactive activities to help educate the patient about an upcoming procedure. All pharmaceuticals will be linked to documents describing the medication's purpose, side effects, interactions, and other information. Patients will be able to access this information at any time, to provide the information to other healthcare providers, and to export this information into their own personal medical record repository.

During the course of therapy, patients will be able to report to the physician's office about their progress with regard to recovery. Physiological data collected with wireless devices and digital images will be transmitted over the Internet to the surgeon's office when appropriate. Additionally, outcomes and patient satisfaction information will be collected through the surgeon's web presence and utilized to improve patient care. Patients will also be able to request prescription refills, schedule follow-up appointments, ask questions, access laboratory results, view educational materials and instructions, and review and settle insurance claims through secure interfaces. The system will automatically remind patients of follow-up appointments and obtain long-term follow-up on patients in research studies. Surgeons will also be able to request follow-up appointment automatically or manually through the system.

When surgeons are on call or not in the office, they will be able to access patients' records through the wireless Internet using a handheld device. When a patient calls for a prescription refill, the physician will receive an alert on this device. If the refill is appropriate, the surgeon will be able to refill the prescription by pressing one button. This process will automatically transmit the prescription to the pharmacy through a secure Internet connection or through a fax, update the patient's electronic medical record, and notify the patient that the prescription has been refilled. If the physician cannot recall the patient, or if the physician is responding to an inquiry from a patient who normally sees another associated physician, the physician will be able to access the patient's record on the handheld device to determine whether the prescription is appropriate. Additionally, office staff and the laboratory will be able to send alerts to these wireless devices. Since the physician will be able to respond with the touch of a button, these methods of communication will be less time consuming and less intrusive than other means of communication.

Application service providers (ASPs) that charge a subscription fee for access and support will provide most of these services. ASPs are responsible for maintaining and upgrading the software and hardware. As a result ASP users do not need to contend with issues outside their area of expertise. Applications for which surgeons may use ASPs include:

- Financial transactions processing
- Insurance claim submission
- Purchasing
- Marketing and web presence
- Electronic medical records
- Secure patient interactions
- Data storage and backup
- Human resource management
- Office accounting functions

6.3 TECHNOLOGIES THAT WILL IMPACT SURGICAL TRAINING METHODS

The potential impact of information technology and the Internet on surgical training is also difficult to predict but will probably be substantial. Current surgical training is mainly composed of graduated and supervised experience based upon actual patient encounters. Experience is limited to patients who present during the time the trainee is present in a particular location. Most institutions currently do not have a mechanism for capturing clinical experiences or storing them in a central data repository for future study.

One of the major benefits of electronic medical records and central data repositories is the potential for education that they will provide. Surgeons in training will have access to a vast library of past clinical experiences. Entering information about a current clinical situation into a query tool will allow them to review prior cases with similar characteristics. They will be able to review past imaging studies, surgical video, and longitudinal outcome data and be able to use this information to help broaden their "clinical" experience. Additionally, they will be able to obtain real-time outcome statistics for comparison to current situations.

Data "mining" of past clinical experiences will be an important new form of clinical research. When used to evaluate a large number of clinical experiences with significant descriptive data, it will allow researchers and training physicians to identify trends and correlations that were not previously apparent.

Interesting and rare cases can be identified, stripped of identifying information, and placed in an online educational "library." These could be exchanged between institutions or archived in an Internet-based archive for use by individuals around the world. Through the use of XML (extensible mark-up language) or similar technology, these cases could be converted "on-the-fly" to interactive educational modules that would allow physicians in training to complement their clinical experience.

Currently, didactic sessions, anatomical dissection, and self-study of the medical literature and textbooks are the main supplements to clinical experience in surgical education. The shear volume of medical information and the logarithmic expansion of medical knowledge make mastery and integration of new information a difficult and stressful task. After developing an understanding of the vocabulary and a knowledge framework, effective physicians will need to develop skills that allow them to efficiently retrieve and manage relevant information.

One of the primary online educational resources essential for surgical training are tools that allow physicians to search the medical literature and access full text versions of this information. Examples of services that are currently available include PubMed from the National Library of Medicine (*http://www.nlm.h.gov/*), which allows the user to search the medical literature (MEDLINE indexed journals) and view abstracts of specific articles. The full text of these articles can be ordered from the site and can be delivered by mail, fax, or over the Internet. Another example is MDConsult (*http://www.mdconsult.com/*), which provides full text access to nearly 40 textbooks and 50 medical journals for a subscription fee. MDConsult also provides additional value by adding context to the medical literature through services such as reviews of information from the lay press with links to relevant full text articles from the literature, reviews of clinical topics, and practice guidelines.

Access to other databases that include information about pharmaceuticals, clinical trials, genetic information, basic science research, legal information, and administrative regulations will also be a critical source of current information that will supplement other educational materials. Knowledge of the available resources—as well as familiarity with the techniques to access this information—will be one of the most important skills that future physicians will need. Ideally, an interface that unifies access to important knowledge bases will be developed.

Internet-based videoconferencing will be an important platform for didactic sessions. Experts from around the world will be able to lecture and share information directly with interested trainees anywhere in the world without the need for and the disruption of travel. Individuals will be able to interact with and provide feedback to the experts through the Internet. Videoconferences will be archived and accessible by the trainee at any time and from any location with an Internet connection.

Similar to practicing surgeons, videoconferencing in the operating room will allow trainees to potentially learn from experts outside of their geographic area and will allow experts to have broader exposure to people within the field. Trainees could be monitored and mentored by experts from a distance, or conversely trainees could observe experts performing surgery and be able to interact with the surgeon during the case. Additionally, surgical skill could be assessed through tele-proctoring of surgeons by anonymous and objective experts as a component of certification or in lieu of multiple choice and oral examinations.

Surgical simulation and simulation of patient encounters will be another important method of surgical training and certification. The Internet will facilitate these technologies by allowing individuals to develop and contribute scenarios for use by trainees at other locations. Due to the significant expense required for development and maintenance, simulators may be developed as an ASP model, whereby an institution develops, administers, and maintains the simulator and charges subscription fees for access. Simulators will be an important tool for practicing surgical procedures and learning new procedures. Objective criteria can be developed to rate surgical skill, monitor progression, and compare the individual to other simulator users.

6.4 CONCLUSION

The Internet and other information technologies will significantly transform and improve the practice of medicine. Exact predictions of these changes are difficult, but it behooves the practicing physician to learn about and become involved in the development of these new applications.

7
Virtual Reality and Surgical Simulation

Charles V. Edmond, Jr., M.D., F.A.C.S.
University of Washington, Seattle, Washington

7.1 INTRODUCTION

Technological change in the surgical arena has proceeded at a rapid pace over the past 20 years, and even more remarkable advances are in sight over the next decade. Advances in imaging technology, minimal access surgery, computer-aided surgical devices, and surgical simulation will drive these changes.

Surgical simulation, unlike any other technology, has the potential to be the most compelling of the advanced technologies. With the cost of high-end computing resources decreasing and CPU and graphical capabilities exponentially increasing, a development team is limited only by its imagination. Simulation technology provides a multifaceted core from which developers can create a multitude of applications directed not only at the acquisition and maintenance of surgical skills, but also knowledge development through computer-based training. Furthermore, the simulator provides an environment in which the feasibility of new surgical procedures, instruments, and devices (computer-aided surgical systems) can be "mocked up" prior to deployment, resulting in a tremendous cost savings for both patient and developer.

Training in a virtual environment can be implemented at all levels of surgical education. Simulation enables a shift from the current "see one, do one, teach one'' paradigm of medical education to one that is more experienced-based. With simulators, hands-on experience is possible at an earlier stage in training, before direct patient involvement and its associated risk. Simulation can increase the availability of experience to the student and conserve the use of scarce tutoring resources. It can enable achieving larger case numbers and exposure to a wider variety of pathology in a compressed period, resulting in an acceleration of the learning curve. Potentially, the level of preparation can improve with a decrease in the cost and time of learning medical procedures, an urgency for teaching institutions that face mounting cost pressures to provide competitively priced services while also strapped with the requirement of educating surgeons. Medical training is expensive, with costs accumulating over a lifetime long after medical school and residency training. Simulation can play a significant role in continuing medical education by assisting, through standardized training and certification programs the dissemination of new procedures and technology that offer better and more cost-effective standards of care.

With the advent of medical digital imaging standards (i.e., DICOM) and the increasing appearance of medical image information infrastructures (i.e., PACS), the creation of patient-specific models from routine medical imaging exams will be available as simulations for training in the future. These simulations will include the latest instruments and computer-aided surgical devices allowing the surgeon to preoperatively plan and rehearse, or experiment with, competing surgical approaches.

This chapter will focus on the current state of the art of surgical simulation in otorhinolaryngology–head and neck surgery, including an overview of surgical simulators and expert systems. The development of the first endoscopic sinus surgical simulator will be discussed.

7.2 BACKGROUND

Computer generated simulators have been used for a number of years to train pilots. For decades, flight simulators have provided crewmembers experience that would be too difficult, too expensive, or even impossible to obtain otherwise. Today, simulation has become indispensable to maintain the operational readiness of our military forces through many roles: instruction and training, skills maintenance and evaluation, and mission rehearsal [1].

Although simulation is a mature technology in aviation, it is not as straightforward to build simulators for medical applications. Existing aviation simulators permit navigation within a virtual environment among mostly fixed objects (such as buildings and terrain) and some rigid moving objects (such as aircraft and ships). Medical procedures, on the other hand, involve complex interactions with anatomy that one can stretch, retract, cauterize, and cut. Anatomy has dynamic physiological behavior, complex shape, and internal structure that are difficult to simulate. Moreover, current technical hurdles do not have any apparent immediate solutions. In particular, the computing requirements of representing soft tissue manipulations are formidable—defying available speed on a supercomputer. Current attempts at simulating soft tissue motion avoid the use of finite element modeling because of its computational demands. The use of crude models and numeric approaches, which are substituted for the more intensive finite element analysis approach, drastically sacrifices realism for speed.

7.3 SIMULATORS

Recently developed virtual reality training systems for surgical simulation address the complexities that are inherent in the interaction of anatomical behaviors, shapes, and structures. A virtual environment training system is usually composed of a computer host, a graphics processor, integrative modeling, rendering and animation software, and display, input, and tracking devices. The form of presentation and feedback to a user may include sensations of touch, sight, force, and audition, all joined together to provide realistic virtual worlds. Current and developmental computer-generated surgical simulators may be divided into the categories of immersive and nonimmersive technologies.

7.3.1 Immersive Simulators

The immersive computer-generated simulators create visual immersion by generating three-dimensional images that are presented to the individual within a head-mounted display (HMD). The HMD achieves the illusion of immersion into virtual reality (VR) by providing the visual information of the VR world to the eyes, while simultaneously blocking visual contact with the outside world. Since sight is our most controlling sense, it is given primary consideration in VR. This approach accomplishes much of the effect of immersion into the VR environment.

We can increase complexity and therefore the sense of presence by adding auditory cues. However, with normal stereo sound systems, precise location of the origin of sound is not possible, since these systems provide cues that indicate that the sound source is to the right or left of the listener or that the sound source is immediately in front of the listener. In contrast, an immersive system permits the listener to localize the origin of sound in the VR precisely. This type of sound is known as true three-dimensional sound. Sound in an immersive system mimics the processes of normal hearing in the real world.

7.3.2 Nonimmersive Simulators

Nonimmersive computer-generated surgical simulators rely on real world props to enhance the physical fidelity, rather than complete immersion. Standard cathode ray tube (CRT) video monitors and even holographic displays are commonly used as the interface to virtual worlds in nonimmersive simulators.

7.3.3 Comparison of Immersive and Nonimmersive Simulators

Both immersive and non-immersive simulators carry specific advantages and disadvantages. Of course, the type of simulator environment that is best for a particular application will depend on multiple factors, including task characteristics, user characteristics, design constraints imposed by human sensory and motor physiology, multimodal interaction, cost, and the potential need for visual, auditory, and haptic components.

The level of detail of the anatomical model and the degree of interactivity will vary based on the goals of the simulator. Low levels of detail may be appropriate for simple tasks focusing on developing better eye-hand coordination, whereas higher degrees of image fidelity may be warranted when the task requires the subject to develop enhanced spatial awareness or situational awareness skills.

Interactivity is undoubtedly one of the real strengths and centerpieces of the simulator. The teaching tool's power relates directly to the level of interactivity. Greater levels of interactivity will support increasingly more powerful teaching tools. Ideally, the simulator would be capable of matching the level of detail with the desired degree of interactivity to produce the most effective transfer of training for a given skill level. At the upper end, an increase in simulated detail and interactivity demands increased processing power, which even at today's computational rates is still the rate-limiting step.

These constraints are reflected in the performance of the simulator's latency and frame refresh rates. Latency is a measure of the interval between the instant when the user initiates an action and the instant when the computer registers the action. Short latency intervals avoid user-induced errors that occur when the user overcompensates or undercompensates for a given action because of the delay between the initiation of the action and the apparent result. Frame-refresh rate is the number of frames that the computer can generate in a given amount of time on the display system. A rate of 30 frames per second (fps) is considered "real time," since the eye does not distinguish one frame from the next. As a result, all simulation systems strive to achieve this level of performance [2].

7.3.4 Haptic Sensations

Creating three-dimensional graphics and adding sound to the virtual environments have been the focus of the majority of the VR systems. The physical aspects of exploration and interaction have been largely ignored [3]. The task of developing technologies that generating sophisticated haptic (i.e., tactile, force, and proprioceptive) sensations is one of the most difficult challenges that re-

Virtual Reality and Surgical Simulation

searchers are encountering in this field [4]. Future VR systems must target both the visual and physical sensory modalities before this technology will allow users to take full advantage of their innate sensory and motor skills.

In theory, a force feedback system should allow the user to perform natural gestures and interactions within the simulated space while the VR system creates feedback forces that feel realistic and convincing [3]. Tactile simulation and force feedback simulation are not equivalent. Tactile simulation replicates the texture of an object for the skin's touch receptors. In a tactile simulation, sandpaper should feel rough and porcelain should feel smooth. Proprioception, the sensory component of force feedback, shares some features of tactile senses, but it is different. Tactile simulation allows someone to feel the smoothness of a porcelain figurine, while force feedback puts the figurine in the user's hand (from a perceptual viewpoint). If a user grasps a figurine in a VR simulator that uses force reflective system (a type of force feedback), the VR computer measures the closure of the user's hand and limits the closure at the calculated boundary of the figurine. The net result is that the VR figurine appears solid.

Rosenberg describes the force feedback human interface system as a closed loop. The cycle begins when a user makes a gesture within the virtual environment. Sensors that are attached to the input devices track the user's physical motions and relay this information to the host computer. The computer then calculates the haptic sensations that the user should feel as a result of the physical motion as well as the defined contents and structure of the simulated environment. The computer signals a set of actuators that then produces haptic sensations. Actuators produce real physical forces, which make their way to the user's body through a mechanical transmission. When the user perceives these synthesized forces and reacts to them, the cycle is complete.

7.4 EXPERT SYSTEMS AND VIRTUAL ENVIRONMENTS

The incorporation of an expert system multimodal input into a VR system provides an intelligent simulation tool for medical training by increasing the functionality of the simulator to another level. The expert system uses a multilayered approach to recognize the student's voice (i.e., "Where is the frontal recess?") and gestural commands (i.e., injecting the uncinate) and events in the virtual environment (i.e., navigation through the nasal cavity). The expert system then infers context from these cues and matches this context against steps in the surgical procedure. Students can query the system for both task and procedural level assistance and receives automatic feedback when they perform the surgical procedure incorrectly. The interface adds an interpretation module for integrating speech and gesture into a common semantic representation, and a rule-based expert system uses this representation to interpret the user's actions by matching them against components of a defined surgical procedure. While speech and gesture have been used before in virtual environments, Billinghurst and Edmond were the first to couple it with an expert system, which infers context and higher-level understanding [5].

7.4.1 Multimodal Input

Employing multimodal input within medical interfaces is an ideal application for the surgical setting, since the surgeon's hands are engaged and the surgeon relies heavily upon on vocal and gestural commands. Voice and gesture compliment each other and, when used together, create an interface more powerful than either modality alone. Cohen showed how natural language interaction is suited for descriptive techniques, while gestural interaction is ideal for direct manipulation of objects [6,7].

Users prefer using combined voice and gestural communication over either modality alone when attempting graphics manipulation. Hauptman and McAvinny used a simulated speech and gesture recognizer in an experiment to judge the range of vocabulary and gestures that were unused in a typical graphics task [8]. In this protocol, the modes of gesture only, voice only, and gesture recognition were tested. Users overwhelmingly preferred combined voice and gestural recognition due to the greater expressiveness possible.

Combining speech and gesture context understanding improves recognition accuracy. By integrating speech and gesture recognition, Bolt discovered that neither had to be perfect if together they converged on the user's intended meaning [9]. In this case, the computer responded to user's commands by using speech and gesture recognition in the concurrent context.

7.4.2 Expert System

An expert system is necessary to effectively integrate voice and gestural input into a single semantic form. This unified representation can then be matched against procedural knowledge contained in the expert system to make inferences about user actions. In this way, the system can recognize when the user performs specific actions, and then the system can provide automatic intelligent feedback (Figure 7.1).

In our interface, we use a rule-based system, which encodes expert knowledge in a set of *if-then* production rules [6]. For example, if *FACT-I*, then *DO-THIS*, where *FACT-I* is the event necessary for rule activation and *DO-THIS* is the consequence of rule activation. The user's speech and actions in the virtual environment generate a series of facts, which are passed to the expert system fact database and matched against the appropriate rules. This then generates intelligent response. Rule-based expert systems have been successfully applied to a wide variety of domains, such as medical diagnosis [10], configuration of computer systems [11], and oil exploration [8].

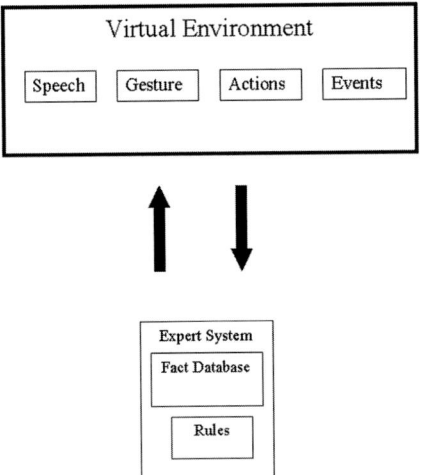

FIGURE 7.1 Demonstration of the user's speech and actions in the virtual environment generates a series of facts that are passed to the expert system fact database and matched against the appropriate rules. The process yields an intelligent response.

7.4.3 Natural Language Processing

Natural language processing (NLP) techniques provide a theoretical framework for interpreting and representing multimodal inputs. NLP is traditionally concerned with the comprehension of written and/or spoken language, but these methods may be modified so that NLP can understand multimodal inputs and create inferences about user actions from these inputs. In effect, NLP methods determine the representation scheme that is used in our expert system, while the expert system determines how these representations are manipulated in an intelligent way. Previous multimodal interfaces show how voice and gesture can be integrated into a common semantic form [8], but our work extends beyond this by using low-level semantic knowledge as the basis for higher-level pragmatic understanding. To do this we draw on established NLP techniques, such as conceptual dependency representations and scripts.

7.4.4 Simulation and Training

By extending this rule-based approach and adding procedural knowledge, the same expert system can be used as a sinus surgery trainer. The sinus interface supports training of a standard anterior-to-posterior approach to the paranasal sinuses. In constructing the expert system database, the complete surgical procedure was broken down into a number of self-contained steps, each of which was

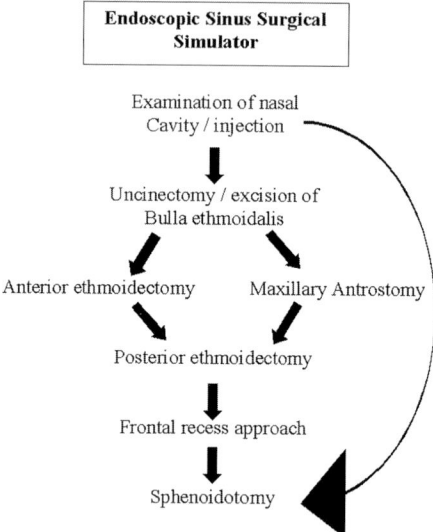

FIGURE 7.2 Example of sequence of surgical steps (procedural knowledge) encoded into a rule-based expert system.

also comprised of several tasks. In this example, some of these steps need to be performed in a specific sequence, while other steps are not sequence-dependent. For example, in order to perform maxillary antrostomy an uncinectomy must first be performed (i.e., in a specific sequence), while the frontal recess can be addressed at any time after the uncinectomy and anterior ethmoid air cells have been opened. The complete set of surgical steps and the relationships between them are shown in Figure 7.2. To identify which stage the user is attempting in the operation, the expert system combines information from the user's multimodal input with the state of the virtual world and compares these data to sets of rules designed to recognize context. Each set of rules corresponds to the onset of a different step in the surgical procedure and, when activated, causes the rest of the user interaction to be interpreted from within that surgical context. This contextual knowledge is then used to improve speech and gesture recognition. When the interface is used for training, activation of a particular context causes activation of the set of rules corresponding to the tasks contained in that surgical step. These rules differ from those used to recognize context in that they correspond to actions that need to be performed in definite sequence. In this way the user's progress can be monitored through the operation in a step-by-step fashion as well as at a task-by-task level.

Response to incorrect actions depends on the training level chosen at the program outset. At the very least, the system prevents the user from performing a task-level action out of sequence and gives auditory warning when they try to do so. While the system cannot constrain instrument movement, it can prevent tissue dissection and removal in virtual world simulation; this block effectively stops the user from progressing further.

Since the entire surgical procedure is encoded in the expert system database, the interface can also respond to requests for help during training. If users become confused, they can ask "What do I do now?" and the system will respond by vocalizing the next task or step in the operation. Alternatively, if the users say, "Show me what to do now," the rules for the next task are used to send commands to the virtual environment so that the instrument moves in the correct manner. At the same time the system describes what it is doing so the user receives visual and auditory reinforcement.

7.5 ENDOSCOPIC SINUS SURGICAL SIMULATOR

Madigan Army Medical Center, in collaboration with Lockheed Martin Tactile Defense Systems (Akron, OH), Ohio State Supercomputer Center, Ohio State School of Medicine, University of Washington School of Medicine–Human Interface Technology Lab, Immersion Corporation and Uniformed Services University of the Health Sciences, has been working on the development of a prototype nonimmersive simulator for training in endoscopic sinus surgery (ESS) (Figure 7.3). Endoscopic sinus surgery is an important, yet approachable procedure for simulation. ESS simulation has more limited tissue interaction requirements than most other surgical procedures. The anatomy of the sinus region is primarily rigid to a good approximation. Dissection is localized in space and time, making the computational requirements more manageable. ESS simulation is therefore less dependent upon the immature technology of the modeling of dissectible and deformable objects. Moreover, the training requirements of learning the intranasal anatomy and spatial awareness are more important than the psychomotor tasks of tissue removal and are consequently less reliant upon realistic simulation of the tissue interaction.

7.5.1 Virtual Patient

The initial patient model for this project was the visible male from the Visible Human Data (VHD) project conducted by the National Library of Medicine. The image data set consists of cryo-slice images photographed in the transverse plane at 1 mm slice intervals. The photographic data is digitized at a 0.33 pixel size. The data set also included CT and magnetic resonance imaging (MRI) scans. These data are the raw input for the segmentation, surface reconstruction, and visual texture development steps.

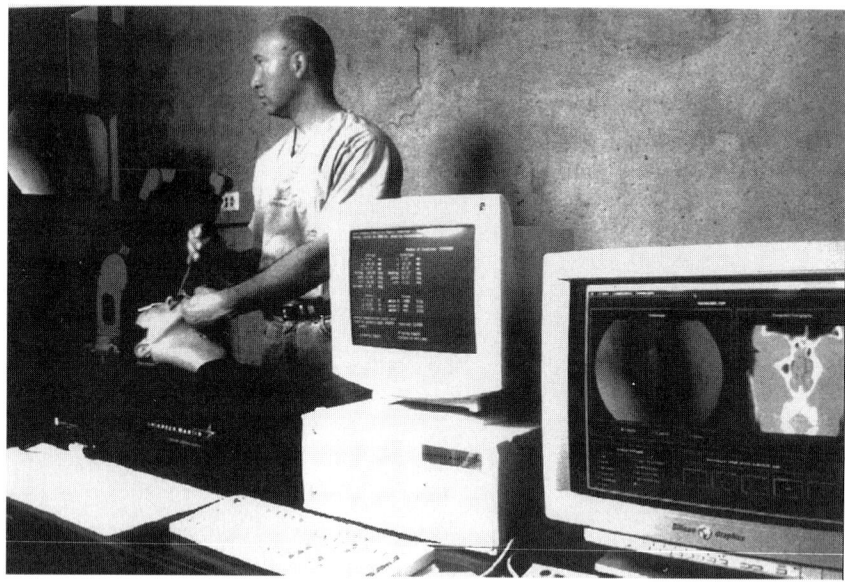

FIGURE 7.3 Madigan Endoscopic Sinus Surgical Simulator.

7.5.2 System Overview

The system has three computer systems linked by an Ethernet interface. An Onyx 2 computer (Silicon Graphics, Mountain View, CA) serves as the simulation host platform. It contains the virtual patient model and is responsible for the simulation of the endoscope image, the surgical interactions, and the user interface. The Onyx is configured with two R10000 CPUs, IR graphics hardware, and a soundboard. The second computer, a 333-MHz Pentium PC (Intel Corporation, Santa Clara, CA), is dedicated to the control of the electro-mechanical hardware. A third computer allows voice recognition and provides virtual instruction while training.

7.5.3 Tracking and Haptic System

The haptic system is comprised of a high-speed Pentium computer and an electro-mechanical component. It tracks the position and orientation of the endoscope through a mechanical apparatus external to the mannequin's head and tracks another surgical instrument via a second mechanical apparatus inside the mannequin's head. The haptic system also monitors the status of the instrument's scis-

Virtual Reality and Surgical Simulation

sors-like grip and of the foot switch. As the user manipulates these physical replicas of an endoscope and a surgical instrument, the connected electromechanical hardware senses their position and orientation in all six degrees of freedom. The haptic system PC reads and transfers the complete state of both tools to the simulation computer. The haptic system applies force in three axes to the distal tip of the surgical tool, simulating haptic cues associated with surgery. The haptic system does not apply force to the endoscope replica (Figure 7.4).

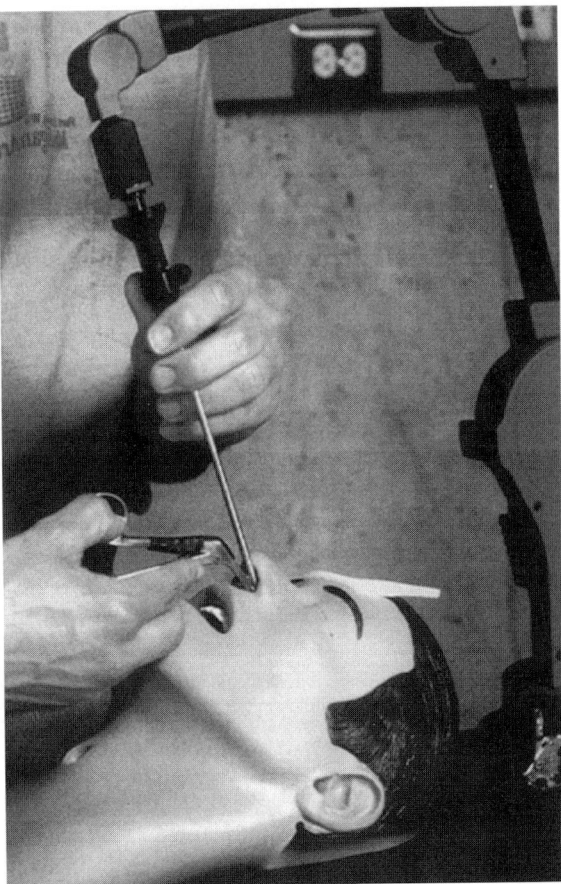

FIGURE 7.4 Physical model with endoscope. The endoscope and forceps are connected to the electromechanical system, which tracks their position and orientation in all six degrees of freedom.

7.5.4 Image Synthesis

Our goal has been to simulate the endoscopic image as closely as possible. The image fidelity demands of the endoscopic imagery are significant and differ sharply with flight simulation and conventional virtual reality applications. Unlike simulating terrain on a flight simulator, the close proximity of the anatomical structures causes a high percentage of the polygons that represent the sinuses to fall simultaneously within the viewing frustum. This places a heavy load on the simulation computer and graphics hardware. All illumination originates from the endoscope creating an image with a high degree of depth attenuation. Fortunately, shadowing is unnecessary because of the co-linearity between with the imaging optics and the light source. The anatomy is moist and reflective, creating numerous conspicuous specular highlights, which yield important depth cues. We have applied high-quality visual texture to the geometry of the virtual patient, generated from the surface reconstruction of the VHD project.

7.5.5 Surgical Interaction

Since a fully realistic simulation would be a difficult undertaking, we have implemented dissection in a limited way: tissue appears to vanish when dissected. This simplification does not compromise training value significantly.

The simulator also models the complex interaction of specific steps of ESS. The injection of a vaso-constrictor to reduce bleeding is one step in the performance of an anterior ethmoidectomy. During simulation, recursive algorithms search to find vertices inside the virtual needle tip, averaging their original color with blood red to simulate the puncture. In a similar fashion, vertices in the volume surrounding the needle's tip are averaged with white to simulate the blanching.

The simulator supports 15 different tools and 3 endoscopes (zero, 30, and 70). The instructor interface provides control of the simulation state, instrument selection, and patient selection. The right side of the instructor interface displays a CT image. The simulator tracks the surgical instruments in the patient coordinates and in real time retrieves the coronal CT image of the plane nearest to the tip of the selected surgical tool, marking its position within the image with a graphic cursor.

7.5.6 Curriculum Design

The sinus simulator takes medical simulation several major steps forward in its evolution. Aside from its technical accomplishments, the integration of a well-thought-out curricular framework allows it to take advantage of virtual reality without sacrificing the benefits of more traditional computer-aided instruction.

Virtual Reality and Surgical Simulation

Three levels of interaction are available for training:

Model 1 introduces the student into an abstract environment, allowing the student to gain the required hand-eye coordination with the endoscope and the special skills needed to maneuver the instrumented forceps without requiring the student to concentrate on anatomy (Figure 7.5).

Model 2 introduces the student to the anatomy but still utilizes the training aids from Model 1. This model gives the student the help of hoops for the initial passes through the anatomy, targets for injection areas, and labels on the anatomical structures with which interaction is necessary. The educational advantages of simulation can best be achieved with a model of this kind (Figure 7.6).

Model 3 introduces the student to a more realistic environment. There are no longer any training aids to guide the student through the procedure. For navigation of the scope, the student must rely on what was learned when navigating through the hoops in Model 2. For injection, the student must remember where injection of the vasoconstrictor is useful. For dissection, the student has no labels to indicate the anatomy of interest; as a result, the student must rely on what was learned in Model 2 to perform the procedure (Figure 7.7).

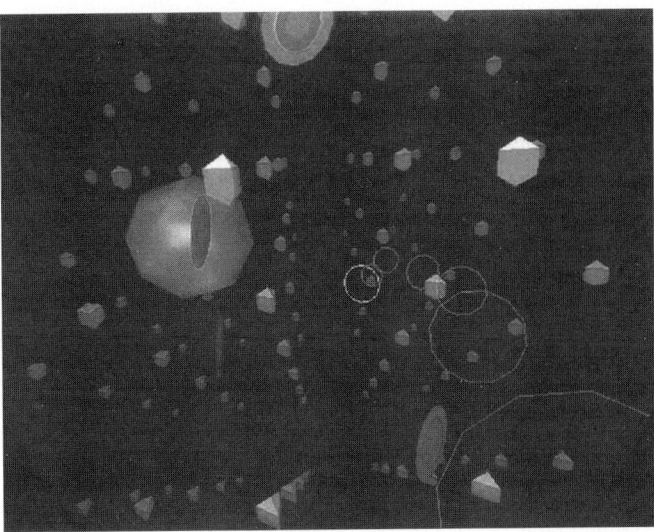

FIGURE 7.5 The Madigan Endoscopic Sinus Surgical Simulator includes a variety of skill levels for the support of student surgical education. The display system for the novice stage is shown.

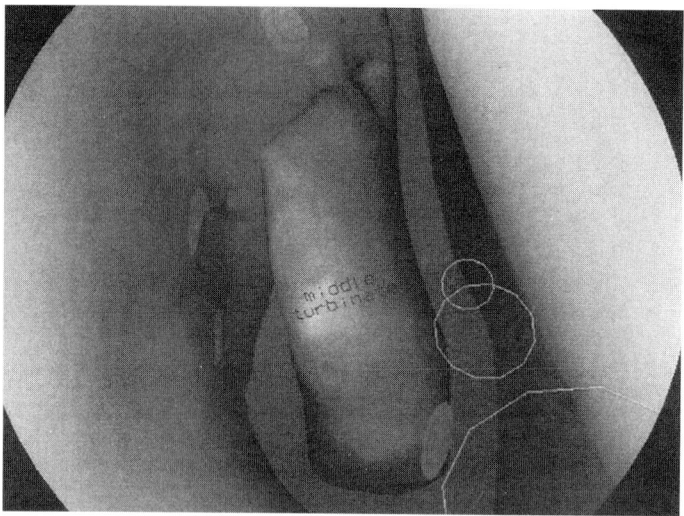

FIGURE 7.6 The Madigan Endoscopic Sinus Surgical Simulator includes a variety of skill levels for the support of student surgical education. At the intermediate stage, visual cues, including "hoops" and direct labels, are presented. The displayed hoops are targets through which the user must pass the virtual telescope.

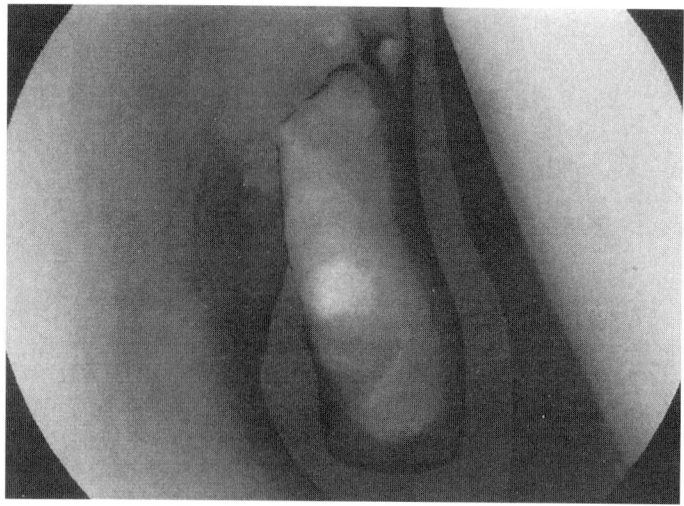

FIGURE 7.7 The Madigan Endoscopic Sinus Surgical Simulator includes a variety of skill levels for the support of student surgical education. At the advanced stage, the virtual surgical field has the appearance of the real world nasal cavity. The visual aids that have been incorporated into the less complex levels have been dropped at this level.

7.5.7 Virtual Instructor

A virtual instructor named Martin was created for the simulator. Martin provides hands-free control of the simulator so that a simulator user can train without assistance from another person. Martin serves two purposes. He acts as the "surgical technician" providing the student surgeon instruments at the student's voice command, and he has built-in intelligence in the form of procedural knowledge. Martin tracks the progress of the student and can provide the student with recommendations for the next surgical sequence.

Martin recognizes a wide variety of voices and responds to over 60 commands. He has a vocabulary of over 180 words and recognizes multiple words for the same command. For example, a user may say "hummer" or "microdebrider" to select the same tool. The sequence of events that causes the simulator to react to spoken commands is as follows. The student surgeon issues a command that is transmitted as corresponding string over the Ethernet connection to the simulation computer. A background task in the simulation computer decodes the string, places the command into shared memory, and forwards the string to the audio server. The real-time software acts on the command. The audio server fetches the appropriate file and plays it through the speakers. The student hears and sees the response, closing the loop.

7.5.8 Endoscopic Sinus Simulator Evaluation

The Madigan sinus surgical simulator was evaluated by the Human Interface Technology Lab at the University of Washington. In general, two types of evaluations were performed during development. Formative evaluations provided design specifications input to the development team, and summative evaluation assessed the success of that effort by formally analyzing the system's effectiveness.

The findings of the evaluation team suggest that the simulator represents a valid and useful implementation of the target endoscopic sinus surgery tasks. In addition, the thoughtful integration of an organized curriculum perspective makes this system uniquely valuable among emerging medical simulation systems [12].

7.6 TRANSFER OF TRAINING

The use of VR and related techniques for medical training is clearly embryonic. Nevertheless, a significant portion of any development team's time and resources should be dedicated towards determining training efficacy and cost-effectiveness. Computer-based simulation in its present state is expensive and unproved. Assessments of training effectiveness can conserve scarce resources, which may be better expended on other projects.

The basic measure of training efficacy is percent transfer of training. In aviation, the transfer effectiveness ratio (TER) has been used to monitor the efficiency of training simulations. Research has suggested that such simulations can yield a TER of .48, indicating that one hour in a simulator saves approximately one-half hour in the air [13]. The TER also addresses which method of training provides the greatest learning in the least amount of time. If one training technique costs much less than another but takes a lot longer for a student to reach a certain level of proficiency, a TER experimental design can determine the cost-effectiveness of each training program per hour of training device operation [14]. It is clear that if surgeons cannot perform efficiently in virtual environments, then further pursuit of this technology may be fruitless.

The author recently completed a pilot study evaluating the transfer effectiveness of the sinus surgical simulator. The results, which will be formally presented in an upcoming publication, demonstrate positive effect of the Madigan sinus surgical simulator on the development of critical surgical skills.

7.7 SUMMARY

In the twenty-first century, simulators have the potential to play a tremendous role in the training and credentialing of surgeons. The magnitude of the role will depend on advances that are made in creating more realistic visual imagery, development of haptic sensations that are realistic and convincing, and production of training systems that are affordable. Developers of these systems must continue to assess transfer of training and continue to seek out and explore the emerging technologies (including artificial intelligence, tele-proctoring, tele-mentoring, and tele-presence) that can be used to either enhance the functionality of the simulators or as adjuncts to conventional training.

ACKNOWLEDGMENTS

This work is supported by the U.S. Army Medical Research and Material Command under cooperative agreement DAMD 17–95–2-5023. The author wishes to express his gratitude to Dave Heskamp and Jeff Miller of Lockheed Martin Tactical Defense Systems, Akron, OH; Douglas Sluis, Ph.D., of ATL Inc., Bothell, WA; Donald Stredney and Dennis Sessana of Ohio Supercomputer Center, Columbus, OH; Roni Yagel, Ph.D., and Naeem Shareef of the Department of Computer and Information Science, OSC, Columbus, OH.; Suzanne Weghorst, Peter Oppenheimer, Chris Airola, and Mark Billinghurst of the University of Washington—Human Interface Technology Laboratory, Seattle, WA; and Michael Levin and Louis Rosenberg, Ph.D., of Immersion Corp., San Jose, CA. The above individuals have contributed significantly to the success of our project.

REFERENCES

1. Edmond C, Heskamp D, Sluis D, Stredney D, Wiet G, Yagel R, Weghorst S, Miller J, Levin M. ENT Surgical Training Simulator. Stud. Health Technology Informatics, 1997, No. 39, pp. 518–528.
2. Edmond C, Wiet G, Bolger B. Virtual environments surgical simulation in otolaryngology. Otolaryngol Clin North Am. April, 1998.
3. Rosenberg L, Stredney D. A haptic interface for virtual simulation of endoscopic surgery. In: Health Care in the Information Age. Amsterdam, The Netherlands, IOS Press, 1996, pp. 371–387.
4. Aukstakalnis S, Blatner D, eds. Silicon Mirage: The Art and Science of Virtual Reality, Berkeley, CA: Peachpit Press, 1992.
5. Billinghurst M, Savage P, Oppenheimer P, Edmond C. Expert surgical assistant: an intelligent virtual environment with multimodal input. In: Health Care in the Information Age. Amsterdam, The Netherlands, IOS Press and Ohmsha, 1996.
6. Cohen PR, Dalrymple M, Pereira FCN, Sullivan JW, Gargan Jr., RA, Schlossberg JL, Tyler SW. Synergistic use of direct manipulation and natural language. Conference on Human Factors in Computing Systems (CHI ''89). Austin, TX, IEEE, ACM, 1989, pp. 227–233.
7. Cohen PR. The role of natural language in a multimodal interface. UIST Proceedings, 1992, pp. 143–149.
8. Hauptman AG, McAvinny P. Gestures with Speech for Graphics Manipulations. Int J Man-Machine Studies, 38:231–249, 1993.
9. Bolt RA. ''Put-that-there'': voice and gesture at the graphics interface. Computer Graphics 14(3):262–270. In: Proceeding of ACM SIGGRAPH, 1980.
10. Buchanan BG, Shorlife EH. Rule based expert systems: The MYCIN Experiments of the Stanford Heuristic Programming Project. Reading, MA: Addison Wesley, 1984.
11. Weimer D, Ganapathy SK. A synthetic visual environment with hand gesturing and voice input. Conference on Human Factors in Computing Systems (CHI '89). Austin, TX, IEEE, ACM, April 30–May 4, 1989, pp. 235–240.
12. Weghorst S, Airola C, Oppenheimer P, Edmond C, Patience T, Heskamp D, Miller J. Validation of the Madigan endoscopic sinus simulator. Stud. Health Technology Informatics 50:399–408, 1998.
13. Johnson R, Bhoyrul S, Way L, Satava R, McGovern K, Fletcher D, Rangel S, Loftin B. Assessing a virtual reality surgical skills simulator. Health Care in the Information Age. Amsterdam, The Netherlands, IOS Press, pp. 608–617.
14. Kozak JJ, Hancock PA. Transfer of Training from VIZ Ergonomics.

8

Digital Imaging in Otorhinolaryngology–Head and Neck Surgery

Eiji Yanagisawa, M.D., F.A.C.S.
Yale University School of Medicine, Yale–New Haven Hospital, and Hospital of St. Raphael, New Haven, Connecticut

John K. Joe, M.D.
Memorial Sloan-Kettering Cancer Center, New York, New York

Ray Yanagisawa, B.A.
Woodbridge, Connecticut

8.1 INTRODUCTION

Digital imaging represents one of the most significant recent technological advances in both the consumer and professional markets. The downside to writing about any groundbreaking technology is that, by the time the article makes it into print, the subject matter may have become passé. Despite this caveat, the continuing implementation of digital imaging in the field of medicine warrants discussion about its clinical applications in otolaryngology and head and neck surgery.

8.2 FUNDAMENTALS OF DIGITAL IMAGING
8.2.1 Image

Photodocumentation of still images has traditionally been captured onto 35 mm negative or slide film, and moving images have traditionally been recorded on VHS, SVHS, Hi8, or 3/4 inch videotape [1–4]. Such analog video input captures images as a continuous stream of varying signal strengths on videotape.

In contrast, a digital camera utilizes a charge-coupled device (CCD) in place of film. A CCD is a silicon chip composed of individual pixels that transform light into voltage in a manner similar to the transformation of chemical emulsions into silver grains on film [5]. A computer within the camera converts this voltage into binary data as a series of ones and zeroes. These discrete binary units provide the fundamental difference between a digital image and the continuous spectrum of values of an analog signal.

By placing a red, green, or blue filter in front of the CCD, the chip is able to digitize the individual color components of an image for color representation. The resolution of a camera refers to its density of light-sensitive picture elements, or pixels. The degree of recorded detail varies directly with the resolution of the recorded digital image; that is, the greater the resolution of a digital image, the higher degree of recorded detail. A greater resolution allows image enlargement with less degradation of picture quality from discrete separation between adjacent points in the image (a phenomenon called pixelation) [6]. The gold standard for image quality is the typical 35 mm Kodachrome slide, which contains silver grains at a density of approximately 2500 lines per inch, or 4096×2736 pixels per frame. Data from the dermatology literature indicate that the minimum resolution needed to recognize relevant details of patient images is 768×512 pixels [5]. Although a higher resolution image provides greater detail, the resulting greater file size presents several downsides as well. A higher resolution image requires more memory for storage, more powerful processors for manipulation, and faster networks for transmission.

8.2.2 Compression

To compensate for the greater hardware requirements necessary for higher resolution, an image may be compressed by one of two methods to decrease its file size [5,6]. One approach retains all image information and is commonly called ''lossless.'' The other approach is termed ''lossy,'' since various amounts of redundant color data are discarded. Lossy compression is commonly used in digital cameras at the time of this writing. Reducing the size of the image file through compression is ideal if memory space is a concern or if network data transmission rates are slow. Even with compression, however, the tradeoff between maximal

Digital Imaging

resolution for optimal image quality and the smallest possible file size remains a dilemma.

8.3 TECHNIQUES OF DIGITAL IMAGING

There are three primary approaches to creating digital images [7]. The first is to convert a photograph or slide into a still digital image using an image scanner connected to a computer. The second is to convert an analog signal from a video camera or videotape into streaming digital video with an image capture board installed in a computer. This method is limited by the relatively low resolution of the analog video signal. Using this method, the senior author (EY) has produced excellent images for his publications [1–4,8,9]. He uses 3/4-inch prerecorded videotapes, a Macintosh computer, Avid Media Suite Pro video editing software, Adobe Photoshop, and a Sony digital dye-sublimation printer. The third method is to capture the image directly with a charge-coupled device digital camera. This method bypasses conversion and starts with a digital image at the time of capture.

8.4 HARDWARE REQUIREMENTS

Components of a digital imaging system include a digital camera, computer, annotation software, removable memory storage, digital video recorder, color printer, and digital projector.

8.4.1 Digital Cameras

Digital still cameras, like conventional film-based cameras, come in point-and-shoot and single lens reflex (SLR) models [5,10–12]. Utilizing fixed lenses and a built-in flash, point-and-shoot cameras are inexpensive, easy to use, and generally smaller and lighter than SLR cameras. The disadvantages of point-and-shoot models include less flexibility in controlling the features of the camera and lower resolution. In contrast, SLR cameras have modified the typical film-based 35 mm camera by replacing the film advance system with the CCD and processing hardware and a LCD (liquid crystal diode) screen. SLR-derived digital cameras are usually larger and more expensive but produce superior quality images.

For medical use, one should choose a megapixel digital camera, which produces high-quality images. Some of the digital still cameras commercially available at the time of this writing are illustrated in Figure 8.1. The Olympus C-3030 camera is shown in Figure 8.1A. This model is a 3.3 megapixel camera with 2048 × 1536 resolution (approximately $990 at the time of this writing). The Nikon Coolpix 950 (approximately $650) is a 2.11 megapixel camera with 1600 × 1200 resolution (Figure 8.1B). The Sony Mavica MVC-FD95 digital still

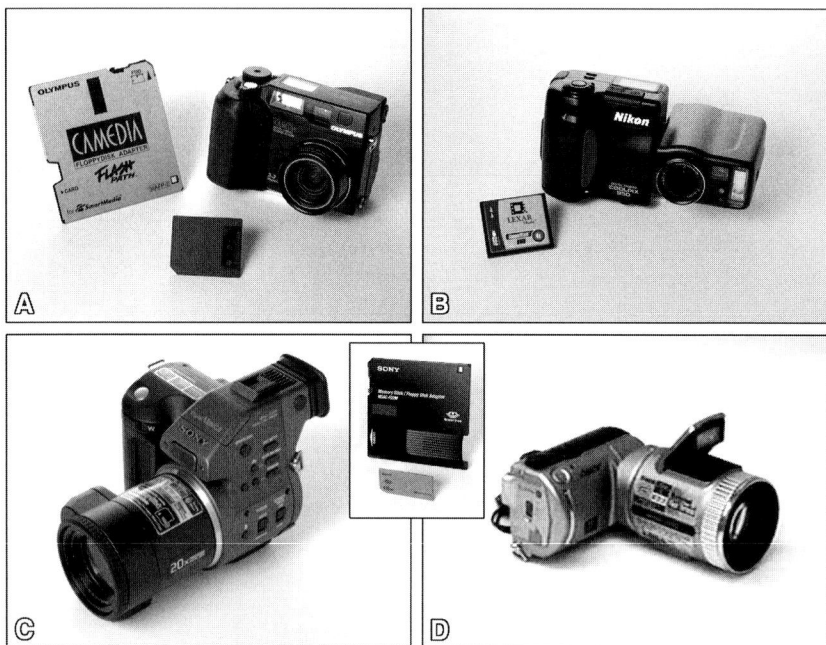

FIGURE 8.1 Digital still cameras: (A) Olympus C-3030 digital camera with a Smart Media card and a floppy disk adapter; (B) Nikon Coolpix 950 digital camera with a Compact Flash card; (C) Sony Mavica FD-95 digital camera; (D) Sony Cyber-shot DSC-F505V digital camera. The insert between C and D shows a Sony Memory Stick with a floppy disk adapter.

camera (approximately $900) is illustrated in Figure 8.1C. It has a 1600 × 1200 pixel resolution, a Carl Zeiss lens, and 10× optical/20× digital zoom. Figure 8.1D shows the Sony Cyber-shot DSC-F505V digital still camera (approximately $900), which has a 5× optical/10× digital zoom.

These digital still cameras include models with which we are familiar. Other digital still cameras available at the time of this writing include the Epson Photo PC 3000Z (3.3 megapixel camera), the Kodak DC290 Zoom (2.1 megapixel camera with 1792 × 1200 resolution), the Sony Mavica MVC-FD73 (640 × 480 resolution), the Sony Mavica MVC-CD1000 (2.1 megapixel with 1600 × 1200 resolution), the HP Photo Smart 315 (2.1 megapixel with 1600 × 1200 resolution and 2.5 digital zoom), and the HP Photosmart 912 (2.24 megapixel with 1600 × 1280 resolution and 3× optical/2× digital zoom). The aforemen-

Digital Imaging

tioned list of digital still cameras is intended to be comprehensive. In addition, the authors do not wish to state and/or imply an endorsement for any particular model.

Although some current digital still cameras are able to record several seconds of moving video segments, other digital cameras are dedicated to the capture of longer segments of digitized streaming video images (Figure 8.2). The camera pictured in Figure 8.2A is an analog Stryker 888 3-chip CCD camera utilized by otolaryngologists for documentation of sinonasal or laryngeal endoscopy. Although this Stryker camera captures an analog signal, the images may be recorded onto either an analog or digital video recorder. In contrast, the cameras illustrated in Figures 8.2B–D represent digital camcorders (also called DV or DVCAM camcorders) that capture a digitized signal. The Canon ZR-10 digital video camcorder (approximately $900) is shown in Figure 8.2B. The Sony DCR-PC100 Mini-DV video camcorder (approximately $1,800) is pictured in Figure 8.2C.

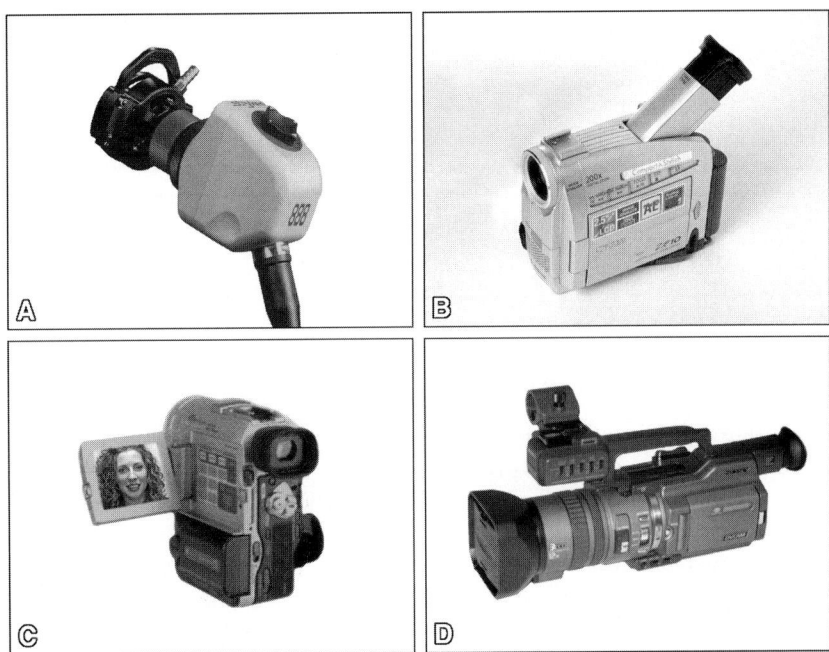

FIGURE 8.2 Digital video cameras and camcorders: (A) Stryker 888 3-chip CCD camera; (B) Canon ZR-10 digital video camcorder; (C) Sony DCR-PC100 Mini-DV video camcorder; (D) Sony professional DSR-PD150 DVCAM camcorder.

Although the cameras previously described represent models manufactured for consumer use, Figure 8.2D illustrates a representative Sony DVCAM DSR-PD150 camcorder (approximately $4,000) for the professional market.

8.4.2 Computer

The computer utilized in a digital imaging system may be either a PC or a Macintosh, although compatibility of images across both platforms is ideal to ensure the widest possible audience. Because higher resolution images tend to result in larger file sizes, the computer should utilize the largest processing power, hard disk memory capacity, and monitor size that are reasonably affordable.

Digital cameras transfer images to the computer by many ways. Some cameras require direct connection through a serial or SCSI cable. Others use removable cards or diskettes that are placed into an appropriate receiver on the computer, and some even use infrared remote transfer of the data. Some cameras function best with an external card reader [12]. Before acquiring a digital camera, users are encouraged to understand the method and process through which digital images are transferred from the camera to the computer.

8.4.3 Software

Proprietary software is necessary to import images captured with a digital still camera or digital video camcorder onto a computer's hard drive. Image processing software usually comes with most digital cameras. Once transferred onto the computer, captured images may then be annotated or manipulated using this software. The speed at which images are transferred from the camera to the computer depends on the type of connection established between the two. Newer camera models use faster connections, e.g., USB (universal serial bus).

8.4.4 Removable Storage Media

Removable storage media are necessary with some cameras to store captured images prior to their download onto a computer. These storage cards allow for the camera to function without a physical connection to the computer when images are captured. Different models of digital image storage cards are currently available, and representative types are illustrated in Figure 8.3. Figure 8.3A shows the Olympus Camedia floppy disk adapter for a Smart Media card. A Smart Media card is pictured in Figure 8.3B. This type of storage media is used by several models of digital still cameras, and cards with different amounts of memory are available, including 8, 16, 32, and 64 MB. Cards with greater amounts of memory storage allow for a larger number of images that may be captured prior to download. Figure 8.3C illustrates the Sony floppy disk adapter for a Sony Memory Stick. The Memory Stick, shown in Figure 8.3D, is the proprietary memory stor-

Digital Imaging

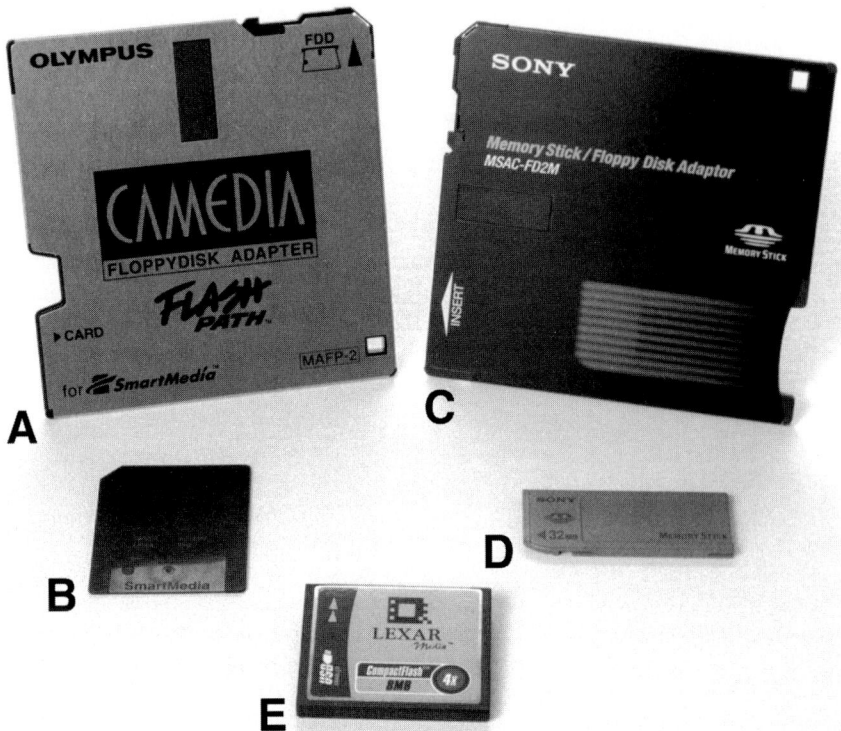

FIGURE 8.3 Digital image removable storage memory cards: (A) Olympus Camedia floppy disk adapter for Smart Media cards; (B) 8 MB Smart Media card (also available in 16, 32, and 64 MB cards); (C) Sony floppy disk adapter for Sony Memory Stick; (D) 32 MB Sony Memory Stick (also available in 16 and 64 MB sticks); (E) 8 MB Compact Flash card (used by Nikon Coolpix series cameras) (also available in 16, 32, 48, 64, and 128 MB cards).

age card used by Sony digital still cameras. It is also available with a variety of memory sizes, including 16, 32, and 64 MB. The Compact Flash card pictured in Figure 8.3E represents another type of storage media. The Nikon Coolpix digital still cameras use this type of card, which is available with a variety of sizes of memory, including 8, 16, 32, 48, 64, and 128 MB.

One current problem with removable storage media for digital still cameras is the lack of a uniform standard. As shown in Figure 8.1, different camera models utilize different types of proprietary memory cards, which are not cross-compatible. This lack of uniformity can be both confusing and expensive for consumers and professionals, who may use more than one model of digital still camera.

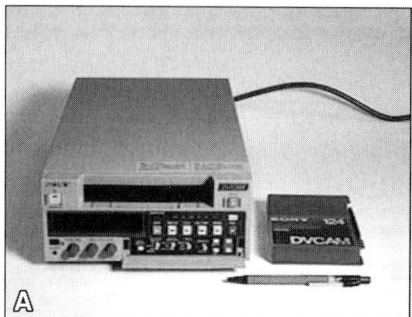 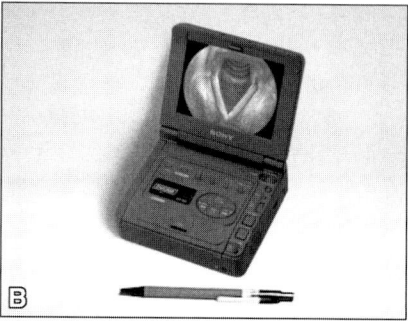

FIGURE 8.4 Digital video recorder/player: (A) Sony DSR-20 DVCAM video recorder with a 60 minute DVCAM videotape (accepts both 60 and 40 minutes tapes); (B) Sony DSR-V10 Video Walkman mini-recorder (accepts only 40 minutes mini DVCAM tape).

8.4.5 Digital Video Recorder/Player

Digital DV or DVCAM camcorders support the recording of digital images in their built-in recorder. The images may be reviewed on the built-in LCD screen. These devices may also be connected to an external monitor for the review of the digital images stored in the devices. Finally, an LCD projector may be used to project the images on a larger screen.

The newest storage medium for digital video camcorders includes a mini-DVCAM tape. DVCAM tape is utilized in digital video recorders/players, representative models of which are illustrated in Figure 8.4. Figure 8.4A demonstrates the Sony DSR-20 DVCAM recorder (approximately $3,500), which is useful for medical documentation on a 60- or 40-minute DVCAM tape. The Sony DSR-V10 Video Walkman mini-recorder (approximately $2,300) is shown in Figure 8.4B. Both models offer digitized capture of video images arising from either an analog or a digital source. Digital recorders from a digital signal offer video images of higher quality than are available with conventional analog videotape. Both models are portable, and the Sony DSR-V10 has a built-in LCD screen for viewing image capture.

8.4.6 Color Printers

Color printers are commonly available in various types (ink jet, dye sublimation, color laser) in a wide selection, whose features and prices vary greatly. As is the case with all hardware devices, printers with more features have decreased in cost as technology has progressed over time. Figure 8.5A illustrates the Olympus P-330 digital printer (approximately $400), a model that is able to print images

Digital Imaging

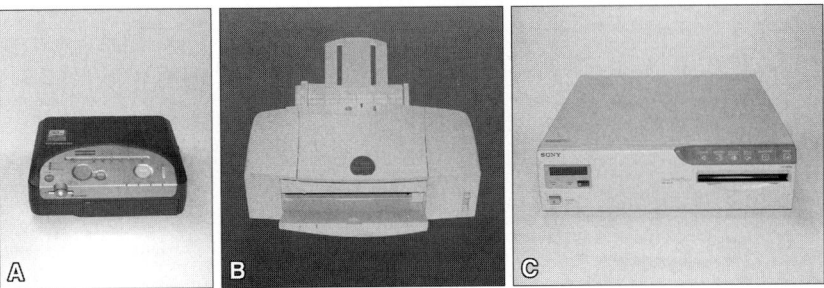

FIGURE 8.5 Digital color printers: (A) Olympus P-330 digital printer; (B) Canon BJC-8200 bubble jet printer; (C) Sony UP-5500 dye-sublimation professional digital printer.

from digital image storage cards without the need for an initial download from computer. Some printers are able to print directly from storage cards, but generally they tend to be more costly than conventional printers. However, these digital printers offer convenience, obviating the need for a computer. Figure 8.5B illustrates a Canon BJC-8200 bubble jet printer (approximately $300), an example of a conventional printer, which requires that a computer download capture images before printing. Such ink jet printers generally offer inexpensive prints of adequate quality. Publication quality pictures may be obtained by using a professional photo paper.

Dye sublimation color printers are expensive but produce superior quality images that are most suitable for publication. The senior author uses the Sony UP-5500 digital color printer (approximately $8,000), a professional dye sublimation color printer (Figure 8.5C). Much less expensive dye sublimation printers are now available from various other companies.

8.4.7 Digital LCD Projector

To present images in a conference setting, one may use a digital projector. Some of the currently available models are presented in Figure 8.6. Figure 8.6A shows the Sony VPL-PX31 LCD projector (2800 ANSI lumens) (approximately $7,500). Figure 8.6B illustrates the Sony VPL-PX1 SuperLite™ Portable LCD projector (1000 ANSI lumens) (approximately $4,500). The Sony VPL-CX1 SuperLite™ LCD projector (550 ANSI lumens) (approximately $2,500) is shown in Figure 8.6C, and Figure 8.6D demonstrates the Mitsubishi X70UX XGA LCD projector (1100 ANSI lumens) (approximately $4,500). There are many other models available from companies such as Epson and NEC.

Technological advances in terms of image brightness and projector portability continue to improve. Some digital LCD projectors project images directly

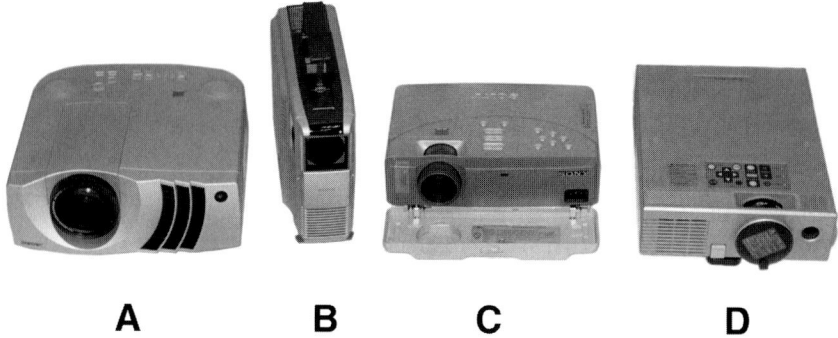

FIGURE 8.6 Digital LCD projectors: (A) Sony VPL-PX31 LCD projector; (B) Sony VPL-PX1 SuperLite™ Portable LCD projector; (C) Sony VPL-CX1 SuperLite™ LCD projector; (D) Mitsubishi X70UX XGA LCD projector.

from storage cards. The availability of such an LCD projector may obviate the need for slide carousels, or even a computer, in presentations.

8.5 ADVANTAGES OF DIGITAL IMAGING

There are numerous advantages of digital imaging [5–13]. In terms of quality, early digital cameras were criticized for inferior photograph quality compared to 35 mm film cameras. However, as technology has improved, current megapixel cameras produce images comparable to that of 35 mm film. With regard to convenience, digital images are immediately available for preview on the LCD screen. Images may then be assessed in terms of quality and content at the time of capture, without the delays that are inherent in film development [10]. Images of unsatisfactory quality may be discarded, saving memory space. Cost issues tend to favor digital photography. Although there is the initial cost of hardware to establish the digital system, there are no ongoing costs for film purchase or development [10]. There are costs involved in printing digital images, but most conventional ink jet printers offer inexpensive, good quality hard copies of captured images. Dye sublimation and color laser printers offer superior image quality, but at a higher cost. In terms of image manipulation, software programs allow for easy annotation of images through the addition of graphics or text. Photographic artifacts may be removed, and color balance, brightness, or contrast may be optimized [5]. Some models of digital still cameras allow in-camera editing of images without the need for download to a computer.

Digital Imaging

The clinical advantages of digital imaging include photodocumentation for the medical record and data archive. Physical findings on examination may be documented and stored as part of a patient's chart. Digital images may also facilitate patient counseling. Archiving digital images on removable storage media allows for compact storage with easy and rapid retrieval of images. The standard 1.44 MB floppy disk is nearly universal and provides an inexpensive medium for sharing captured images with patients. Although the cost for storing images (in terms of cents per MB) is greater for a floppy disk than for other higher capacity media (such as CD-R or CD-RW), cost per disk is less for floppy disks, and the convenience of floppy disks should not be discounted.

The efficient data archive possible with digital images also has educational applications. Interactive CD-ROMs utilize digitized images for the instruction of medical students, residents, or practitioners. Computer software programs significantly improve the speed and efficiency by which images may be cataloged and retrieved in comparison with the traditional method of sifting through numerous videotapes, photographs, and/or slides.

Digitized images may be easily duplicated and disseminated without degradation in image quality [7]. The distribution of data over a hospital network or the Internet allows for rapid and economical teleconferencing. Compression improves the speed by which images may be transmitted for remote viewing or instruction. The increasing availability of greater bandwidth communications provides for near-instantaneous transmission of images.

8.6 DISADVANTAGES OF DIGITAL IMAGING

Although digital cameras have made significant technological advances over the past several years, there are still shortcomings to this technology. The control and flexibility of photographic features available with traditional film cameras are not yet uniformly available on consumer level digital still cameras. The power requirements for most digital cameras, whose LCD viewscreens require substantial power, result in significantly shorter battery life compared to film cameras. The internal memory within current digital cameras are so limited that, unless large capacity removable storage cards are used, few high-resolution images may be captured before they must be downloaded to the computer.

The implementation of any new technology often requires establishing new infrastructure. Many conference rooms are not yet equipped for the presentation of digital images, necessitating the conversion from a digital medium to traditional 35 mm slides [10]. Not all health care environments have the resources or infrastructure necessary to implement a digital system [2,3]. For those who wish to establish a digital system, competing technologies provide greater choice of formats, but deciding upon a particular system may be difficult. Once a digital system has been purchased, professional and technical staff must become familiar with this new technology [10].

The ease with which digital images may be manipulated to enhance picture quality raises new concerns regarding the ethics of publication and presentation [5,12]. Digital images may be tampered with for falsification to an extent not feasible with previous media.

Finally, in light of the ease of transmission of digital images over a network or the Internet, attention should be paid to issues of security and patient confidentiality [6].

8.7 CLINICAL APPLICATIONS IN OTOLARYNGOLOGY–HEAD AND NECK SURGERY

Digital imaging has many potential uses in the field of otolaryngology. Figure 8.7 illustrates a side-by-side comparison of image quality of analog video images and digital computer images. The high quality of the captured digital images is evident in Figures 8.7A and B. Such high-quality digital images are immediately available for review at the time of capture without the need for film development. Images may be annotated by the addition of labels, such as the patient's name and the date of examination. The images may then be stored on a 1.44 MB floppy disk in the patient's chart. A copy may also be presented to the patient. The images may be downloaded to a computer for archive, and representative images may be then projected for presentation and education. If necessary, images may be shared with consulting colleagues by electronic transmission.

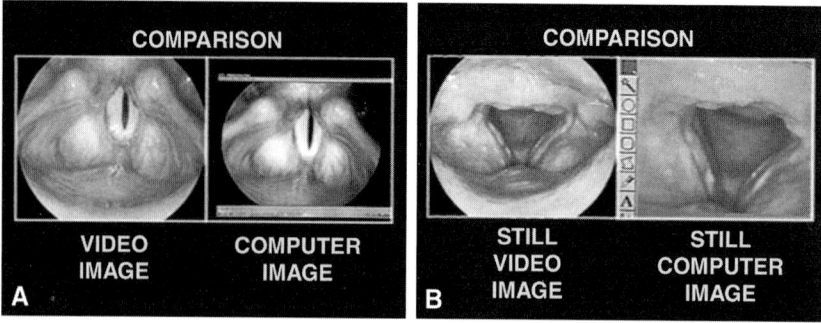

FIGURE 8.7 Comparison of analog video and digital computer images: (A) comparison between laryngoscopic video and computer images; (B) comparison between laryngoscopic still video and still computer images.

Digital Imaging 129

Figure 8.8 demonstrates some examples of the clinical applications of digital imaging in otolaryngology and head and neck surgery. As shown in Figures 8.8A, B, and C, facial plastic surgeons may catalog preoperative and postoperative images of patients for comparison, counseling, and education. Captured images provide much more illustrative information than either descriptive text or coarse drawings. Figure 8.8D demonstrates the right auricle with herpetic lesion. Figure 8.8E shows a close-up view of this lesion. The captured image may be zoomed in or out in the digital camera itself by using the zoom button of the camera. The image can also be moved to the right or to the left or centered. The intraoral digital image can be taken using the cheek retractors as shown in Figure 8.8F. Any lesion of the head and neck may be recorded. Digital images may be

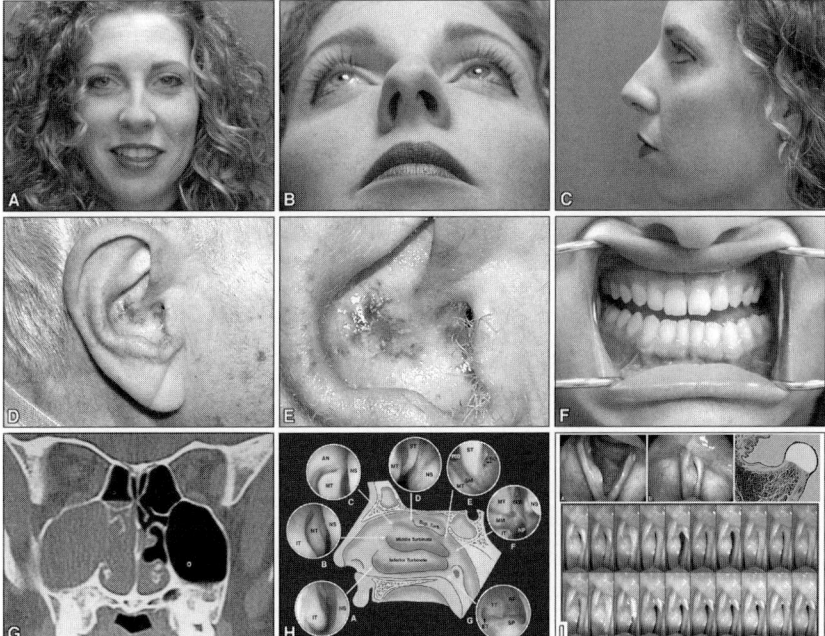

FIGURE 8.8 Clinical applications in otolaryngology–head and neck surgery: (A–C) photographs of the face (frontal, basal and lateral views); (D) digital photograph of the auricle with herpetic lesions; (E) close-up view of the same patient showing the details of the skin lesion; (F) digital image of teeth; (G) preoperative CT scan of sinuses; (H) computer graphics of endoscopic sinonasal anatomy and laryngostroboscopic view of vocal fold cyst (adapted from Ref. 8); (I) Computer graphics of endoscopic sinonasal anatomy and laryngostroboscopic view of vocal fold cyst (adapted from Ref. 8).

used to document intraoperative findings and surgical specimens. This may prove helpful for medicolegal documentation. As shown in Figure 8.8G, preoperative sinus computed tomography (CT) scans may be photographed by digital still cameras. Figures 8.8H and I show computer graphics prepared for publication in textbooks [8].

Two types of digital imaging systems useful for functional endoscopic sinus surgery (FESS) are illustrated in Figures 8.9A and B. These types of computer-aided surgery systems provide improved localization for maximimal safety during FESS.

The Kay Digital Strobo Recording System (DVRS) illustrated in Figure 8.9C is useful for laryngology. Voice disorders may be evaluated with high-quality stroboscopic images superimposed with electrophysiological information. During laryngostroboscopy, any given segment of the image may be captured

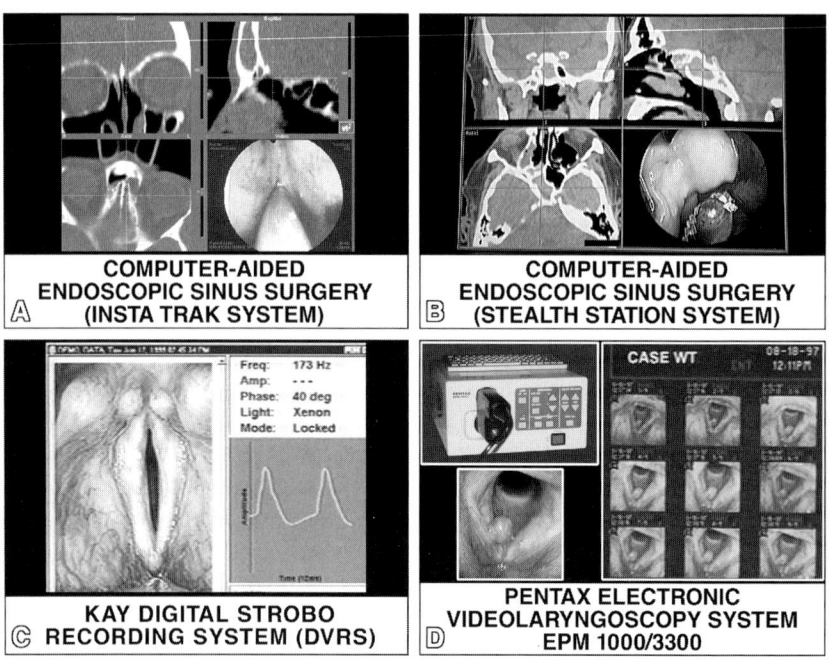

FIGURE 8.9 Clinical applications in otolaryngology-head and neck surgery: (A) computer-aided endoscopic sinus surgery (Insta Trak system); (B) Computer-aided endoscopic sinus surgery (Stealth Station system) (adapted from Ref. 14); (C) Kay Digital Strobo Recording System (DVRS); (D) Pentax Electronic Videolaryngoscopy System EPM 1000/3300.

Digital Imaging

for a detailed study. The Pentax Electronic Videolaryngoscopy System EPM 1000/3300 shown in Figure 8.9D also provides high-quality digital images of the larynx.

8.8 DESCRIPTIONS OF CURRENT DIGITAL IMAGE CAPTURE SYSTEMS

The features of digital image capture devices continue to improve while their costs continue to decrease. Two of the most up-to-date systems currently available are presented here. Their descriptions serve not as product endorsement but rather convey the state of technological capability at the time of this writing. In selecting a digital image capture system, one should choose the system that allows fast capture time.

Figure 8.10 illustrates the Stryker SDC Pro digital capture device (approximately $14,000), which can be used to record still images or video segments. Housed within the device are a CPU (central processing unit) and hard drive that can capture digital images or streaming video onto a write-able compact disk

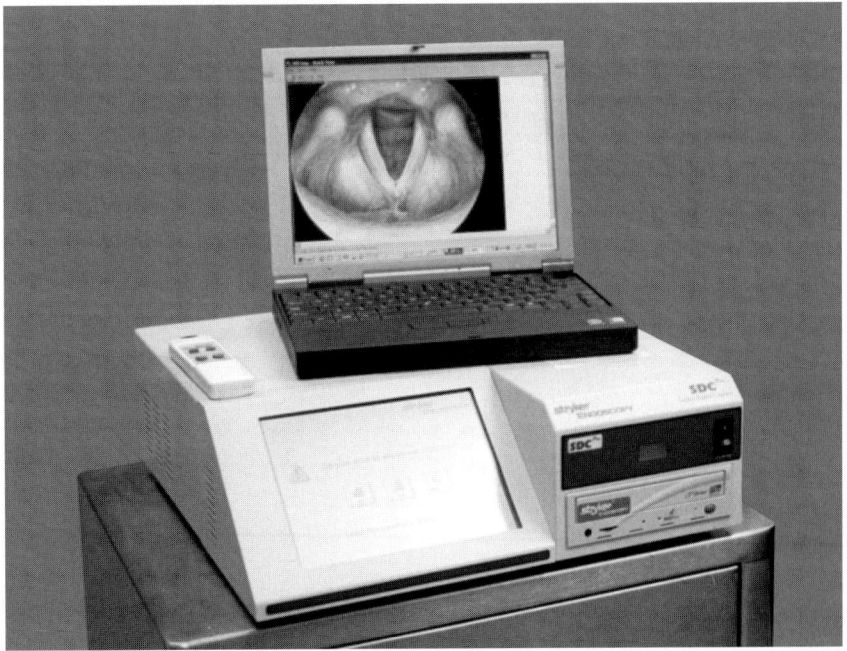

FIGURE 8.10 Stryker SDC Pro digital capture device.

(CD-R). The CD has become the de facto standard for data storage, since it may be accessed from almost any computer system using either a Macintosh or Windows-based operating system. A single CD may hold approximately 650 images captured in bitmap (BMP) format, or approximately 12,000 images in compressed Joint Photographic Expert Group (JPEG) format. Alternatively, a single CD may record up to 20 minutes of continuous video. Alternatively, a CD may contain a mixture of both still images and digital video.

Included with the Stryker SDC Pro system is the SDC Image Pro software package for digital annotation of captured still images or video segments. Image quality may be adjusted digitally using a variety of image control functions, and the results are immediately displayed on the console. Still images and video segments are conveniently organized by patient name and date of examination for later retrieval or for import into other software programs, such as Microsoft PowerPoint. The SDC Pro system has an image capture time of less than one second.

Shown in Figure 8.11, the Sony DKC-CM30 digital still camera (approximately $2,000) captures still images and does not capture video segments. A C-

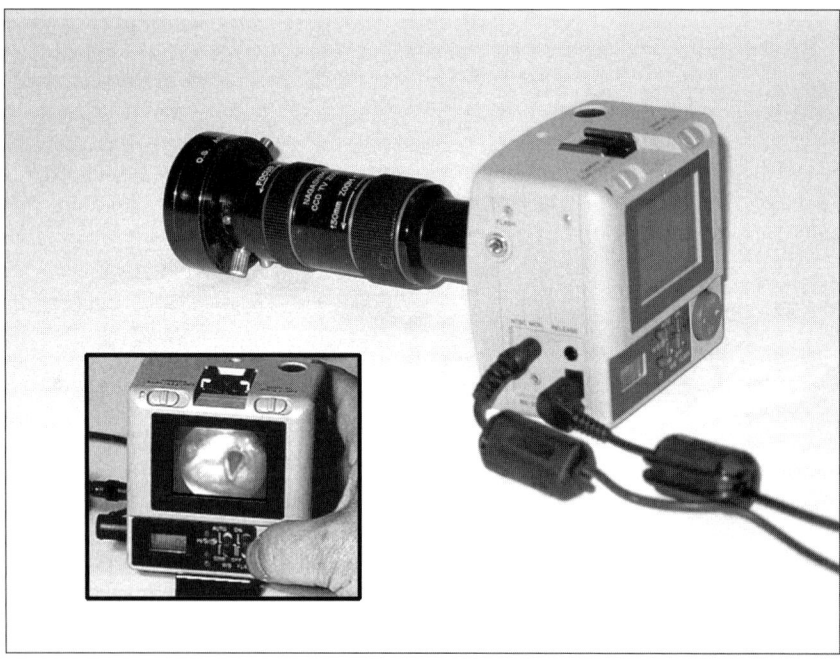

FIGURE 8.11 Sony DKC-CM30 digital still camera with a Nagashima endoscope attached. The insert shows a digitized laryngeal image on the LCD viewscreen located on the back of the camera.

mount lens may be attached to the camera to accept a variety of rigid telescopes for endoscopic examination. The number of images that may be taken depends on the resolution selected. Up to 30 images may be captured in high resolution, or up to 120 images may be captured in standard resolution. The inset image of Figure 8.11 illustrates a digitized laryngeal image on the LCD viewscreen on the back of the camera. Since the capture time of the Sony DKC-CM30 is slow, this camera is not currently recommended for digital photography of moving subjects.

8.9 CONCLUSIONS

The convenience and features of digital imaging systems will likely result in their continued integration into health care delivery as technology improves and prices fall. The ease with which images may be manipulated and transmitted mandates attention to the ethical presentation and distribution of these images. Furthermore, the storage and transmission of digital images requires a uniform and flexible network, which permits ease of operation. A digital system for image capture, storage, and distribution is currently a useful adjunct to traditional film-based systems, but the replacement of film by digital media may not be too far in the future.

ACKNOWLEDGMENTS

The authors would like to thank Dr. Michael Willett and Dr. Ken Yanagisawa for their assistance during the preparation of this chapter.

REFERENCES

1. Yanagisawa E, Yanagisawa R. Laryngeal photography. Otolaryng Clin North Am 24:999–1022, 1991.
2. Yanagisawa E, Yanagisawa K. Otologic photography and videography. In: Hughes GB, Pensak ML, eds. Clinical Otology, 2nd ed. New York: Thieme, 1997.
3. Yanagisawa E, Yanagisawa K. Otolaryngologic photodocumentation in the office setting. In: Krouse JH, Mirante JP, Christmas DA, eds. Office-Based Surgery in Otolaryngology. Philadelphia: Saunders, 1999.
4. Yanagisawa E. Videolaryngoscopy and laryngeal photography. In Ferlito A, ed. Diseases of the Larynx. London: Arnold, 2000.
5. Ratner D, Thomas CO, Bickers D. The uses of digital photography in dermatology. J Am Acad Dermatol 41:749–756, 1999.
6. Korman LY. Digital imaging in endoscopy. Gastrointestinal Endoscopy 48:318–326, 1998.
7. Tse CC. Anatomic pathology image capture using a consumer-type digital camera. Am J Surg Path 23:1555–1558, 1999.

8. Yanagisawa E. Color Atlas of Diagnostic Endoscopy in Otorhinolaryngology. New York: Igaku Shoin, 1997.
9. Yanagisawa E. Atlas of Rhinoscopy—Endoscopic Sinonasal Anatomy and Pathology. San Diego: Singular/Thomson Learning, 2000.
10. Belanger AJ, Lopes AE, Sinard JH. Implementation of a practical digital imaging system for routine gross photography in an autopsy environment. Arch Pathol Lab Med 124:160–165, 2000.
11. Delange GS, Diana M. 35 mm film vs. digital photography for patient documentation: Is it time to change? Ann Plast Surg 42: 15–20, 1999.
12. Spiegel JH, Singer MI. Practical approach to digital photography and its applications. Otolaryngol Head Neck Surg 123:152–156, 2000.
13. Van As CJ, Tigges M, Wittenberg T, Op de Coul BM, Eysholdt U, Hilgers FJ. High-speed digital imaging of neoglottic vibration after total laryngectomy. Arch Otolaryngol Head Neck Surg 125:891–897, 1999.
14. Yanagisawa E, Christmas DA. The value of computer aided (image-guided) systems for endoscopic sinus surgery. ENT J 78:822–826, 1999.

9

The Neuroradiology Perspective on Computer-Aided Surgery

S. James Zinreich, M.D.
Johns Hopkins Medical Institutions, Baltimore, Maryland

9.1 INTRODUCTION

The evolution of various neuroimaging modalities has significantly improved both the diagnosis and treatment of central nervous system anomalies and diseases. The excellent visual display of brain and spine anatomy afforded by both computed tomography (CT) and magnetic resonance (MR) imaging has improved not only the identification and diagnosis of central nervous system pathology, but also the surgical interventions used to treat such pathologies. With software advances, digitized imaging information can easily be reconstructed to provide a three-dimensional display. The three-dimensional images can be viewed from virtually any orientation and segmented to display "hidden" areas. Furthermore, images obtained from various modalities can be superimposed upon each other to provide a functional understanding of both the morphology and underlying pathology of the evaluated area. All of this information can be made available to the referring clinician/surgeon for evaluation and treatment planning. Prior to surgery, such information may be easily studied to gain familiarity with the regional anatomy and establish a surgical approach as well as define the extent of a surgical procedure. Nevertheless, once in the surgical suite, a surgeon would still have to rely on the information assessed prior to surgery and could only be guided by memory and the acuity of one's vision. Unfortunately, in neurosurgical procedures, a person's visual capability is unable to precisely delineate the boundary between normal and abnormal pathology, a boundary more sensitively displayed by MR imaging. Thus, the ultimate wish and need is for MR imaging (MRI) to be available within the surgical suite and able to provide guidance of the surgical procedure. This need established the field of frameless stereotactic surgery.

Perhaps the most significant neurosurgical advance that has surfaced within the past decade is the development and evolution of various frameless image-guided surgical systems. Computer-aided image guidance dramatically improves the surgeon's visualization of the operative field both before and during surgery, thereby reducing both the invasiveness and potential morbidity of a host of neurosurgical procedures.

9.2 EVOLUTION OF COMPUTER-AIDED SURGERY

The development of current computer-aided surgery (CAS) systems began with the pioneering work that resulted in frameless stereotactic image-guided neurosurgery. Although the concept of stereotaxy was introduced in the early part of the century, Spiegel et al. [1] were the first authors to describe a device that was used in humans that relied on a fixed frame relative to external landmarks. The advent of computed tomography enabled three-dimensional morphological maps of the brain, which in turn encouraged the increased use of stereotactic frames in surgical procedures. However, the frames are cumbersome (in some cases painful for the patient), and they often restrict the surgeon's access to the surgical field. Positioning this instrumentation requires significant time and effort from the neurosurgeon, and recently third-party payers have not consistently reimbursed for this additional time.

Thus, the development of methods that would provide stereotaxy without the use of a frame was begun. During a neurosurgical procedure, the head is totally immobilized in a mechanical clamp (Mayfield frame). From a perspective of registration, the ''fixation'' of the anatomical area and the lack of pulsations and breathing motion made neurosurgical procedures ideally suited for the introduction of image guidance (also known as surgical navigation).

Basic navigational systems consisted of two components: (1) the sensor that integrates the patient's position and morphological area of interest and (2) the information contained within the computer hardware/software. The sensor is used to co-register the patient with the patient's information in the computer and subsequently is used as a ''pointer'' during surgery. The sensor tip is represented on the computer screen by a set of crosshairs, and therefore the tip of the ''pointer'' in the surgical field is easily tracked on the computer screen. This process represents a crucial interaction that includes the registration process as well as a tracking process, which is used to track surgical instruments. A separate sensor can also be attached to the patient and is able to update the computer information with regards to patient motion.

Watanabe and colleagues [2] were the first to develop the "Neuronavigator" device, which consisted of a probe attached to a multijointed sensing arm capable of converting the motion of the probe tip into a digital signal. The Neuronavigator computer was able to interpret the relative position of the probe tip from this information; as a result of this process, the computer displayed the probe tip information (as cross hairs) on the computer monitor. Before surgery, fiducial markers were strategically placed on the patient's head and face, and a CT scan was performed. The CT data were then entered into the computer system via a video digitizer. In the operating room, proprietary software was then used to combine the CT data with the actual position of the patient on the operating table. In an early report on 12 patients undergoing neurosurgical procedures, an average accuracy of 3.0 mm was reported [2].

Guthrie and colleagues [43,44] described a stereotactic neurosurgical operating arm, which was similar to Watanabe's unit. In a report describing their experience with shunt catheter guidance, removal of a subdural hematoma, and resection of tumors, the reported accuracy was 4 mm. In 1989, stereotaxy evolved even further when Zinreich et al. [3] introduced the Viewing Wand image-guided neurosurgery system (ISG, Mississauga, Ontario, Canada), a smaller and more versatile unit that was quickly accepted by neurosurgeons.

9.3 REGISTRATION

Neurosurgical procedures have paved the way for the development of various registration techniques, and the evolution of these techniques paralleled the development of CAS. The two major types of registration techniques are the combined use of anatomical and surface points and the use of fiducial markers.

The anatomical landmark method of registration uses the patient's distinguishable facial features as landmarks. With the Viewing Wand (ISG, Mississauga, Ontario, Canada), the viewing wand probe is placed on the lateral canthal area of the right eye, while the mouse is simultaneously used to place the crosshairs over the same landmark on the three-dimensional (3D) computer-generated image. The location of the crosshairs is then registered into the computer. The contralateral, lateral, canthal, and left and right nasal alar regions are similarly entered [4,5]. The probe is placed at approximately 40 additional locations, and the computer matches the patient's facial contour to the identical contour pattern of the reconstructed 3D image. This provides a precise correlation of each point in the CT scanned volume with its corresponding x, y, z coordinate within the reconstructed information on the computer screen.

The registration process that uses external fiducial markers sends the precise location and orientation of the object to the computer that contains the 3D representation of the anatomical region to be evaluated, so that the image of the probe tip on the computer screen displays the actual position of the probe tip on or in the object. When each registration marker on the patient is touched with the tip of the probe, the corresponding marker's representation on the computer image is identified by a mouse-driven cursor on the screen (Figure 9.1). This process provides a point-pair file that contains the real space and image space locations for each of the markers or anatomical landmarks. To visually check the registration, widely separated anatomical points on the surface of the patient's head are touched and the indicated locations on the computer screen are confirmed.

When compared with the anatomical landmark-surface fit registration method, fiducial marker methods are more accurate and reproducible for neurosurgical procedures. In one study, fiducial registration resulted in greater accuracy when measured by a computer comparison of the calculated position to the true position on the scan as indicated by the system operator. For CT scans obtained in 21 cases, the fiducial registration error was on average 2.8 mm, compared to 5.6 mm for the anatomical landmark-surface fit algorithm method [6].

After the registration process, the computer displays the root mean square (RMS) value. This value is an expression of the standard deviation for each individual point of the registration set compared to the whole. Clinical observations

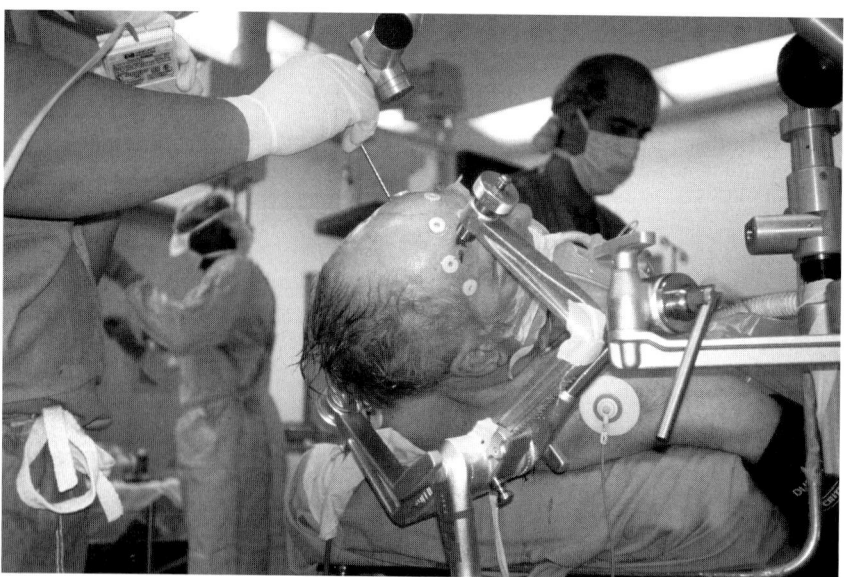

FIGURE 9.1 Patient positioned in a Mayfield frame with external fiducial markers in place for the presurgical registration process.

Neuroradiology Perspective

have suggested that lower RMS values correspond to more accurate registration. Registration accuracy can be subsequently corroborated by placing the probe tip on the center of one of the markers on the patient's face and visually checking its corresponding position on the computer screen.

One of the more recent advances in registration technique is the development of an automatic registration method for frameless stereotaxy, image-guided surgery, and enhanced reality visualization. Grimson et al. [7] reported on this system in 1996. Their method automatically registered segmented clinical reconstructions from CT or MR to provide the surgeon with a "live" view of the patient, thus enabling the surgeon to visualize internal structures before the actual procedure, as well as interactively viewing extra or intracranial structures noninvasively. The functionality and ease of use of this system is yet to be evaluated.

9.4 SENSORS

A critical aspect of the registration process is the sensor used to gather patient positional information for both the registration process as well as the tracking and updating of the surgical field. The evolution of sensor technology has been relatively slow in comparison with the development of graphical and computational workstations used in CAS. With the advance of high-performance, low-cost personal computers, software development has no longer been a restrictive factor in the advancement of CAS. The type of sensor used for tracking the surgical field and instrument is dependent on the procedure being performed; therefore, the sensor type may be considered procedure-specific. Early sensor technology was based on mechanical systems; more recently, optical and electromagnet sensor technology has been introduced.

9.4.1 Mechanical Sensors

Kogusi and Watanabe et al. were among the first to describe a mechanical articulated arm for position sensing (Figure 9.2) [8–13]. In this approach, mechanical sensors are articulated passive robotic arms that use various types of angle encoders at each joint. Optical encoders or potentiometers at each of the rotational areas pass information about the relative angles of the arm segments to the computer via analog to digital conversion. Surgical probes are attached to the arm at the last joint (Figure 9.3). Using the angles from the encoders in conjunction with known geometric information about the arm, a computer solves the spatial position and orientation of the device trigonometrically. Registration to the image set is accomplished by locating markers present on the patient during the CT scanning procedure and the operating room. This device provides minimal encumbrance for setup and use, with little imposition on the operative field. Other groups have also reported success with mechanical digitizing arms [14]. The

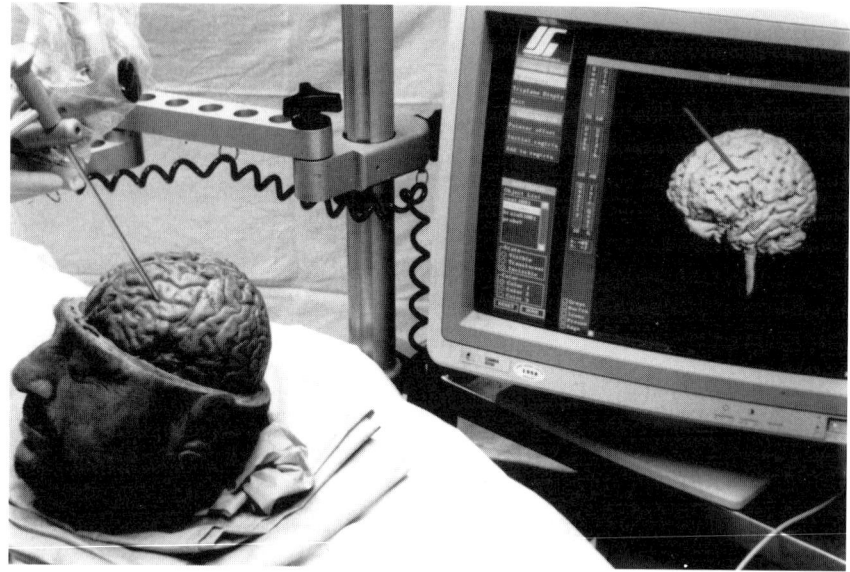

FIGURE 9.2 Laboratory model displaying the accuracy of a mechanical sensor prior to its introduction for use in neurosurgery.

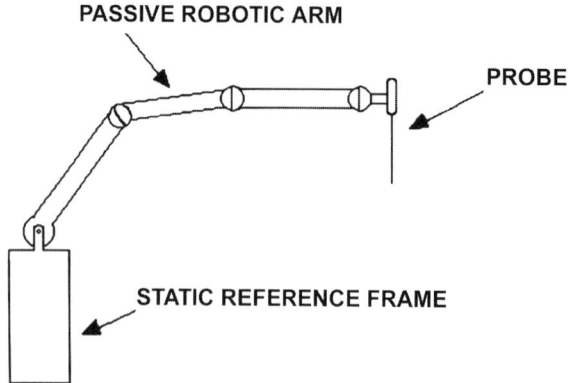

FIGURE 9.3 Mechanical sensor configuration

Neuroradiology Perspective

accuracy and clinical experience of the articulated arm has been previously reported [15]. Due to its size, the mechanical arm has been clinically limited to cranial procedures. Attempts at using the mechanical arm for spinal procedures as well as endoscopic sinus surgery procedures were reported; however, the need to also be able to track body movement in these procedures precluded the use of this sensor [16]. Since most neurosurgical procedures continue to be performed with the patient's head fixed in a Mayfield frame, the mechanical sensor continues to be used at several institutions. Its dependability and accuracy of approximately 2 mm meet the needs of the surgical procedure.

9.4.2 Optical Sensors

When a mechanical sensor is used for registration in neurosurgical procedures, in which the patient is not immobilized, an additional registration process must be performed during the procedure in the event that patient repositioning is necessary. Inadvertent patient movement also requires repeat registration. This problem has been addressed by the development of optical sensors, which are able to "track" potential motion and eliminate the need for additional registration steps during the procedure. These optical tracking sensors are quickly replacing mechanical sensor use in neurosurgery. This type of system uses dynamic frames of reference that track the movement of instruments used during surgery as well as motion of the operative field while the computer screen shows the registered anatomical area undergoing the surgical procedure. In these optical systems, strobing infrared light-emitting diodes (LEDs) mounted at known locations on the proximal tip of the surgical tools are triangulated by two or more infrared cameras. The cameras in turn are mounted on a boom approximately 1 or 2 m above the surgical field equidistant from one another (Figure 9.4). When compared with the mechanical sensor, this system is advantageous from the perspective that it is able to track the movement of several objects (several instruments as well as the patient's body movement); however, the location of the camera system can be intrusive, and the camera system needs to be able to detect the flashing light from the LEDs (i.e., maintain direct "line of sight"). Excessive lighting in the operating room may interfere with the camera's detection of light bursts from the LEDs. Objects placed in the path of the camera's detection also disrupt the tracking capability of the sensor.

During spinal surgery, a dynamic reference frame is used to track motion during surgeries that have the potential for patient movement. Surgical instruments equipped with LEDs are tracked in relation to the dynamic reference frame. In their experience with a similar system using LEDs mounted on a probe, Tebo et al. [17] reported accuracy rates comparable (95% of errors approximately 3 mm) to those obtained with conventional frame-based systems and with those of the mechanical arm–based system.

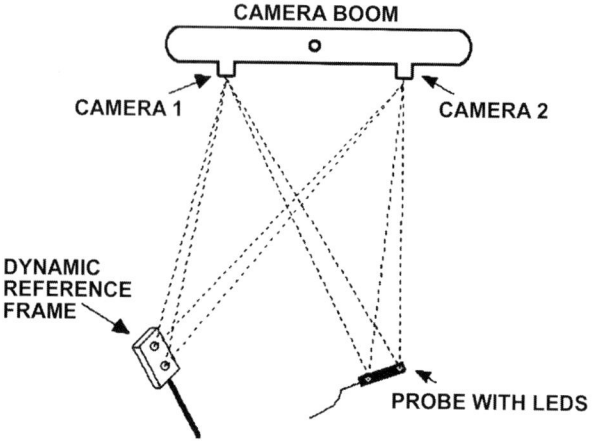

FIGURE 9.4 Optical sensor configuration

9.4.3 Electromagnetic Sensors

Any optical sensor system requires the maintenance of a line of sight between LEDs and the cameras above the operative field. This disadvantage led to the development of electromagnetic sensors, which were first applied to cardiac surgery (Figure 9.5) These latter sensors are able to track a nonlinear path, but they

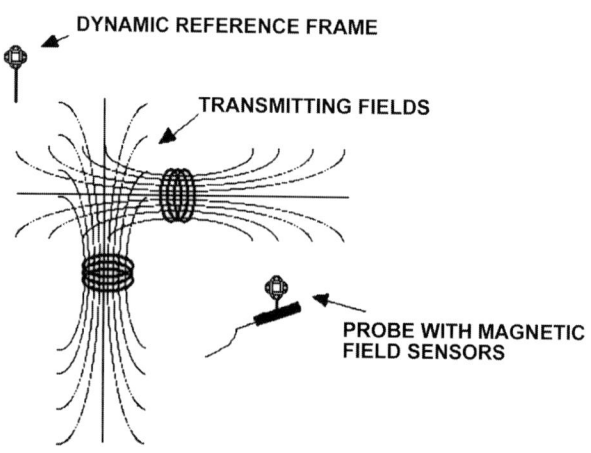

FIGURE 9.5 Electromagnetic sensor configuration

Neuroradiology Perspective

are susceptible to environmental conditions (most notably the presence of metals). Their ability to "pinpoint" a particular site accessible with a catheter or a flexible endoscope is a considerable advantage, since other sensors are only effective when attached to a rigid, linear instrument or "pointer."

9.4.4 Characteristics of the Ideal Sensor

All sensor systems continue to be in use, as each approach to sensor technology addresses the needs and requirements of a specific surgery. A "universal" sensor is not available. The optimal sensor systems should have the following characteristics:

> Miniature size (<3 mm in diameter)
> Easily incorporated with or attached to the surgical instruments
> Not interfere with the surgical field
> Not require "special attention" from the surgeon during procedure
> Not traumatize and/or cause discomfort to the patient
> Avoid the need of elaborate and expensive devices to keep sensors attached to the patient's body
> Reusable
> Inexpensive

9.5 IMAGING MODALITIES AND APPLICATIONS

Perhaps the paramount advantage to using CAS is its ability to afford the surgeon with a three-dimensional representation of neurosurgical anatomy during the surgical procedure. Conventional neuroimaging modalities (CT, MRI, ultrasound, fluoroscopy) alone can only provide a two-dimensional display of these areas. Thus, the only three-dimensional model the surgeon is able to create is a mental one based on his or her interpretation of two-dimensional images. Current computer hardware/software algorithms are able to provide the surgeon with frequent 3D reconstructions of CT and MRI information about patient anatomy before and during surgery (Figure 9.6). The combination of this advanced computer technology with novel radiographic innovations has enabled the integration of near real-time, high-contrast, and high spatial resolution volumetric images with frameless stereotactic, interactive localization methods [18].

Because each imaging modality provides a unique display of patient anatomy, a full spectrum of radiographic techniques is utilized in CAS procedures. No imaging modality displays every aspect of patient anatomy perfectly—CT, MRI, fluoroscopy, endoscopy, and ultrasound each has advantages and disadvantages in terms of contrast resolution of soft tissue vs. bone, spatial orientations, fields of view, image displacement, and section thicknesses. The technical, economic, and safety factors associated with the practical implementation of each

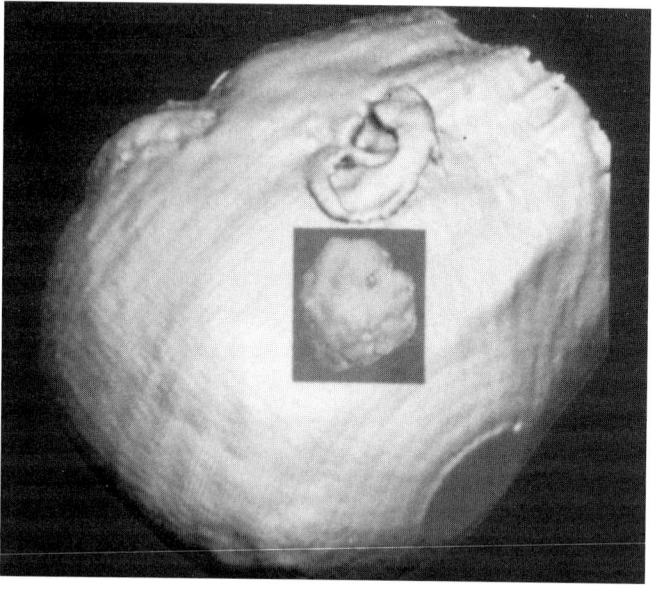

(A)

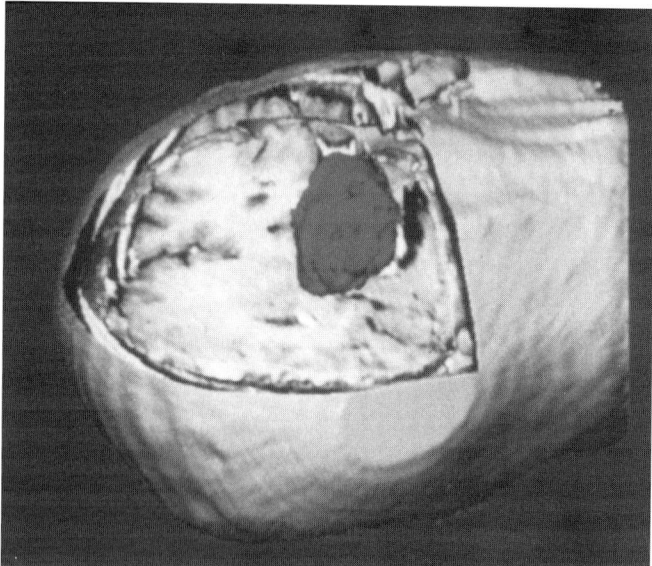

(B)

FIGURE 9.6 Three-dimensional surface rendered images of MRI data reveal the location of an intracranial mass and its relationship to the soft tissues covering the calvarium. Note the ease of determining the surgical approach from these images.

Neuroradiology Perspective

modality in the operating room as well as the type of image needed for a particular procedure determine which modality is integrated most frequently with CAS systems.

Spinal surgeries, including facet block injections, vertebroplasty, interbody fusion, pedicle screw insertion, and therapeutic radiation procedures, require the imaging of both bony and soft tissue structures within the spine [19]. Various methods of CT, MRI, fluoroscopy, and ultrasound are used in CAS systems to guide surgical spinal procedures; however, no single modality has been universally recognized as the "gold standard" for use with image-guided spinal surgery. The ideal navigational system for spinal surgery should incorporate more than one imaging modality—it is hoped that the combination of MRI and CT fluoroscopy can be perfected to provide an optimal display of both the soft tissue and bony framework of the spine. Intraoperative MRI also shows promise as a tool for the advancement of spinal procedures.

Several modalities are used in CAS systems during both brain biopsy and open brain surgical procedures; however, CT and MRI are generally favored over other modalities (fluoroscopy, endoscopy, ultrasound) due to their superior image quality. A variety of CAS systems have been developed, tested, and implemented for use during brain biopsies, skull base surgery, the excision of malignant and benign tumors, and the treatments of intracranial hemorrhage, cavernous hemangioma, and arteriovenous malformation. Because of its superior representation of soft tissue structures, delineation of tumor margins, and ability to display patient anatomy in any orthogonal plane, MRI has emerged as the preferred imaging modality for use in image guided intracranial procedures.

9.5.1 Ultrasound, Endoscopy, and X-Ray Fluoroscopy

Both ultrasound and endoscopy have the advantage of providing real-time images during surgery; however, the image quality of each modality is suboptimal. It is difficult to distinguish tissue types on ultrasonographic images, and the overall clarity of the images is highly dependent on the skill of the operator. Endoscopic images have a considerably limited field of view and show only surface information and can only be obtained using invasive probes.

X-ray fluoroscopy affords excellent bony detail, a wide field of view, and easy accessibility. These systems are also easily transported and relatively inexpensive. As with CT, however, x-ray fluoroscopy exposes both patient and operator to a significant dose of radiation, and the soft tissue discrimination is poor.

9.5.2 Computed Tomography

CT affords both an excellent display of bony detail as well as superior contrast between bone and soft tissue. It also provides good localization of interventional instrument tips during intraoperative navigation. These features represent its primary strengths as a modality for use in CAS. While not as good as MR in representing normal soft tissue anatomy and tumor margins, intraoperative CT guidance has been shown to reduce the likelihood of postoperative complications and generally facilitates the surgical procedure by enhancing the surgeon's perception of the operative field with three-dimensionally reconstructed CT images.

Additional benefits offered by newer developments in CT technology include the potential for real-time imaging, reconstruction, and display offered by fluoroscopic CT, and the flexibility and compatibility with other modalities afforded by mobile CT systems.

9.5.2.1 Real-Time CT Fluoroscopy

Although real-time CT fluoroscopy is most frequently utilized to guide abdominal, thoracic, and other musculoskeletal percutaneous biopsy procedures, a few investigators have used the modality for selected neurointerventional procedures [20]. CT fluoroscopy affords real-time visualization of the needle trajectory from skin entry to target point—prior to this technique, only intermittently obtained static images could be used to depict the relationship of the needle to the targeted lesion. CT fluoroscopy provides continuous visualization of the biopsy procedure, which has been found to significantly reduce both the potential for erroneous needle placement and the length of time needed to perform the procedure with radiographic guidance [21,22].

Katada et al. [21] reported their initial experience with a real-time CT fluoroscopy system used to guide 57 nonvascular interventional procedures, 11 of which were intracranial. The cerebral parenchyma, cerebral ventricles, and hematoma were clearly visualized, and real-time monitoring of the entire process of the puncture could be observed when the location of the lesion allowed the use of a transfrontal approach. When a transparietal approach was necessary, only the arrival of the needle at the target site could be monitored in real time. These investigators determined that both the puncture precision and efficiency of the procedures were improved.

Although CT fluoroscopy is generally recognized to improve the localization and efficiency of biopsy procedures, its significant radiation exposure to both patient and operating room staff remains an issue. Gianfelice et al. [23] reported their experience using a ''spot-check'' technique that only utilized fluoroscopy at intermittent points during the procedure, including immediately before the needle insertion. This reduced total radiation exposure time to 11 seconds, without compromising the visual benefit of the technique. In a trial that measured radiation exposure resulting from CT fluoroscopy, Nawfel et al. found that modifications in CT scanning techniques similar to those employed by Gianfelice et al., as well as the use of a lead drape placed adjacent to the scanning plane substantially reduced radiation doses [23,24]. Several investigators report the use of a needle holder to reduce the radiation dose absorbed by the physician's hands; however, this does limit the tactile feedback from the puncture needle [21,24,25]. Over the past two decades, several advances in the development of robots have occurred. These devices, if trained to have some "tactile" sensation, could have a significant role in the application of CT fluoroscopy. CT coordinates can easily direct the robots and, thus, reduce the radiation dose delivered to the interventional neuroradiologist and staff performing the procedure.

9.5.2.2 Mobile CT

Recently developed mobile CT scanning systems eliminate the need for patient transport to the CT suite if scans are needed during a neurosurgical procedure. These portable CT scanners are equipped with a translating gantry, which permits multislice computed tomographic scans to be obtained of a patient who is positioned in an immobile holder such as an operating room table. The scanner weighs approximately 460 kg and has wheels, which allow for transport to different areas of the hospital. Electrical wall outlets provide a power source and charge the internal battery of the scanner. A computer used to acquire, display, and archive the computed tomographic images is also part of the system [26].

Hum et al. [27] recently reported on their preliminary experience with a mobile CT scanner used intraoperatively for complex craniocervical operations and spinal tumor resections. These investigators found that intraoperative CT scanning facilitated ventral clival and craniocervical decompressions, promoted more complete tumor resections, and verified correct graft and instrument placement before surgical closing. Butler et al. [26] describe their experience with an identical mobile CT scanner, which was utilized during intracranial procedures as well as at the bedside of neuro ICU patients for whom transport is a problem. Although neurosurgical procedures were relatively longer because of the additional time needed to initially position the patient on the table adapter and position the gantry for image acquisition during surgery, the authors found overall efficiency increased as personnel became more accustomed to using the system. They concluded that, in general, the mobile CT scanner improved the efficiency of the procedure. The mobile CT scanner also proved beneficial for bedside imaging of ICU patients receiving mechanical ventilation or invasive monitoring.

Matula et al. [28] reported on their experience with mobile CT-guided neuronavigation system used in 20 microsurgery and neuroendoscopy cases. In all cases, the investigators found that the mobile CT system they used provided optimal intraoperative control of brain tumor resections. In 20% of cases, the intraoperative updates of the neuronavigation data sets identified residual tumor tissue that would not otherwise have been identified. In addition, these procedures could be performed on the original CT scanning table, thereby eliminating the difficulty of moving the patient out of the operating room for scanning.

Although the convenience of mobile CT scanners is attractive, this modality does have some limitations. Surgical instrumentation (radiolucent head devices and cranium pins) that is compatible with intraoperative CT is essential, but such instrumentation is not readily available. When intraoperative CT is contemplated, titanium cranium pins are currently used in lieu of stainless steel pins; although titanium produces fewer artifacts than stainless steel, it does still produce some artifactual signal distortion in images that are coplanar with the pins [26]. Another consideration regarding the use of mobile CT scanners is the additional time that the radiology personnel must devote to their operation and maintenance. In 1999, participants in a comprehensive workshop exploring the technical requirements for computer-aided spinal procedures were less than enthusiastic about mobile CT scanners for spinal surgery, citing reduced image quality, slower acquisition time, and difficult integration with other modalities[19]. Finally, as with any CT system, the significant initial and/or maintenance costs and inevitable radiation exposure to staff and patient remains an issue.

9.5.3 MRI and Intraoperative Image Guidance

The evolution of radiographic modalities and image-processing technologies has made intraoperative image guidance possible through the integration of digitized images with previously described registration/tracking methods. Navigation of surgical instruments is tracked and displayed on 3D images, providing the surgeon with a view of surgical interaction with anatomical structures that would otherwise be "hidden" deep within the brain. This type of image guidance uses three-dimensional reconstructions of CT and/or MR images obtained prior to surgery. The major limitation of these systems is their inability to represent anatomical changes that commonly occur during neurosurgical procedures. The act of opening the skull, as well as the resection or biopsy of brain lesions or leakage of CSF during surgery, may cause significant changes in brain anatomy that are not represented by initially obtained CT or MRIs [29–32]. In addition, CAS systems that use previously obtained images cannot detect the development of potential surgical complications until they become clinically evident. These limitations led to the development of near real-time intraoperative imaging techniques.

Several imaging modalities have been explored for use in intraoperative image guidance, but MRI has become the preferred modality for near real-time intraoperative image guidance. The high spatial and temporal resolution of MRI as well as its superior contrast resolution are essential for intraoperative imaging [31]. In addition, MRI images can be obtained and display in any orthogonal plane [31]. During intracranial procedures, MRI is unmatched in its ability to define soft tissue structures and tumor margins, vascular abnormalities, communication between fluid containing structures, and subtle tissue abnormalities. Until recently, however, the closed magnet systems characteristic of MRI prevented physician access to the patient. This disadvantage, along with the electromagnetic environment and its resultant incompatibility with surgical instruments, precluded

Neuroradiology Perspective

any investigation of potential role of MRI as an intraoperative imaging modality. The development of the mid-field strength, open configuration MRI unit presented new opportunities. Specially designed open MRI systems (Signa SP, GE Medical Systems, Milwaukee, WI) allow neuroradiologists and surgeons to perform interventional and intraoperative procedures with near real-time MR imaging guidance [29]. During operative MR scanning, a series of fast-sequence MR scans are obtained and displayed at external consoles and on two 5-inch (diagonal width) liquid crystal display monitors mounted in the gap of the magnet. In this way, the surgeon may interactively localize, target, and monitor the procedure in near real time. Intraoperative MRI provides dynamic monitoring of anatomical and tissue changes as well as potential complications that may occur as a result of surgery.

Intraoperative MR imaging was first used in biopsy procedures. Black et al. in 1997 [33] reported on their experience with 63 stereotactic biopsies, 16 cyst drainages, 66 craniotomies, 3 thermal ablations, and 3 laminectomies, using a 0.5 T intraoperative MRI system (GE Medical Systems, Milwaukee, WI) in collaboration with Brigham and Women's Hospital in Boston. This system provided near real-time imaging and tracking through the use of LED-based optical tracking of surgical instruments combined with manipulation of MRI planes. This provided continuous interactive feedback between surgical maneuvers and corresponding image formation [33]. The authors concluded that MRI has distinct advantages over other modalities in localization and characterization of tumor margins. This tracking method is not appropriate for use with flexible instruments such as catheters, guidewires, and flexible endoscopes. When these types of instruments are used, a nonoptical tracking method is appropriate, such as a coil-based tracking method with miniature coil attached to the instruments. For neurosurgical applications, Black et al. concluded that procedures performed under interactive MRI guidance have several advantages, including elimination of the need for fiducial markers and registration, superior capabilities in localization of lesions and dynamic tracking of changes in fluid and tissue compartments, precise plotting of the best trajectory of a surgical approach, as well as dynamic guidance and verification of operative execution, accurate identification of normal structures, and superior tissue characterization.

Several other investigators have also obtained good results using similarly designed intraoperative MRI units. Knauth et al. [34] found that a more complete resection of intracranial lesions could be accomplished using intraoperative MRI guidance. Samset and Hirschberg [35] reported favorable results using intraoperative MRI equipped with an optical tracking technique as well as an additional surgical navigation system. These authors found that the combination of these two technologies yielded better results than the use of either by itself. Real-time MRI images may have limited contrast resolution and/or a poor signal-to-noise ratio, and they are only available in one plane. On the other hand, intraoperative

MRI affords a continuous display of the operative procedure. Since the images are continually updated, they depict soft tissue changes, including tissue edema, brain shift, and even early intraoperative surgical complications. The surgeon can use this information to identify incipient problems and take appropriate corrective actions. Of course, repetitive intraoperative MRI images also serve to monitor the progress of the procedure. Surgical navigation devices support the 3D reconstruction of high-quality images in any orthogonal plane, and the combination of the two systems (intraoperative MRI and surgical navigation) provides mapping between the image space and the surgical space, which makes patient reregistration in the field unnecessary when images are updated [35].

Intraoperative real-time MR scanning, although not currently available for guidance of spinal procedures, does hold future potential for reducing the invasiveness and improving the general outcome of these surgeries. The vertical gap configuration of open magnet units allows the patient to sit upright, raising the possibility of new modes of radiographic evaluation and dynamic spinal surgery [33].

Although the initial experiences with intraoperative MRI are exciting, the challenges of realistically incorporating this complex technology into surgical practice cannot be ignored. One of the major issues with the use of an MR magnet in the operating room is the necessity for surgical instruments that are compatible with the magnetic field. Titanium and ceramic probes, forceps, headholders, and other tools have been developed and continue to evolve in order to meet this need; however, even the use of these nonmetallic materials does not completely eliminate the presence of artifacts [31].

All authors stress that state-of-the-art magnet design, high-resolution image quality, and incorporation of navigational methods are critical for the optimal utilization of intraoperative MRI. If these criteria are not met, the benefit derived from intraoperative MRI will be diminished, and it becomes questionable as to whether the significant cost and effort involved in the implementation of intraoperative MRI is justified. Tronnier et al. [30] point out the necessity for an analysis of the cost-effectiveness of implementing intraoperative MRI systems. Cost-analysis methods should include duration of surgery, maintenance costs of the system, and the length of hospital stay as well as patient variables (namely, life tables relating to both length and quality of life).

Accuracy issues for this technology should not be dismissed. One study has even reported systematic error with the use of MRI in stereotactic procedures due to spatial distortion resulting from magnetic field warping, susceptibility artifacts, and chemical shift effects [36]. To address these issues, the authors developed a method of image fusion between MRI and CT using a chamfer matching technique, which resulted in more precise stereotactic localization of anatomical structures.

Neuroradiology Perspective

9.6 IMAGE RESOLUTION

The ability of the computer hardware/software program to maintain a high degree of resolution when reconstructing and manipulating images is vital to the utility of any CAS system. Image resolution determines a lower boundary on a system's accuracy; that is, system accuracy cannot exceed the resolution of the scan data set. On a practical level, system accuracy is the net result of several factors.

Image resolution in these systems may be classified into two types. Understanding the subtle differences between in-plane and out-of-plane resolution is critical for a better understanding of CAS technologies, image resolution, and system errors.

In-plane resolution, which reflects the x and y dimensions of individual pixels, is determined by imaging parameters as well as hardware limitations. Typically, MRI array sizes are 256×256, with a field of view (FOV) from as little as a few centimeters up to 40 cm. For head and neck imaging, approximately 25 cm is typical for a FOV. This FOV results in a pixel size of approximately 1 mm $\times$ 1 mm. For the typical CT scan, a pixel matrix size of 512×512 is common, and similar FOV boundaries are employed. These parameters lead to a corresponding reduction in pixel dimensions. Although it is possible to achieve decreases in pixel size, this objective cannot be accomplished without greater imaging scan time, greater radiation exposure (CT only), and/or decreased tissue contrast; however, the above-mentioned parameters have been found to be adequate for stereotactic procedures.

Out-of-plane resolution has also been referred to as slice thickness. This type of resolution is usually less than that of in-plane resolution, with slice thickness of 1.5–3 mm common in MRI and 3–4 mm in CT. These measurements can be reduced, but only at the cost of greater scanning times, greater radiation exposure (CT only), and/or decreased tissue contrast. Both in-plane resolution and out-of-plane resolution are important because it is necessary that the slice spacing be the same as or less than the slice thickness to achieve the best 3D data set for stereotactic procedures.

Another important consideration is software interpolation between pixels; this process can produce larger pixel arrays with smaller dimensions both in-plane and out-of-plane. Such algorithms must be used with caution because the computer will make an educated guess at the derived pixel values. The computer then smoothes out sharp edges that are representative of actual anatomy—this smoothing may lead to a decrease in resolution or a less accurate depiction.

Pixel intensity level errors can also affect accuracy. Some pixels can be read as higher or lower than their actual value due to image noise. This issue can be addressed by signal averaging, but this technique risks increased imaging time or decreased resolution. A much greater problem is partial volume averaging, which occurs when two or more substances with different imaging characteristics occupy the same voxel (the imaging data set's unit volume that corresponds to each pixel in the displayed image). The resulting voxel value is then an average of all the intensities produced by each substance, weighted by the percentage of the voxel they occupy. These averaged voxels can cause errors during 3D reconstruction because they are classified into incorrect tissue categories. This incorrect categorization affects both the reconstructed boundaries and volumes of affected structures [37].

9.7 ACCURACY

Stereotactic neurosurgical procedures demand a very high standard of accuracy. Surgeons must be able to rely on the information provided by the system to guide them with precision. Localization errors could have quite a drastic effect on the outcome of such procedures. Thus, it is imperative to have a clear understanding of the nature and sources of errors in these systems.

The two principal terms to describe accuracy, bias and skew, are described by Maciunas et al. [38] Bias is the average measure of how well a device reaches a desired target point in space. An unbiased device will have errors that measure symmetrically around the correct target point; that is, its errors will have a mean close to the true value. The measure of the spread or a number of trials around their average value is defined as precision. A precise device will have errors that are clustered close to some center point [37]. Statistically speaking, precision is analogous to standard deviation, such that lower precision will produce a higher standard deviation in measured values. Both these terms are encompassed by the term accuracy. A device must be both unbiased and precise to be accurate.

There is also a distinction between the accuracy of the stereotactic device itself and the accuracy obtained when the device is used during the surgical procedure. This has been defined as the difference between mechanical accuracy and application accuracy [9]. While mechanical accuracy depends solely on the quality of the apparatus construction and refers to the device's ability to reach a known location within its area of operation, application accuracy is a measure of the device as it is used in a real-world setting. This, then, encompasses such contributing factors as imaging error, reconstruction error, point selection error, registration error, perception error, and movement error, as well as errors associated with the localizing device [37]. Application accuracy is more significant than mechanical accuracy because it better represents the magnitude of errors likely to be encountered during surgery. Device manufacturers, however, often report on mechanical accuracy when describing the accuracy of their particular system.

When the accuracy figures associated with a particular system are reported, physicians should demand that the 50th percentile accuracy figure as well as the

95th percentile accuracy figure be presented. This would prevent authors from simply expressing their very best accuracy data, which is usually achievable in less than 5% of their patient population.

9.8 SOURCES OF ERROR

To detect and compensate for sources of errors when using stereotactic devices, a thorough knowledge of potential pitfalls is necessary. This knowledge is also helpful in designing protocols and procedures that will minimize the effects of these errors.

Factors that are intrinsic to the imaging data set may greatly influence surgical navigation accuracy. A study by Galloway et al. showed that CT slice thickness greatly influences the accuracy of each of the four most commonly used frame stereotactic systems [9]. Higher application accuracies are obtained when thinner CT slices are used. It seems reasonable to anticipate that these results may be extrapolated to MRI. Geometric distortions caused by scanner hardware or software can lead to errors in the acquired dataset. However, proper calibration and maintenance of the scanner will minimize this problem. Other factors, such as patient movement or artifacts from foreign objects (metal fillings or a prosthesis), can also degrade the quality of images and affect accuracy.

Another source of error is the 3D reconstruction process. Any chosen method involves some subjective way of evaluating the boundaries of structures to be included in the 3D objects. The process of object creation and display requires smoothings and interpolations (typically of the software) and can cause inaccuracies. Thus, discrepancies between real and reconstructed objects and structures can occur [39]. These types of errors can affect a stereotactic system in two ways. First, position identification inaccuracies on the reconstruction during registration could result in errors in the data fit to the patient. In addition, ambiguities in display of the 3D data on the screen may make the viewer perceive the location incorrectly even if the system may correctly identify the location of the probe tip. The use of the original cross-sectional radiographic information as well as the multiplanar reconstructions can reduce these ambiguities.

The data derived from the localizing device are also subject to several factors, including changes in temperature, aging, bending of the pointing device, bending or maladjustment of the sensor array, and poor lighting or acoustic conditions that can influence accuracy. This is particularly true of surgical instruments that are used as pointing devices, because these instruments undergo constant use and stress. Periodic checks on these instruments are mandatory. In the case of endoscopes used as localizing pointers, this problem can be more complex because the actual localizing point is arbitrary. Using the end of the scope as the stereotactic localizer will show where the lens is; however, that may not necessarily represent the area of interest because the FOV provided is 1–1.5 cm distal to the endoscope tip. If a point in advance of the lens is to be used, i.e., the focal point, it is necessary to precisely indicate where that point is. These problems, while not insurmountable, need to be addressed.

Another source of potential error is the transfer of imaging data from CT or MR scanner to the surgical unit. In the recent past, a magnetic tape was used for this purpose, and the reliability of both the equipment as well as the technician was paramount in affording a successful transfer. The replacement of magnetic tapes with optical disks has made the task less time consuming; however, it did not eliminate the possibility of human error. Data transfer may seem a trivial task, but it is often the rate-limiting step in determining whether a surgical case will be performed with CAS technology. Fortunately, the potential for data transfer errors has been largely eliminated by the replacement of the intermediate transfer medium (tape, optical disk) by an electronic/tele-technique that automatically performs the transfer task. This saves time in the "preparation" of the case.

Improper positioning of the sensor tip and/or cursor while choosing points to be registered or localized may result in inaccuracies. The exact location cannot always be determined when selecting points from radiographic images, primarily because of imaging limitations. There may be some disparity between the position pointed to with the probe and the position that appears on the screen.

Another source of stereotactic inaccuracy can arise from intraoperative movement of the patient. Either the stereotactic device and patient anatomy must be locked in the same frame of reference, or there must be some method that can follow or compensate for patient movement.

Local errors can also be caused by intraoperative tissue changes resulting from surgical alterations or reactions to manipulations. Some of these local errors can be visually or mentally compensated for by an experienced surgeon, who might then be able to predict the magnitude and character of the movement. Although this is rather imprecise, it is often all that can be done because tissue changes of this type are quite difficult to model; however, this is a subject of much research [40].

9.9 PRACTICAL CONSIDERATIONS

The use of state-of-the-art CAS systems is far from standard in most hospitals. Two important considerations for the realistic incorporation of CAS system into a clinical setting are its ease of use and its cost-effectiveness.

Even if the information conveyed by the CAS system is unique and of extremely high quality, the system will be discarded if it is difficult to use or disrupts normal operative flow. The CAS system should be easy enough to handle by the surgeon and other operating room personnel without the need of an independent operator.

Neuroradiology Perspective

In terms of cost-effectiveness, CAS systems necessarily entail additional costs to both the hospital and the patient. In addition, many systems necessitate additional radiographic studies to meet the imaging requirements for the dataset. This may result in greater radiation exposure to the patient as well as scheduling issues for the hospital personnel. However, as experience with these systems increases, these additional costs and/or disadvantages can be reduced or eliminated. For example, with more experience, surgeons could identify prospective patients earlier so that specific CAS imaging requirements (the stereotactic dataset) could be obtained at the initial radiographic examination. Of course, the additional costs of technician time and new equipment to process the data and prepare for surgery cannot be eliminated. Although the cost of the equipment, as well as maintenance and upgrades, is significant, that cost can be amortized over a large number of patients. There is also the additional time in the operating room to consider. Anon et al., describing their experience with the ISG Viewing Wand System, estimated that using this system added approximately 10 minutes of operating room time [4,5]. At this point it is still too early to determine a cost versus benefit ratio for the use of stereotactic systems for neurosurgical procedures.

9.10 FUTURE DIRECTIONS

Future advances in the field of CAS and real-time intraoperative imaging promise to revolutionize many other diagnostic and therapeutic surgical procedures. Intraoperative MRI, although still in its earliest stages of development, has evolved quickly to improve the accuracy and efficiency of a plethora of neurosurgical procedures. The rapidity of intraoperative MRI's initial development predicts that the challenges associated with its implementation will be quickly surmounted. The interest in and production of MR-compatible surgical tools continues to grow—in 1994, very few manufacturers offered such tools; now more than 50 companies produce instrumentation compatible with intraoperative MRI [41]. In addition, the discovery of the technology's unique benefits for a growing number of procedures will surely give rise to necessary cost-benefit analyses.

CAS systems have the potential not only to improve the outcome of currently practiced neurosurgical procedures, but also to spur the innovation of new surgical techniques that would be impossible without CAS. For example, the delivery of heat via laser to neoplasms, scar tissue, and cancerous tumors has been proven effective in the treatment of these entities; however, this technique has not been widely used due to the inability to monitor both the temperature deposition during the procedure and the progress of therapy [32]. Temperature-sensitive MRI sequences have the capacity to monitor and control the energy delivery during such procedures, a function necessary to ensure the safety of normal brain structures surrounding the tumor [42]. Other interstitial thermal therapies, such as cryotherapy and highly focused ultrasound, may also benefit from intraoperative MR imaging [32].

Both the evolution of current CAS systems and the innovation of novel procedures within the field of CAS promise to expand the role of the neuroradiologist during neurosurgical procedures. The generation of multiple images and their availability during the procedure makes it possible for the neuroradiologist to offer objective opinions about the advisability of a surgical approach, the completeness of a biopsy or resection, and the assessment of any intraoperative complications [29]. Ideally, a closed-circuit, two-way audiovisual system will one day be widely available to support the interaction of the neuroradiologist in the reading room and the surgeon in the operating room [29].

Clearly, the future of neurosurgery is heading towards "knifeless" resection of intracranial pathology. The future neurosurgical medium—whether it will be cryotherapy, heat, or electromagnetic waves—may not even require a formal incision; such modalities may require at most a very small, keyhole-sized craniotomy. Thus, the guidance needed from imaging modalities will be of even greater importance. Given the fact that most cross-sectional imaging data is digitized, the "fusion" of several modalities will afford guidance during the initial surgical approach as well as monitoring of the effect and extent of therapy.

The appearance and design CAS equipment is sure to change as well. The most important of these changes will be the development of new sensor technology, the utility of which will not be dependent on an external monitoring system or external environmental conditions. In parallel with these developments, evolution of currently used imaging equipment that will push these devices toward greater mobility and accessibility as well as an expanded role in direct therapy may also be anticipated.

REFERENCES

1. Spiegel EA, Wyeis HT, Marks M, Lee A. Stereotactic apparatus for operations on the human brain. Science 1947; 106:349–355.
2. Watanabe E, Watanabe T, Manka S, Mayanagi Y, Takakura K. Three-dimensional digitizer (neuronavigator): new equipment for computed tomography-guided stereotactic surgery. Surg Neurol 1988; 27:543–547.
3. Zinreich SJ, Dekel D, Leggett B, Greenberg M, Kennedy DW, Long DM, Bryan RN. 3D CT interactive "surgical localizer" for endoscopic sinus surgery and neurosurgery. 76th Annual Meeting of the Radiological Society of North America, Chicago, 1990.
4. Anon JB, Klimek L, Mosges R, Zinreich SJ. Computer-assisted endoscopic sinus surgery: an international review. Otolaryngol Clin North Am 1997; 30:389–401.
5. Anon JB, Lipman SP, Oppenheim D, et al. Computer-assisted endoscopic sinus surgery. Laryngoscope 1994; 104:901–905.

Neuroradiology Perspective

6. Golfinos JG, Fitzpatrick BC, Smith LR, Spetzler RF. Clinical use of a frameless stereotactic arm: results of 325 cases. J Neurosurg 1995; 83:197–205.
7. Grimson WEL, Ettinger GJ, White SJ, Lozano-Perez T, Wells WM III, Kikinis R. An automatic registration method for frameless stereotaxy, image-guided surgery, and enhanced reality visualization. IEEE Trans Med Imaging 1996; 15:129–140.
8. Day R, Heilbrun MP, Koehler S, McDonald P, Peters W, Siemionow V. Three-point transformation for integration of multiple coordinate systems: applications to tumor, functional, and fractionated radiosurgery stereotactic planning. Stereotact Funct Neurosurg 1994; 63:76–79.
9. Galloway RL, Maciunas RJ, Latimer JW. The accuracies of four stereotactic frame systems: an independent assessment. Biomed Instrum Technol 1991; 25:457–460.
10. Heilbrun MP. Clinical frontiers of interactive image-guided neurosurgery. Introduction. Neurosurg Clin North Am 1996; 7:xv.
11. Heilbrun MP. Computed tomography-guided stereotactic systems. Clin Neurosurg 1983; 31:564–581.
12. Heilbrun MP, Koehler S, McDonald P, Siemionow V, Peters W. Preliminary experience using an optimized three-point transformation algorithm for spatial registration of coordinate systems: a method of noninvasive localization using frame-based stereotactic guidance systems. J Neurosurg 1994; 81:676–682.
13. Kosugi Y, Watanabe E, Goto J, Watanabe T, et al. An articulated neurosurgical navigation system using MRI and CT images. IEEE Trans Biomed Eng 1988; 35:147–152.
14. Zamorano LF, Nolte LP, Kadi AM, Jiang Z. Interactive intraoperative localization using an infrared-based system. J Neurosci Res 1993; 15:290–298.
15. Sipos EP, Tebo SA, Zinreich SJ, Long DM, Brem H. In vivo accuracy testing and clinical experience with the ISG Viewing Wand. Neurosurgery 1996; 39:194–202, discussion 202–204.
16. Kato AT, Yoshimine T, Hyakawa T, Tomita Y, Ikeda T, Mitomo M, Harada K, Mogami H. Armless navigational system for computer-assisted neurosurgery. J Neurosurg 1991; 74:845–849.
17. Tebo SA, Leopold DA, Long DM, et al. An optical 3D digitizer for frameless stereotactic surgery. IEEE Computer Graphics and Applications 1996; 16:55–64.
18. Jolesz FA. Image-guided procedures and the operating room of the future. Radiology 1997; 204:601–612.
19. The Joint Working Group on Image Guided Spinal Procedures. Technical requirements for image-guided spine procedures: workshop report April 17–20, 1999. Imaging Acience and Information Systems (ISIS) Center, Radiology Departments, Georgetown University Medical Center, Washington, DC, 1999.
20. Kanno T, Nonomura K, Shanker K, Katada K. Early experience with real-time CT fluoroscopy for an intracranial lesion. Stereotact Funct Neurosurg 1997; 68:49–53.
21. Katada K, Kato R, Anno H, Ogura Y, Koga S, Ida Y, Sato M, Nonomura K. Guidance with real-time CT fluoroscopy: early clinical experience. Radiology 1996; 200:851–856.
22. Goldberg SN, Keogan MT, Raptopoulos V. Percutaneous CT-guided biopsy: improved confirmation of sampling site and needle positioning using a multi-step technique at CT fluoroscopy. J Comput Assist Tomogr 2000; 24:264–266.

23. Gianfelice D, Lepanto L, Perreault P, Chartrand-Lefebvre C, Milette PC. Value of CT fluoroscopy for percutaneous biopsy procedures. J Vasc Interv Radiol 2000; 11: 879–884.
24. Nawfel RD, Judy PF, Silverman SG, Hooton S, Tuncali K, Adams DF. Patient and personnel exposure during CT fluoroscopy-guided interventional procedures. Radiology 2000; 216:180–184.
25. Kato R, Katada K, Anno H, Suzuki S, Ida Y, Koga S. Radiation dosimetry at CT fluoroscopy: physician's hand dose and development of needle holders. Radiology 1996; 201:576–578.
26. Butler WE, Piaggio CM, Constantinou C, Niklason L, Gonzalez RG, Cosgrove GR, Zervas NT. A mobile computed tomographic scanner with intraoperative and intensive care unit applications. Neurosurgery 1998; 42:1304–1311.
27. Hum B, Feigenbaum F, Cleary K, Henderson FC. Intraoperative computed tomography for complex craniocervical operations and spinal tumor resections. Neuorsurgery 2000; 47:374–380, discussion 380–381.
28. Matula C, Rossler K, Reddy M, Schindler E, Koos WT. Intraoperative computed tomography guided neuronavigation: concepts, efficiency, and work flow. Comput Aided Surg 1998; 3:174–182.
29. Schwartz RB Hsu L, Wong TZ, Kacher DF, Zamani AA, Black PM, Alexander E 3rd, Stieg PE, Moriarty TM, Martin CA, Kikinis R, Jolesz FA. Intraoperative MR imaging guidance for intracranial neuorsurgery: experience with the first 200 cases. Radiology 1999; 211:477–488.
30. Tronnier VM, Wirtz CR, Knauth M, Lenz G, Pastyr O, Bonsanto MM, Albert FK, Kuth R, Staubert A, Schlegel W, Sartor K, Kunze S. Intraoperative diagnostic and interventional magnetic resonance imaging in neurosurgery. Neurosurgery 1997; 40: 891–902.
31. Jolesz, FA. Interventional and intraoperative MRI: a general overview of the field. J Magn Reson Imaging 1998; 8:3–7.
32. Moriarty TM, Kikinis R, Jolexa FA, Black PM, Alexander III E. Magnetic resonance imaging therapy: intraoperative MR imaging. Neurosurg Clin North Am 1996; 7: 323–331.
33. Black PM, Moriarty T, Alexander III E, Stieg P, Woodard EJ, Gleason L, Martin CH, Kikinis R, Schwartz RB, Jolesz FA. Development and implementation of intraoperative magnetic resonance imaging and its neurosurgical applications. Neurosurgery 1997; 41:831–845.
34. Knauth M, Wirtz CR, Tronnier VM, Aras N, Kunze S, Sartor K. Intraoperative MR imaging increases the extent of tumor resection in patients with high-grade gliomas. Am J Neurorad 1999; 20:1642–1646.
35. Samset E, Hirschberg H. Neuronavigation in intraoperative MRI. Comput Aided Surg 1999; 4:200–207.
36. Alexander E III, Kooy HM, van Herk M, Schwartz M, Barnes PD, Tarbell N, Mulkern RV, Holupka EJ, Loeffler JS. Magnetic resonance image-directed stereotactic neurosurgery: use of image fusion with computerized tomography to enhance spatial accuracy. J Neurosurg 1995; 83:271–276.
37. Zinreich SJ, Tebo BS, Snyderman CH, Carrau RL, Anon JB. Intraoperative stereotaxis for endoscopic sinus surgery: a technical review. In: Myers EN, Bluestone

CD, Brackman DE, Krause CJ, eds. Advances in Otolaryngology—Head and Neck Surgery, Vol. 11. St. Louis: Mosby-Year Book, Inc., 1997:181–199.
38. Maciunas RJ, Galloway RL, Latimer JW. The application accuracy of stereotactic frames. Neurosurgery 1994; 35:682–695.
39. Hildebolt CF, Vannier MW, Knapp RH. Validation study of skull three-dimensional computerized tomography measurements. Am J Phys Anthropol 1990; 82:283–294.
40. Mendis KK, Stalnaker RL, Advani SH. A constitutive relationship for large deformation finite element modeling of brain tissue. J Biomech Eng 1995; 117:279–285.
41. Jolesz FA, Morrison PR, Koran SJ, Kelley RJ, Hushek SG, Newman RW, Fried MP, Melzer A, Seibel RMM, Jalahej H. Compatible instrumentation for intraoperative MRI: expanding resources. J Magn Reson Imaging 1998; 8:8–11.
42. Anzai Y, Lufkin R, DeSalles A, et al. Preliminary experience with a technique for MR-guided thermal ablation of brain tumors. Am J Neurorad 1995; 16:39–48.
43. Guthrie BL, Kaplan R, Kelly PJ. Freehand sterotaxy: neurosurgical stereotactic operating arm. Proc Neurosurg Soc Am 1989; 59–61 (abstr).
44. Guthrie BL, Kaplan R, Kelly PJ. Neurosurgical stereotactic operating arm. Proc Congr Neurolog Surg 1989; 232 (abstr).

10
Moving Stereotaxis Beyond the Dura: A Neurosurgical Perspective on Computer-Aided Otorhinolaryngology

**Richard D. Bucholz, M.D., F.A.C.S., and
Keith A. Laycock, Ph.D.**
Saint Louis University School of Medicine, St. Louis, Missouri

10.1 INTRODUCTION

The critical need for accuracy during cranial procedures compelled neurosurgeons to be the first to employ computers during surgery. The accuracy afforded by navigational technology and computer-aided surgery (CAS) techniques directly addresses the problems of traversing the complex and vulnerable structure of the brain. Neurosurgeons gladly suffered the pains of development of early surgical guidance techniques to avoid spatial errors in navigation which could have permanent, devastating consequences for their patients, and they have been at the forefront of subsequent development and refinement.

This chapter will examine current research within the neurosurgical field on the accuracy and functionality of such systems that might be germane to the use of CAS in procedures performed by otorhinolaryngologists. Emphasis will be made on the importance of visualization and the state of the art in navigational systems used within neurosurgery.

10.2 IMAGING AND VISUALIZATION

The history of modern neurosurgical cranial interventions starts with the Scottish surgeon Sir William Macewen in the 1880s. Although no modalities capable of imaging the brain were available, Macewen was able to localize tumors with astonishing precision using his detailed knowledge of physiological principles and disease processes (Macewen, 1881). Shortly after he performed the first successful intracranial procedures, the concept of a stereotactic device was proposed by Zernov (1890).

Stereotaxis is a hybrid word, consisting of the Greek *stereos*, meaning solid, and either the Greek *taxis*, meaning ordered or arranged, or the Latin *tactus*, meaning touch. The concept of stereotaxis consists of the careful touching, or intervention, into a solid object using a carefully ordered process. The role of the stereotactic device was to bring order to this three-dimensional (3D) navigational process. The desire to have something other than the surgeon's intuition guide a cranial procedure resulted from the high incidence of unintended iatrogenic trauma incurred during early cranial procedures and the perception that these complications occurred due to incursions into normally functioning brain tissue. Since available computational power was extremely limited, these early navigational systems used mechanical devices to restrict the motion of the surgeon to a carefully selected path. The surgical path was determined by the preoperative selection of a particular target and entry point. Because these selections have to be referenced to some sort of reference system superimposed upon the patient's anatomy, a plane of origin had to be established as the first step in a stereotactic procedure. Almost all traditional stereotactic systems established this base plane by the application of a frame or ring, which defined the x- and y-coordinates for the subsequent point selections. The z-axis was usually perpendicular to this plane, and any point in the anatomy of the patient can be precisely described using three numbers consisting of the respective x-, y-, and z-coordinates. The association between these early stereotactic instruments and the use of the frame is clearly identified by referring to this technique as framed stereotaxis. (In comparison, more modern stereotaxis systems are frameless navigational systems.)

An important feature of such framed stereotactic systems is that the reference system (i.e., the frame) has to be established prior to the imaging that is used to select the entry and target points. The ability to make these selections was extremely limited in the first half of the twentieth century as the only preoperative imaging data available consisted of plain radiographs. Because radiographs do not show the location of the brain without the introduction of contrast, pneumoencephalography was commonly performed prior to a stereotactic procedure to show the location of the ventricles, and especially the third ventricle. Fortunately, the third ventricle has two points, the anterior and posterior commissures, which

A Neurosurgical Perspective

are easily identified on lateral skull radiographs. By locating these points, the position of the third ventricle can be determined accurately. Atlases of human cranial anatomy were then developed, based upon these points, which could indicate the position of structures around the third ventricle with some degree of accuracy, but which failed miserably at locating structures such as the cortex that were lateral to the midline. The net result was that early stereotactic procedures only allowed precise approach to deep structures located near the midline in patients whose anatomy was not affected by the presence of space-occupying lesions. Inasmuch as the vast majority of cranial procedures involve manipulation of soft tissue not identifiable by such means in patients with anatomy distorted by tumor, stroke, or trauma, stereotactic surgery was relegated to a small faction of neurosurgeons who selected targets close to the midline to restore lost neurological function.

It is an interesting historical point that the first atlases employed phrenological maps based upon the contours of the human scalp to allow approach to laterally based structures such as the cortex, which was a much more interesting target for correction of psychological disturbances. This concept of using the contour of the head would be reborn in the twenty-first century to guide more complex procedures.

For the remainder of neurosurgeons, guidance could only be obtained by exposing large amounts of normal anatomy, and using this exposed anatomy, combined with the surgeon's knowledge of anatomy, to reach the desired area. This reliance on visualization of anatomical landmarks also limited the use of cranial endoscopy, as the limited visualization seen through an endoscope was often inadequate for orientation.

The advent of modern image-guided surgery is wholly dependent upon the availability of high-quality 3D imaging. Until the advent of computed tomography (CT), there was simply no reason to employ computers in the operating room, because there was no means of visualizing a patient's anatomy other than through surgical exposure. Currently a surgeon is able to obtain comprehensive information about the proposed surgical field by choosing from a range of imaging modalities. Today, plain radiographs have been replaced by CT and magnetic resonance imaging (MRI). The two-dimensional (2D) images acquired with these modalities can be manipulated by now relatively inexpensive computer technology into 3D virtual models of the patient's anatomy to provide clear 3D views of both bone and tissue surrounding the target site. These visualization techniques have thereby markedly increased the range of applications for stereotactic techniques. Furthermore, volume-rendering protocols, which permit rotation of 3D virtual models, enable the surgeon to determine the best surgical approach. Preoperative images can also be supplemented by the use of intraoperative imaging, allowing the surgeon to evaluate the progress of the operation and decide if changes to the surgical plan are necessary due to movement of tissue.

Image guidance directly supports the development of endoscopy and related minimally invasive surgery techniques as it enables the surgeon to view the operative site directly without the need for extensive exposure of normal anatomy. It should be stressed, however, that even with the most advanced CAS navigation and visualization apparatus available today, procedures of this type still carry risk and require the input of a trained surgeon to enable the best possible outcome. In the hands of a well-trained surgeon, the use of CAS can markedly reduce the risk associated with critical interventions when compared to the situation before CAS navigation was widely adopted.

This chapter will discuss the critical concepts behind navigational systems, including registration techniques, types of digitizers, atlases, and instrumentation, before discussing common applications of this technique within neurosurgery. Attention will be given to a description of stereotactic radiation techniques, which may have direct bearing upon management of skull base neoplasms.

10.3 REGISTRATION

The fundamental concept underlying all CAS surgical navigation is that of *registration*. This is the method for mapping images of a specific patient to one another and to the physical space of the patient. Registration has been traditionally performed by identifying and aligning points, called fiducial points, seen on the sets of images to their location on the patient in physical space in a process termed paired-point registration. Registration can also be used to relate image data sets on the same patient obtained using different imaging modalities. This process is termed image fusion and produces a hybrid image that is an amalgamation of the information present on the parent images.

Paired-point–based methods (including stereotactic frames, fiducial markers, and anatomical landmarks) have now been supplemented with curve and surface matching methods, moment and principal fixed axes methods, correlation methods, and atlas methods (Maurer and Fitzpatrick, 1993).

10.3.1 Paired-Point Methods

The most straightforward method for achieving co-registration of coordinate spaces is to use a set of markers that are visible in the patient's image data set and that can be pointed to by a localization device or digitizer (see below). While only three points (in a nonlinear arrangement) are required to relate two 3D objects to each other, using more points improves the accuracy of the subsequent registration and lessens the risk of failure that may arise when one of the markers moves in relation to the others or becomes obscured and undetectable by the digitizer. For cranial surgery the most common problem is movement, since fiducial markers are usually attached to the scalp, and the scalp can move in relationship to the underlying bony skull.

Some investigators (notably in the radiosurgical field) have used clearly defined anatomical features (such as the bridge of the nose or lateral canthus) as reference markers (Adler, 1993). However, there is a certain degree of ambiguity associated with feature-based registration, as any anatomical feature departs from an ideal fiducial, that is, an extremely sharp spot detectable clearly in three orthogonal planes. Therefore most neurosurgeons prefer to use artificial markers, which are applied to the patient prior to imaging. Different types and sizes of artificial fiducial markers are manufactured for use with different imaging modalities, and they may be fixed to the patient's skin using adhesive or embedded directly in the bone (skull-based fiducial markers). Markers applied to the skin cause no discomfort to the patient but may be dislodged between preoperative imaging and surgery and are more prone to localized movement relative to each other. This can have deleterious effects on the accuracy of both registration and target localization. Accordingly, it is normal practice to use 5–10 adhesive fiducial markers in an attempt to compensate for movement-related error. Because of the importance of the distribution of the fiducial markers, the registration program should demonstrate the zone of highest accuracy (Figure 10.1).

In contrast, bone-implanted fiducial markers offer the highest accuracy of any registration technique, including stereotactic frames (Maciunas et al., 1993), since they cannot move relative to the patient's head and, once implanted, remain in place until the surgery is completed. As a result of this reliability, it is usual to use only four skull-based markers on a patient to decrease the amount of pain associated with their attachment. However, the trauma associated with implantation of bone-anchored fiducial markers in the patient's skull militates against their routine usage.

Regardless of the type of marker used for paired-point registration, the resultant accuracy of the registration process depends upon not only the markers but how markers are distributed over the volume being registered. Regardless of their number, markers arranged co-linearly will never allow a 3D registration. Further, coplanar markers will allow registration but will have little accuracy in the z dimension that is perpendicular to the plane of the markers. For the best possible registration, the markers should be spread as widely over the entire 3D volume as possible.

10.3.2 Contour and Surface Mapping

As an alternative to matching isolated detectable points, it is also possible to obtain a registration by matching contours obtained from the surface of the patient. Data from imaging studies depicting a contour can be matched to points

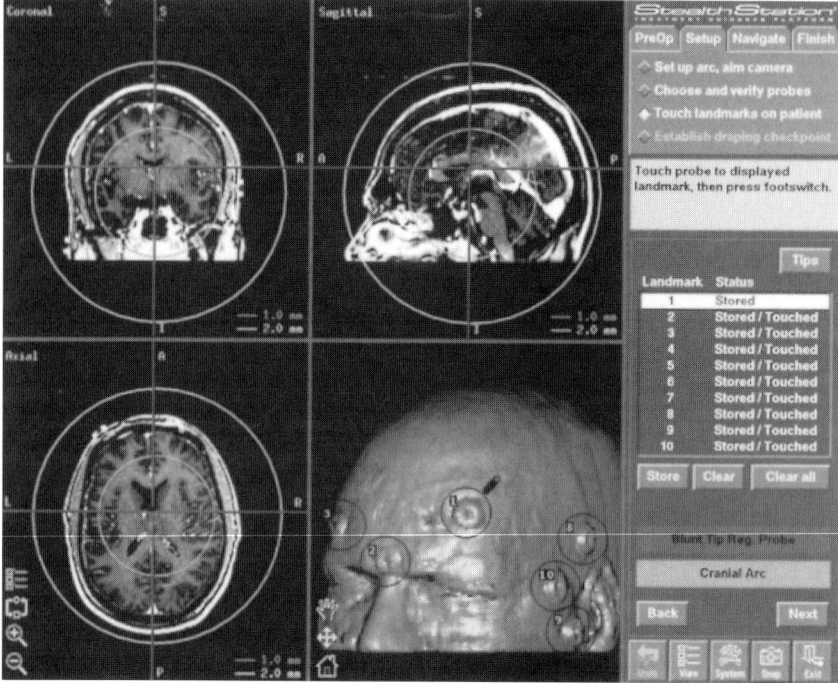

FIGURE 10.1 Display of the StealthStation (Medtronic Surgical Navigation Technology, Louisville, CO) after completion of registration. The system shows a sphere of accuracy, which demonstrates the volume of greatest accuracy based upon the distribution of the fiducial points used during the registration process.

on that contour obtained randomly using the digitizer depicting the curvature of a portion of the scalp. The computer can then align these features, with areas of maximum curvature being the most useful for the process. A further development is to dispense with point matching altogether and simply match large surface areas. The surfaces imaged by positron emission tomography (PET), CT, or MRI can be matched directly with the scalp as imaged in the operating room. This permits rapid registration immediately prior to the surgery, without the need for repeating preoperative diagnostic imaging with fiducial markers in place. This saves both time and money, although care must be taken to ensure that the diagnostic images are of sufficient quality to justify relying on them for surgical planning and guidance. Frequently diagnostic images lack the fine spacing needed between images to allow for accurate intraoperative guidance.

A Neurosurgical Perspective 167

In order to perform surface matching efficiently, it is necessary to isolate the data that derive from the patient's skin surface and remove extraneous background information derived from other surfaces or equipment. This process is known as segmentation. Initially, limited computing capacity meant that the digitized data had to be manually segmented, which was time-consuming and tedious. Automated segmentation is preferred, although there is some variation in the degree to which surface-matching techniques can be automated. The best known surface-matching strategy is that of Pelizzari and Chen (1989), but a number of alternative approaches have been published.

Existing surface-based registration techniques are generally less accurate and less reliable than fiducial marker–based techniques and require considerably more technical support and time. The application accuracy achieved for surface matching is usually in excess of 3.0 mm (West et al., 1997). Further, it is important to note that contour matching is incapable of registering two perfect spheres using their contours; therefore points for the registration process should be obtained wherever there is a departure of normal anatomy away from a sphere, such as the area around the face and nose.

A combination of rapid contour mapping with fully automated segmentation would result in a system permitting frequent, rapid, and accurate updates of the registration information at each stage of the surgical procedure. The technology required for this is still under development.

10.4 NAVIGATIONAL SYSTEMS

For the remainder of this chapter, specific reference will be made to one specific navigational system, the StealthStation (Medtronic Surgical Navigation Technology, Louisville, CO). The StealthStation consists of (1) a UNIX-based workstation, which, by communicating with the other components of the system, displays position on a high-resolution monitor or head-mounted display; (2) an infrared optical digitizer with camera array; (3) a reference light-emitting diode (LED) array (e.g., a reference arc); and (4) surgical instruments modified by the addition of LEDs. Optional components of the system include a robotically controlled locatable surgical microscope and surgical endoscopes modified by the placement of LEDs. A description of the instruments used in this system, called effectors, as well as the views produced by the system follow.

10.4.1 Frames

Prior to the advent of computer technology, intracranial procedures were performed with the assistance of stereotactic frames that were firmly fastened to the patient's head. Such frames allowed accurate guidance of instruments to targets along predetermined trajectories and enabled precise determination of the location of an instrument inside the enclosed 3D space. Position determination was usually expressed in Cartesian coordinates, i.e., each point within the intracranial volume was defined relative to three axes: x, y, and z. Types of frames that are coordinate based include the Leksell, Talairach, and Hitchcock frames. The Leksell is an arc-centered system, enabling easy adjustment of the angles of the arc and probe carrier, while keeping the target point centered. Non-Cartesian frames include the Reichert-Mundinger frame and the popular Brown-Roberts-Wells (BRW) frame, in which targets and trajectories are defined by four angles and a length. The latter frame was developed after computers became available, so that Cartesian scanner coordinates could be readily converted into spherical coordinates.

Use of such frames in conjunction with preoperative 2D images obtained from several perspectives by fluoroscopy, or with stereotactic atlases, enabled the surgeon to plan the trajectories for the procedure with a fair degree of accuracy. However, there were several limitations to the use of these frames. In the first place, the target and trajectory parameters were usually calculated with respect to preoperative image data and did not necessarily take into account intraoperative changes in anatomy. Also, many surgeons find the frames to be cumbersome, and they may impede access to the operative site in certain situations. These limitations lead to the use of devices that can determine position in 3D space without resorting to the use of mechanical calipers; this technology is termed 3D digitizers.

10.4.2 Digitizers

More recent stereotactic systems do not use a frame, but still require a precise coordinate system for the operative space. The location of an instrument or pointing device must be conveyed to the computer so that its position can be related to the imaging data. This localization is provided by a 3D digitizer that is installed in the operating room. The digitizer assigns coordinates to each selected point, enabling co-registration of patients, images, and instruments within the same coordinate system.

10.4.2.1 *Early Approaches*

Among the earliest systems were articulated arms with potentiometers at the joints between the links. These sensors determine the angles of the joints by measuring resistance, enabling the orientation of the distal section and location of the tip to be determined. The first reported use of a passive localization arm of this type for neurosurgical guidance was by Watanabe (1993), who used an arm with six joints. A widely used commercial model is the ISG Viewing Wand (ISG Technologies, Toronto, Canada). Guthrie and Adler (1992) developed a

A Neurosurgical Perspective

similar series of arms in which optical encoders replaced the potentiometers to improve accuracy. These arm-based systems are simple and do not require a clear line of sight. However, they can interfere with the surgeon's movements and are difficult to use with surgical instruments.

Another early approach used ultrasound emitters and microphone arrays in a known configuration to localize the position of the instruments. Position was determined on the basis of the time delay between emission of an ultrasonic pulse produced by the emitter and its detection by each microphone. A version of this technique was applied to an operating microscope by Roberts et al. in 1986, and developments continue to this day. Barnett et al. (1993) developed a system in which ultrasonic emitters are fitted to a handheld interactive localization device (Picker International, Highland Height, OH), and the detecting microphone arrays are fitted to the side-rails of a standard operating table. However, ultrasound-based digitizing systems are limited by their requirement for a clear line of sight between the emitters and detectors, and the systems may be confused by echoes, environmental noise, and the effects of fluctuating air temperature. On the positive side, they are relatively inexpensive, costing no more than half as much as an optical digitizer, can be set up rapidly, and can cover a very large working volume. Also, it is easy to affix the emitters to all kinds of instruments and other equipment.

10.4.2.2 Optical Digitizers

Modern navigation systems make use of light-emitting diodes (LEDs) to track the location of instruments within the operative space. Bucholz first developed navigation systems based on optical digitizers. The LEDs used in such systems emit near-infrared light, which can be detected by at least two charge-coupled device (CCD) cameras positioned in the operating room. Inside the cameras, light from the LEDs is focused onto a layer of several thousand CCD sensor elements, and the infrared energy is converted into electrical impulses. These digital signals may be further processed or converted to analog form. Through triangulation the point of light emission can be calculated with an accuracy of 0.3 mm.

Optical triangulation techniques are highly accurate and robust. A useful comparison of their properties with those of sonic digitizers has been published (Bucholz and Smith, 1993). Like sonic digitizers, optical systems require a clear line of sight, but they are unaffected by temperature fluctuations and do not appear to be compromised by surgical light sources. The infrared light is not visible to the surgical team and causes no harmful effects.

A minor variation on the infrared detection approach uses passive reflectors instead of active emitters, with an infrared source illuminating the operative field. The reflected light is detected in the same way as light emitted by the active systems. Instruments fitted with passive reflectors do not need to have electrical cables attached and are thus easier to sterilize. However, the passive markers are constantly "on," appearing simultaneously to the CCD cameras at all times. This can confuse the navigation system if multiple instruments, which carry a large number of reflectors, are present in operative field at once. Another passive approach substitutes an ultraviolet source as the field illuminator, with fluorescent markers reirradiating the UV light at visible frequency levels. However, there is concern that prolonged exposure to UV in this context may pose a health hazard.

10.4.3 Reference Systems

Because of the limitations of the stereotactic frame, it was immediately apparent that frameless surgical navigation represented a significant improvement. This approach dispensed with frames and allowed the surgeon to wield the instruments freehand. However, an important aspect of stereotactic frames was the mounting of surgical instruments directly to the patient's anatomy through the base ring. With frameless devices there is no connection between the instruments and the patient's anatomy, which can lead to error if the position of the patient is not accurately known.

An important benefit of surgical navigation systems is the ability to change the patient's position following registration. To avoid the need for reregistration, it is necessary to have some means of tracking the head relative to the detection mechanism. This is commonly achieved with a reference device fixed directly to the patient's head or to the head-holder, assuming that the head does not move in relationship to the holder. The reference device has at least three emitters detectable by the digitizer employed in the design of the system; for optically based systems a multiplicity of LEDs serves this function, allowing one or more LEDs to be blocked and still allow the position of the head to be determined prior to localization of the surgical instruments.

10.4.4 Effectors

The term *effector* simply refers to those instruments used by a surgeon to perform surgery on the patient. Although surgical instruments comprise the largest part of this group of devices, it is important to realize that the more general term "effector" can be used to refer to anything to treat the patient surgically. Hence, surgical microscopes, endoscopes, genetic material, drug polymers, and robots are effectors that will soon be part of a routine operation. These new effectors all rely upon precise position in order to produce the maximal benefit for the patient; therefore, integration of navigational technology is critical to their success.

Essential components of a surgical navigation system are the instruments that, through modifications by the addition of LEDs or reflectors, permit localization. The variety and number of such instruments define the functionality of the navigational device. Since the LEDs or spheres must be visible to the camera

A Neurosurgical Perspective

array at all times, they cannot be mounted on the tip of an instrument, as the tip will not be visible to the cameras during surgery. These LEDs or spheres are usually located at a given distance from the tip in the handle of the instrument. If the instrument is linear in geometry, such as a forceps, then the minimum requirement for localization is two LEDs mounted in alignment with its tip. Reflective spheres generally do not localize well if they are placed in a linear alignment, because reflective systems experience difficulty when the views of the spheres partially overlap. For this reason, reflective arrays usually consist of at least three spheres in a nonlinear arrangement. This requirement usually makes LEDs the detector of choice for microsurgical instrumentation.

A bayoneted instrument is commonly employed to allow surgery through a small opening. The offset design of a bayonet instrument allows the handle to be placed off the axis of the line of sight of the surgeon and is therefore an ideal geometry use by a navigational system. Additionally, a suction tube, dissecting probe, curette, drill guide, or ventriculostomy stylet can all be equipped with LEDs and localized.

For instruments with complex 3D shapes LEDs or spheres must be placed off-axis to allow tracking. An example of such placement is the biopsy guide tube attachment used in the StealthStation system, or trackers for suction tubes.

When a specific trajectory into the brain is desired, rigid fixation of instrumentation is preferred to ensure that the instrumentation is aligned along the selected surgical path. Typical situations in which the surgical path is the central key issue include tumor biopsy, insertion of depth electrodes for epilepsy, insertion of ventricular catheters, and functional surgery. This function is carried out by a biopsy guide tube adaptor, which attaches to the reference arc using a standard retractor arm with adjustable tension. The tube is equipped with four LEDs to provide redundancy.

10.4.4.1 Localizing Microscope

An operating microscope can also be tracked relative to the surgical field and the position of the focal point displayed on the preoperative images.

One example of such a device that we have coupled to the StealthStation system is the Moeller "Smart Scope" (Moeller Microsurgical, Waldwick, NJ). The primary modification consists of a bracket containing four LEDs attached to the back of the microscope. The microscope head is then tracked relative to the surgical field. The motor-driven variable focal length of the microscope is reported to the operative computer. By determining the position of the head of the microscope and adding the offset of the focal length, the position of the focal point of the microscope can be precisely calculated and displayed using the preoperative images. The crosshairs displayed by the computer system indicate the position of the focal point of the operating microscope.

Certain microscopes can also be robotically controlled by the system. The microscope is equipped with motors that allow the head of the microscope to be moved in two dimensions. Using these motors, the workstation can drive the scope to focus upon a specific point in the surgical field chosen by clicking on the spot as viewed on the workstation display. The system mouse is used to point to the position of interest, and then, by selecting the microscope drive function from the menu, the microscope will be focused on that structure. Alternatively, the scope can be placed in position manually and tracked using the LEDs.

10.4.4.2 Image-Guided Endoscope

In neurosurgery, endoscopes are primarily used for intraventricular procedures. A rigid straight fiberscope ("INCLUSIVE" endoscope, Sofamor Danek Inc, Memphis, TN) has been modified to work with the StealthStation. The endoscope is inserted into the brain through a modified sheath that is itself introduced into the brain over an obturator. Four LEDS are attached to the endoscope near the camera mount using a star-shaped adapter. The geometric configuration of the LEDs is programmed into the surgical navigational system along with the endoscopic dimensions.

The system also assists in entering the ventricle by allowing the stereotactic placement of the endoscopic sheath through a burr hole. The obturator and sheath are modified to fit over the registration probe of the system. The LEDs mounted in line with the tip of the probe provide continuous positional information for the introducer tip during ventricular cannulation.

10.4.5 Intraoperative Visualization

Surgical navigational systems exist to help the surgeon visualize the current location of surgical instruments within a patient's body. The manner in which this information is transmitted to the surgeon during the operation is critical to the acceptance of the device by busy surgeons. This function is performed by the surgical workstation and is depicted on a growing variety of displays.

The StealthStation utilizes CT or MRI for intraoperative guidance. Images are typically obtained in the axial dimension, and the scanning parameters for each modality are adjusted to achieve roughly cubic voxels. Image files are transmitted from the CT or MRI scanner to the surgical workstation over an Ethernet-based local area network and are then converted to a standard file format.

During surgery, three standard views (the original axial projection and reconstructed sagittal and coronal images) are displayed on a monitor at all times. A crosshair pointer superimposed on these images indicates the position of the surgical instrument, endoscope, or microscope focal point. A fourth window can alternatively display a surface-rendered 3D view of the patient's anatomy or live video from the endoscope or microscope. An alternative view, the naviga-

A Neurosurgical Perspective

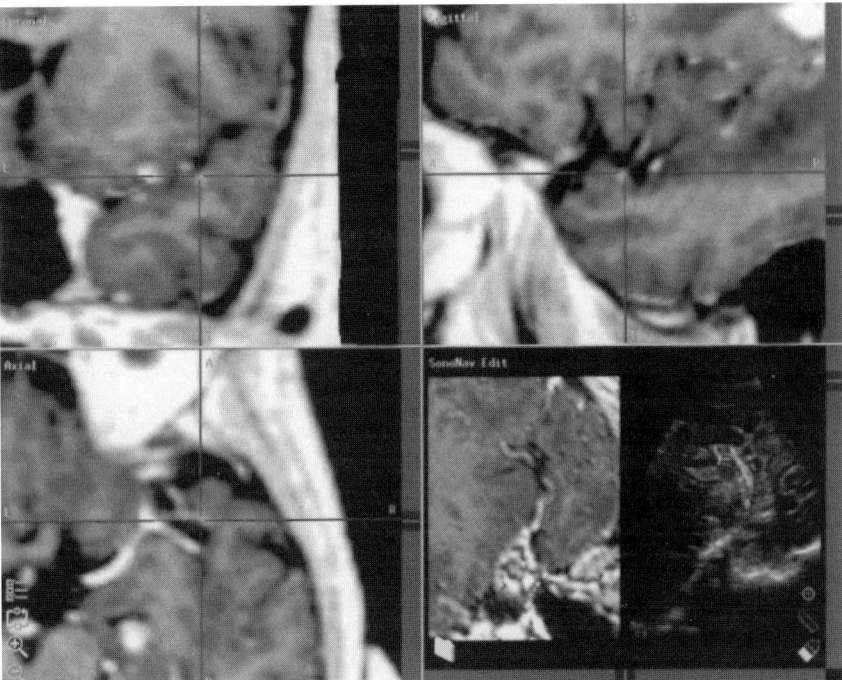

FIGURE 10.2 StealthStation (Medtronic Surgical Navigation Technologies, Louisville, CO) display with the fourth window showing a real-time ultrasound display produced by a color Doppler ultrasound unit reformatted to a preoperative image. Note the correspondence in position of the middle cerebral vessels within the Sylvian fissure.

tional view, produces images orthogonal to the surgical instrument rather than the patient, and is particularly useful for aligning the instrument with a surgical path.

The system can also track an ultrasound probe in real time (Figure 10.2). By applying LEDs on the probe and having the probe go through a registration process, the system can reformat the preoperative dataset to make an image identical in size and orientation to the ultrasound image. This allows the surgeon to detect, and compensate for, movement of soft tissue during the procedure.

10.4.6 Intraoperative System Control

As navigational systems become more complex, the need for the surgeon to interact with the system during a procedure increases. This need will intensify as more complex effectors, such as robots, are brought into the operating room.

Furthermore, as these units proliferate into community hospitals, it will be imperative to make these units capable of being controlled by a small, scrubbed surgical team.

A variety of control techniques have now been developed which allow the surgeon to control the system while scrubbed. One technique involves the use of touch-sensitive flat panel displays that can be placed in a sterile bag and used for controlling the system as well as indicating position. Another solution is to incorporate voice recognition in the head-mounted display worn by the surgeon during a procedure. By placing a boom mike on these devices, voice recognition becomes possible.

As these systems become more advanced it will be important to improve the diversity and utility of the information presented. Rather than being limited to simply showing where a surgeon is within the patient's anatomy, these systems can be employed to compare the patient's anatomy to that of previous patients' functional anatomy. This function is served through the use of an atlas of functional anatomy.

10.5 ATLASES

Stereotactic atlases in printed form have been used for many years to assist in the planning of neurosurgical procedures. Traditional stereotactic atlases are nearly all based on Cartesian coordinates, although individual atlases may differ in certain aspects, such as the point of origin of the coordinates, the orientation of the axes, and the intervals of sampling.

The atlas assigns a set of 3D coordinates to each anatomical feature in a slice, thereby permitting the information from the atlas plates to be incorporated into the planning of the procedure. However, traditional atlases have some limitations that restrict their utility. The first drawback is that the atlas plates are usually based on sections of a single individual, and the anatomical structures shown may differ considerably in size and proportion from those of the patient. This discrepancy may be further exacerbated by the presence of tumors, abscesses, or accidental trauma that seriously distort the normal anatomy, making it difficult to identify or orientate the patient's image data relative to the atlas plate. The second limitation is that the plates in a printed atlas are essentially immutable and cannot easily be resized or warped to match the patient's anatomy.

A promising breakthrough that addresses both these problems is the development of electronic deformable atlases (Figure 10.3). In these atlases, the images obtained from the reference subject are stored in digital form and may be warped and deformed so that designated points coincide with the corresponding points in the image data obtained from the patient. Not only does this enable more precise preoperative planning, it is also valuable if the surgical plan has to be updated intraoperatively to reflect brain shift, or if ambiguous structures are en-

A Neurosurgical Perspective

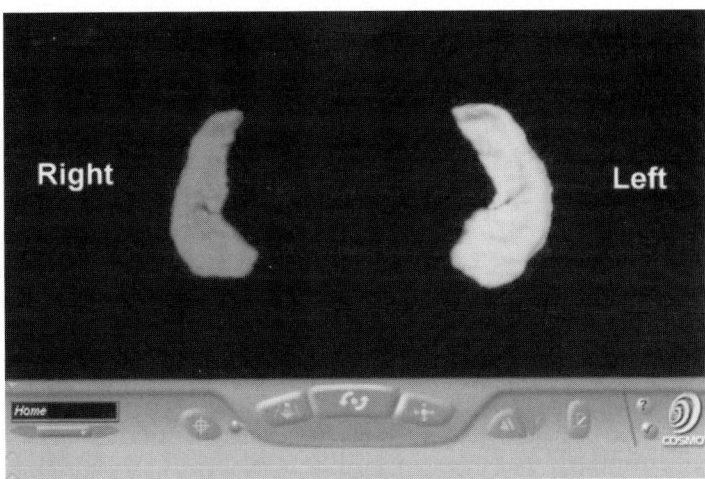

FIGURE 10.3. Deformable atlas applied to the hippocampus. This bilateral structure has been automatically segmented from the overlying tissues by a process that uses an automated protocol.

countered that must be identified before proceeding further. Several deformable atlases have now been produced for neurosurgical applications (Nowinski et al., 1997, 1998), although there is still some skepticism about their value in conservative circles.

10.6 CURRENT APPLICATIONS IN NEUROSURGERY

Computer-aided surgery techniques have been found to be valuable in diverse neurosurgical procedures, including tumor removal and ablation, treatment of arteriovenous malformations, functional neurosurgery for the treatment of epilepsy or tremor-inducing conditions, and implantation of devices for the control of hydrocephalus.

10.6.1 Tumors

CAS is of great value for planning tumor-removal procedures. The actual location of certain types of tumor with distinct margins is usually apparent in preoperative imaging. However, some forms of tumor are not so easily delineated. Also, with deep-seated tumors, it is necessary to plan an approach that avoids causing damage to functional cortex. Postoperative imaging will reveal whether the tumor has been fully excised, and a follow-up surgery can be planned to remove any residual material. However, it is clearly preferable to remove the tumor in a single procedure if possible.

Primary glial neoplasms, especially astrocytomas, have an infiltrating nature that makes them very difficult to resect in their entirety, resulting in a high recurrence rate. Image guidance can facilitate a more complete excision of the tumor, either during the initial surgery or in a subsequent procedure to remove a recurrent growth.

In patients with intracranial meningiomas, finding and delineating the tumor is not normally a problem, as it is usually clearly visible on the patient's image set. Thus, the application of frame-based stereotactic techniques was limited to planning of the craniotomy over the tumor location. However, the advent of freehand surgical navigation systems has permitted more extensive use of CAS in meningioma surgery. In addition to planning the craniotomy location and approach to the tumor, CAS techniques are now used to avoid vascular structures and sinuses and to determine the position of the instruments inside the large, featureless mass of the tumor. Another possible application of CAS for meningioma treatment would be the placement of radioactive seeds directly inside tumors that are otherwise inoperable.

10.6.2 Vascular Malformations

Intracerebral vascular malformations normally require surgical intervention to prevent a future hemorrhage and the attendant neurological deficits. Excision of such malformations is particularly difficult when they occur in eloquent areas of the brain such as those responsible for speech or motor-sensory functions. CAS technology enables the malformation to be modeled in three dimensions and thus permits the optimal resection to be planned, taking into account the relationships of the feeding and draining vessels.

10.6.3 Ventriculostomy

The most common application of the neuroendoscope is in the performance of third ventriculostomies in patients with obstructive hydrocephalus or aqueductal stenosis (Kelly, 1991; Dalrymple and Kelly, 1992; Drake, 1993). Obviously, the ventricles must be large enough to accommodate the endoscope in order for this procedure to be performed, and once the endoscope is successfully inserted it is frequently possible to proceed on the basis of visual guidance. However, computer-based image guidance can ensure a straight trajectory from the burr hole through the foramen of Monroe to the floor of the third ventricle and help avoid unseen branches of the basilar artery. Image guidance is also of particular value in cases of abnormal anatomy, such as patients with myelomeningoceles or small

A Neurosurgical Perspective

foramina of Monroe, or where orientation becomes difficult owing to bloody or blurry cerebrospinal fluid (Muacevic and Muller, 1999). Recent developments in the field of virtual endoscopy promise to aid in the planning and conduct of these procedures (Burtscher et al., 2000).

10.6.4 Functional Neurosurgery

Patients with medically intractable epilepsy are now frequently referred for functional neurosurgery to alleviate their condition. In order to treat the condition surgically, it is first necessary to identify and localize the seizure focus within the brain. Once localized, the region can be eradicated. These processes require accurate spatial localization during preoperative imaging and electro-physiological investigations, and accurate co-registration of the patient data with the surgical field is essential to prevent destruction of uninvolved tissue.

While the advent of CT and MR imaging had a significant impact on epilepsy management, the more recent development of PET, SPECT, functional MRI (fMRI), and magnetic source imaging (MEG) has enabled greater understanding of the underlying neurophysiology and has permitted refinement of treatment protocols. The ability to co-register each of the imaging modalities with the others (and with the patient) is fundamental to the process of determining the nature of the pathology in a given patient.

Video-EEG recordings of actual seizure events also provide vital information for determining which cases are suitable for surgery. Invasive recording techniques are used to evaluate more difficult cases, and placement of the required recording hardware can be facilitated by image guidance. A common approach involves the insertion of depth electrodes into critical mesial structures to localize the seizure origins (McCarthy et al., 1991). Another evaluation technique requires the placement of subdural strip electrodes on the cortical surface. Accurate placement of subdural strips is crucial, and frameless image guidance is potentially of great assistance in the process, though many centers still place the strips without such guidance. A variation on this approach uses subdural grid electrodes, which are similar in construction to the strips but have the contacts arranged in a series of rows and columns embedded in a flexible sheet. At present these are usually placed without stereotactic guidance, but employment of navigational techniques would facilitate more accurate positioning.

Therapeutic procedures for treating seizure disorders associated with structural lesions have been highly successful in producing seizure-free outcomes. A summary of a combined series of 293 lesionectomy cases reported a seizure-free outcome in 66.6% of cases and noted improvement in an additional 21.5% of cases (Engel et al., 1993). These results are comparable to seizure-outcome results achieved with temporal lobe resections and considerably better than can be expected with nonlesional extratemporal resections. Similarly, Piepgras et al. (1993)

reported a series of 102 patients with seizures apparently arising from arteriovenous malformations and found that 83% were seizure free at long-term follow-up.

All such surgical interventions for seizure disorders benefit considerably from CAS, since it is desirable to fully eliminate the causative lesion, while minimizing damage to surrounding tissue. However, it has been found that the optimal resection to achieve a seizure-free outcome may require removal of tissue that lies outside the visible lesion, but which is still involved in the seizure focus according to EEG data (Jooma et al., 1995).

It is likely that the future will see development of noninvasive source localization that will obviate the need for surgical implantation of recording electrodes. However, there will still be a requirement for CAS in therapeutic surgery. Improvements in noncontact registration should enable the registration of patient image data to be accomplished and updated more rapidly. Finally, it is anticipated that real-time electrocorticography and similar recording techniques will enable intraoperative evaluation of the effectiveness of the surgical procedure, ensuring more complete resection of the seizure focus.

10.6.5 Stereotactic Radiosurgery

Another area in which CAS has been of considerable assistance is stereotactic radiosurgery (SRS), in which one or more highly collimated beams of radiation are directed at a tumor. This is usually an outpatient, nonsurgical procedure using the LINAC scalpel or Gamma Knife. For certain types of brain tumor, this treatment is an effective alternative to conventional surgery. However, the radiation does not remove the tumor (although it may shrink it) and resultant scar tissue may make any future surgery more difficult.

A number of technologies may be used in SRS, each with its preferred applications and limitations.

10.6.5.1 Linear Accelerator (LINAC)

The use of conventional LINAC-based radiation therapy is, at best, rarely indicated for the treatment of pituitary microadenomas, but the approach continues to play an important role in the management of macroadenomas. Reports of visual improvement from conventional radiotherapy for pituitary tumors from the 1970s revealed a range of improvement from 41 to 80%. Trans-sphenoidal surgery, however, has shown a rate of visual improvement of approximately 74–90%, which seems superior overall to radiation only. LINAC-based therapy continues to be widely used as an adjuvant treatment. Radiation injury to the optic nerves or optic chiasm is the most feared complication from conventional radiotherapy of pituitary adenomas.

A Neurosurgical Perspective

Although the Gamma Knife has supplanted the use of LINAC in many applications, a recent report found that LINAC treatment of acoustic neuromas gave results comparable to those obtained with the Gamma Knife (Spiegelmann et al., 2001).

10.6.5.2 Gamma Knife

The Gamma Knife was developed by Lars Leksell in Stockholm and was first used to treat a pituitary tumor patient in January 1968. Although ideally suited for irradiation of pituitary tumors, these cases account for only approximately 8% of Gamma Knife cases to date.

The technical features of the device are as follows:

It contains 201 cobalt-60 sources in an approximately hemispherical array.
Each source has a tungsten precollimator and a lead collimator.
Secondary collimation of each beam is accomplished by a helmet.
Sources can be selectively blocked with occlusive plugs to prevent irradiation of specific regions.

Gamma Knife therapy offers numerous advantages over conventional radiotherapy for neurological tumors. It is particularly valuable for treating tumors in close proximity to vital structures that would be damaged by conventional techniques [such as pituitary tumors unsuited to transphenoidal surgery (Hayashi et al., 1999; Landolt and Lomax, 2000; Sheehan et al., 2000), acoustic neuromas (Noren et al., 1993; Pollock et al., 1995; Kondziolka et al., 2000), or tumors adjacent to the optic nerve or brain stem]. The most recent reports indicate that radiosurgery for acoustic neuroma performed using current procedures is associated with lower rates of posttreatment morbidity than in earlier reports (Flickinger et al., 2001).

Intracranial arteriovenous malformations and other nontumoral disorders are also often treated with the Gamma Knife (Lundsford et al, 1990; Guo, 1993). The device is occasionally used to treat meningiomas (Kondziolka et al., 1991; Ganz et al., 1993), but slow-growing tumors of this type are usually removed by conventional surgery unless their location dictates the use of radiosurgery. However, Gamma Knife treatment is useful in conjunction with microsurgery for the treatment of skull base meningiomas, where the proximity of the cranial nerves sometimes makes total resection problematic (Aichholzer et al., 2000; Pollock et al., 2000).

Another possible application of the Gamma Knife is in functional surgery, such as the treatment of intractable epilepsy (Regis et al., 2000) or thalamotomy for essential or multiple sclerosis–related tremor (Niranjan et al., 2000).

Other advantages of Gamma Knife treatment include the following:

Stereotactic radiosurgery of tumors with the Gamma Knife is generally administered in a single session, unlike fractionated LINAC-based radiotherapy, which is administered four to five times per week over a 6-week period.

Because of the nature of the Gamma Knife therapy and the fact that the radiation dose conforms to the tumor shape, there is a steep fall-off of radiation dosage to surrounding tissue such as the brain. Development of secondary tumors or neurocognitive complications is therefore much less likely with Gamma Knife than with conventional radiotherapy.

Gamma Knife radiosurgery is safe as long as the dose of radiation to the optic structures is kept under 10 Gy. Treatment mortality is zero. Long-term follow-up is required.

10.6.5.3 Particle Beam

Proton beam therapy offers certain theoretical advantages over Gamma Knife and LINAC because it makes use of the quantum wave properties of protons to reduce doses to surrounding tissue beyond the target to a theoretical minimum of zero. This is particularly useful when treating unusually shaped brain tumors and arteriovenous malformations. The circular collimators currently in use in photon radiosurgery units result in roughly spherical or elliptical target volumes, and the homogeneous doses delivered also make fractionated therapy possible; no portion of the target in a proton field is likely to receive a complication-producing dose because of superimposition of high-dose areas.

Like the Gamma Knife, stereotactic proton beam therapy was seen as a possible treatment for intracranial arteriovenous malformations (AVMs) and cavernous malformations (CMs) that were otherwise inaccessible. However, recent reports indicate that the therapy is ineffective for the treatment of medium- or large-sized AVMs larger than 3 cm (Seifert et al., 1994), and a retrospective study concluded that although radiosurgery does seem to reduce hemorrhage in such CMs, there is potential for complications and continued lesion progression afterwards (Amin-Hanjani et al., 1998).

10.7 CONCLUSION

As can be seen from this review, the field of CAS has grown dramatically by employing the power of current computers and technology. Based upon the advances made in imaging, CAS has gone from a few applications limited to the midline of the brain to being employed in nearly every cranial procedure. As this technology improves, and as more effectors are built that rely upon precise placement, CAS will become the standard of care for all cranial interventions. This technology will provide the infrastructure upon which the future of neurosur-

A Neurosurgical Perspective

gery will grow, and attention to the concepts and assumptions behind CAS will ensure that the technology is used appropriately.

REFERENCES

Adler JR Jr. Image-based frameless stereotactic radiosurgery. In: Maciunas RJ, ed. Interactive Image-Guided Neurosurgery. Park Ridge, IL: American Association of Neurological Surgeons, 1993. 81–89.

Aichholzer M, Bertalanffy A, Dietrich W, Roessler K, Pfisterer W, Ungersboeck K, Heimberger K, Kitz K. Gamma knife radiosurgery of skull base meningiomas. Acta Neurochirurg 2000; 142:647–652, discussion 652–653.

Amin-Hanjani S, Ogilvy CS, Candia GJ, Lyons S, Chapman PH. Stereotactic radiosurgery for cavernous malformations: Kjellberg's experience with proton beam therapy in 98 cases at the Harvard Cyclotron. Neurosurgery 1998; 42:1229–1236; discussion 1236–1238.

Barnett GH, Kormos DW, Steiner CP, et al. Intraoperative localization using an armless, frameless stereotactic wand. J Neurosurg 1993; 78:510–514.

Barnett GH, Kormos DW, Steiner CP, et al. Frameless stereotaxy using a sonic digitizing wand: Development and adaptation to the Picker Vistar medical imaging system. In: Maciunas RJ, ed. Interactive Image-Guided Neurosurgery. Park Ridge, IL: American Association of Neurological Surgeons, 1993:113–120.

Bucholz RD, Smith KR. A comparison of sonic digitizers versus light-emitting diode-based localization. In: Maciunas RJ, ed. Interactive Image-Guided Neurosurgery. Park Ridge, IL: American Association of Neurological Surgeons, 1993:179–200.

Burtscher J, Dessl A, Bale R, Eisner W, Auer A, Twerdy K, Felber S. Virtual endoscopy for planning endoscopic third ventriculostomy procedures. Pediatric Neurosurg 2000; 32:77–82.

Dalrymple SJ, Kelly PJ. Computer-assisted stereotactic third ventriculostomy in the management of non-communicating hydrocephalus. Stereotact Funct Neurosurg 1992; 59:105–110.

Drake JM. Ventriculostomy for treatment of hydrocephalus. Neurosurg Clin North Am 1993; 4:657–666.

Engel J Jr, Van Ness PC, Rasmussen TB, et al. Outcome with respect to epileptic seizures. In: Engle J Jr, ed. Surgical Treatment of the Epilepsies. New York: Raven Press, 1993:609–621.

Flickinger JC, Kondziolka D, Niranjan A, Lunsford LD. Results of acoustic neuroma radiosurgery: an analysis of 5 years' experience using current methods. J Neurosurg 2001; 94:1–6.

Ganz JC, Backlund EO, Thorsen FA. The results of Gamma Knife surgery of meningiomas, related to size of tumor and dose. Stereotactic Funct Neurosurg 1993; 61:23–29.

Guo W. Radiological aspects of Gamma Knife radiosurgery for arteriovenous malformations and other non-tumoural disorders of the brain. Acta Radiol Suppl 1993; 34:388.

Guthrie BL, Adler JR Jr. Computer-assisted preoperative planning, interactive surgery, and frameless stereotaxy. Clin Neurosurg 1992; 38:112–131.

Hayashi M, Izawa M, Hiyama H, Nakamura S, Atsuchi S, Sato H, Nakaya K, Sasaki K, Ochiai T, Kubo O, Hori T, Takakura K. Gamma Knife radiosurgery for pituitary adenomas. Stereotact Funct Neurosurg 1999; 72 (Suppl 1):111–118.

Jooma R, Yeh H-S, Privitera MD, et al. Lesionectomy versus electrophysiologically guided resection for temporal lobe tumors manifesting with complex partial seizures. J Neurosurg 1995; 83:231–236.

Kelly PJ. Stereotactic third ventriculostomy in patients with nontumoral adolescent/adult onset aqueductal stenosis and symptomatic hydrocephalus. J Neurosurg 1991; 75: 865–873.

Kondziolka D, Lunsford LD, Coffey RJ, Flickinger JC. Gamma Knife radiosurgery of meningiomas. Stereotactic Funct Neurosurg 1991; 57:11–21.

Kondziolka D, Lunsford LD, Flickinger JC. Gamma knife radiosurgery for vestibular schwannomas. Neurosurg Clin of North Am 2000; 11:651–658.

Landolt AM, Lomax N. Gamma knife radiosurgery for prolactinomas. J Neurosurg 2000; 93 (suppl 3):14–18.

Lunsford LD, Coffey RJ, Bissonette D, Flickinger JC. Stereotactic radiosurgery for arteriovenous malformations. Case selection and initial results from the first North American Gamma Unit. Proc Harvard Radiosurgery Update, Boston, 1990.

McCarthy G, Spencer DD, Riker RJ. The stereotaxic placement of depth electrodes in epilepsy. In: Lüders H, ed. Epilepsy Surgery. New York: Raven Press, 1991:371–384.

Macewen W. Intra-cranial lesions, illustrating some points in connexion with the localization of cerebral affections and the advantages of antiseptic trephining. Lancet 1881; 2:541–543.

Maciunas RJ, Fitzpatrick JM, Galloway RL, et al. Beyond stereotaxy: Extreme levels of application accuracy are provided by implantable fiducial markers for interactive image-guided neurosurgery. In: Maciunas RJ, ed. Interactive Image-Guided Neurosurgery. Park Ridge, IL: American Association of Neurological Surgeons, 1993: 259–270.

Maurer CM, Fitzpatrick JM. A review of medical image registration. In: Maciunas RJ, ed. Interactive Image-Guided Neurosurgery. Park Ridge, IL: American Association of Neurological Surgeons, 1993:17–44.

Muacevic A, Muller A. Image-guided endoscopic ventriculostomy with a new frameless armless neuronavigation system. Comp Aid Surg 1999; 4:87–92.

Niranjan A, Kondziolka D, Baser S, Heyman R, Lunsford LD. Functional outcomes after gamma knife thalamotomy for essential tremor and MS-related tremor. Neurology 2000; 55:443–446.

Noren G, Greitz A, Lax I. Gamma Knife surgery in acoustic tumors. Acta Neurochir (Wien) 1993; 58:104–107.

Nowinski WL, Bryan RN, Raghavan R. The Electronic Clinical Brain Atlas. Multi-Planar Navigation of the Human Brain. New York: Thieme, 1997.

Nowinski WL, Yeo TT, Thirunavuukarasuu A. Microelectrode-guided functional neurosurgery assisted by Electronic Clinical Brain Atlas CD-ROM. Comp Aid Surg 1998; 3:115–122.

A Neurosurgical Perspective

Pelizzari CA, Chen GTY, Spelbring DR, Weichselbaum RR, Chen C. Accurate three-dimensional registration of CT, PET, and/or MR images of the brain. J Comput Assist Tomogr 1989; 13:20–26.

Piepgras DG, Sundt TM Jr., Ragoowansi AT, et al. Seizure outcome in patients with surgically treated cerebral arteriovenous malformations. J Neurosurg 1993; 78:5–11.

Pollock BE, Lunsford LD, et al. Outcome analysis of acoustic neuroma management: a comparison of microsurgery and stereotactic radiosurgery. Neurosurgery 1995; 36:215–229.

Pollock BE, Stafford SL, Link MJ. Gamma knife radiosurgery for skull base meningiomas. Neurosurg Clin North Am 2000; 11:659–666.

Regis J, Bartolomei F, Hayashi M, Roberts D, Chauvel P, Peragut JC. The role of gamma knife surgery in the treatment of severe epilepsies. Epileptic Disord 2000; 2:113–122.

Roberts DW, Strohbehn JW, Hatch JF, et al. A frameless stereotaxic integration of computerized tomographic imaging and the operating microscope. J Neurosurg 1986; 64:545–549.

Seifert V, Stolke D, Mehdorn HM, Hoffmann B. Clinical and radiological evaluation of long-term results of stereotactic proton beam radiosurgery in patients with cerebral arteriovenous malformations. J Neurosurg 1994; 81:683–689.

Sheehan JM, Vance ML, Sheehan JP, Ellegala DB, Laws ER. Radiosurgery for Cushing's disease after failed transsphenoidal surgery. J Neurosurg 2000; 93:738–742.

Spiegelmann R, Lidar Z, Gofman J, Alezra D, Hadani M, Pfeffer R. Linear accelerator radiosurgery for vestibular schwannoma. J Neurosurg 2001; 94:7–13.

Watanabe E. The neuronavigator: A potentiometer-based localization arm system. In: Maciunas RJ, ed. Interactive Image-Guided Neurosurgery. Park Ridge, IL: American Association of Neurological Surgeons, 1993:135–148.

West J, Fitzpatrick JM, Wang MY, et al. Comparison and evaluation of retrospective intermodality image registration techniques. J Comput Assist Tomogr 1997; 21:554–566.

Zernov DN. L'encéphalomètre. Rev Gen Clin Ther 1890; 19:302.

11

Role of Computer-Aided Surgery in Functional Endoscopic Surgery

**Stephanie A. Joe, M.D., and
David W. Kennedy, M.D., F.R.C.S.I.**
*University of Pennsylvania Health System, Philadelphia,
Pennsylvania*

11.1 INTRODUCTION

The treatment of sinonasal disease is based on patient symptomatology and diagnostic information obtained from the combination of endoscopy and radiography. Both endoscopic and diagnostic radiographic techniques have rapidly improved in recent years; simultaneously, the characterization of paranasal sinus disease has also progressed in parallel with these technological advances. Computed tomography (CT) scans are routinely used in the initial assessment of sinus disease and for surgical planning. Magnetic resonance (MR) images can provide valuable soft tissue information in more unusual situations. Advanced computer technology allows ready manipulation of the digitally stored images, and advances in digitization of three-dimensional objects have made computer-aided surgery a viable reality. These tools and other advances in surgical instrumentation have assisted in the refinement of sinus surgery and aided in the extension of endoscopic procedures to include more invasive surgical approaches involving both sinus and parasinus pathology.

The adaptation of computer-aided surgery (CAS) for intraoperative localization in otorhinolaryngology has proven to be a beneficial supplement to functional endoscopic sinus surgery (FESS). The senior author has now been using these systems in selected surgical cases since 1988. He has participated in the evolution of these devices from tools that were very difficult to use routinely in the operating room settings. Early systems, which had mechanical arms and unfriendly software, were cumbersome. Today, newer systems are a very solid adjunct to surgery. The technology also supports the teaching of endoscopic techniques.

Sinus surgery is a particularly good application for CAS because of the anatomical "bony box" within which the surgery is performed. As long as the surgery is performed within these confines, anatomical relationships will not shift as tissue is removed, and thus preoperative radiographic studies remain valid for localization and resection margins. However, once the confines of this "box" have been violated, prolapse of tissue and other intraoperative shifting of soft tissue may occur. Thus, for accurate evaluation during intracranial surgery or surgery within the orbit, the value of computer-assisted techniques is much more limited. When working within the confines of the sinuses, CT and CAS allow the surgeon to see beyond the area visualized by the endoscope and provide valuable additional and potentially very accurate information.

Early image-guided systems were adapted from neurosurgery [1–4]. These systems used an attached sensing arm and rigid head frames and required the patient's head to be fixed during the procedure. Because of these rather stringent, technologically based requirements, general anesthesia and frequently a Mayfield head frame were necessary. Additionally, this rigid field restricted patient exposure and surgical access. Furthermore, the localizing probes were unwieldy, and their maneuverability within the delicate confines of the nose and sinuses was problematic, since their attached rigid mechanical arms had only two or three joints. Current systems are significantly less cumbersome and more intuitive. They also allow surgery to be performed under general or local anesthesia. This continued development of CAS systems has facilitated their overall ease of use and accounts for wider appeal.

Major complications still occur during endoscopic sinus surgery, and the surgery remains a leading source of malpractice suits against physicians. In general, the term "major complication" refers to skull base injury with secondary cerebrospinal fluid leak, intracranial complications, intraorbital hematoma, visual loss, other orbital injury, and death [5]. The major complication rate of functional endoscopic sinus surgery is said range from 0.41 to 1.1% [6,7]. It should be remembered that these numbers may be misleading due to underreporting by surgeons. Computer-assisted surgery was designed in part to decrease the risk of such complications [8], although this has not been definitively proven to date.

Furthermore, the role of new technology in surgery must be kept in mind. Advancing technology is important in the diagnosis and treatment of sinonasal disease, but it is not a substitute for education, study of the anatomy through cadaver dissections, or experience.

Endoscopic Sinus Surgery

This chapter will review the indications for CAS in functional endoscopic sinus surgery (FESS) and its advantages and disadvantages. We review the current systems in use at our institution along with their time-tested strengths and weaknesses. Future and alternative navigation systems are also briefly discussed.

11.2 HISTORY

Systems for stereotaxis were first used in neuroanatomy in the early twentieth century and have been used in various surgical applications for much of the subsequent century. Reports of stereotaxis for use in surgery involving the human brain appeared in the middle of the twentieth century [2,9]. Extensive progress in intraoperative stereotactic navigation has occurred since the development of CT in the 1970s. These early CAS systems were used in neurosurgery. They relied upon modified stereotactic frames that required that the patient's head remain rigidly fixed. In the mid-1980s, reports of frameless stereotactic systems began to appear in the surgical literature. In 1988, Watanabe et al. [10] reported on their development of a frameless, three-dimensional digitizer. The hardware of this system included a localizing probe that was attached to a jointed, motion-sensing mechanical arm, which sent positional information in digital format to the system computer. External fiducial markers, which were placed on the patient's head before a CT scan and then maintained through the surgical procedure, served as a system for the correlation of patient position (relative to the mechanical arm) with the corresponding points in the CT scan data set. Before intraoperative localization, each fiducial marker was touched with the localizing probe so that a correlation between points in the real world and virtual world could be established. Future localizations were then based upon extrapolation from this registration information.

Several other similar systems have been described in the neurosurgery literature. (For further information, please see Chapter 2.)

The first CAS system for sinus surgery was developed at Aachen University of Technology in Germany by Schlondorff in the mid-1980s [2]. This system also used a digitizing arm for intraoperative localization. Zinreich and colleagues reported on a similar but more versatile frameless CAS system, known as the Viewing Wand (ISG, Mississauga, Ontario, Canada), in 1989 [2]. Early work with this device during endoscopic sinus surgery led to the creation of other more versatile sensing systems that permitted head manipulation and thus facilitated their greater ease of use during FESS [2,8].

The first reports within otorhinolaryngology of an optical tracking system for use in CAS appeared in the early 1990s. Optical tracking systems incorporate infrared light-emitting diodes (LEDs) into surgical instruments and localizing probes. A camera array, which is situated at a distance from the operating table, can then monitor the relative positions of these instruments and send this digital information to the computer. This positional information is correlated with the stored image data to provide the surgeon with intraoperative localization. These early systems, which were designed for industrial digitization, were large and hence cumbersome. They were also very accurate and very expensive.

In addition to optical tracking, electromagnetic tracking was introduced. These early electromagnetic systems were relatively inaccurate, and the magnetic field was easily distorted by any metallic object within even moderate distances of the electromagnetic sensing and emitting devices. In an electromagnetic tracking system, an electromagnetic emitting source is attached to the patient. Electromagnetic sensors, which are incorporated into the localizing probe and surgical instruments, provides positional information [2,8].

Early CAS systems were plagued by technological limitations, but progress in their development has been rapid. Over time, the problems associated with both early optical and electromagnetic systems have been largely overcome. As a result, the use of CAS in otorhinolaryngology is growing today.

11.3 INDICATIONS

It is sometimes difficult to predict preoperatively which cases would benefit most from the use of CAS [9,11]. Therefore, some surgeons advocate the use of CAS for every case [4,8,9]. However, we find that there are specific situations in which such a system is especially useful. CAS is certainly beneficial in cases with unusual or distorted anatomy. During routine, primary FESS cases, standard landmarks, such as the medial orbital wall and skull base, may be identified with certainty, but massive disease can distort or destroy these and other less consistent anatomical landmarks. In these situations, CAS helps confirm location within the sinus cavities (Figure 11.1). CAS technology is also a guide in revision cases where the usual landmarks have previously been resected, as is frequently the case in patients with diffuse polyposis (Figure 11.2). CAS is also useful in the unexpected bloody field, which is often associated with significant mucosal inflammation. In this scenario, a suction attachment to the sensing probe is ideal. On the other hand, localizing probes without suction are much less helpful. Indeed, in a relatively bloodless field where location and anatomy is more straightforward, there is little call for probes attached to forceps.

CAS is particularly helpful during surgery in the difficult frontal recess. In 1997, Kuhn described the variable pneumatization pattern of the cells in the frontal recess and its effect on intraoperative identification of the frontal sinus [12]. An agger nasi or supraorbital ethmoid cell that extends into the frontal sinus can be close to the skull base and be mistaken for the frontal sinus by endoscopic examination alone. This circumstance, combined with the vulnerability of the adjacent areas, makes it an excellent situation for the use of CAS. The triplanar (axial, coronal, and sagittal) images provided by the computer system are also

Endoscopic Sinus Surgery

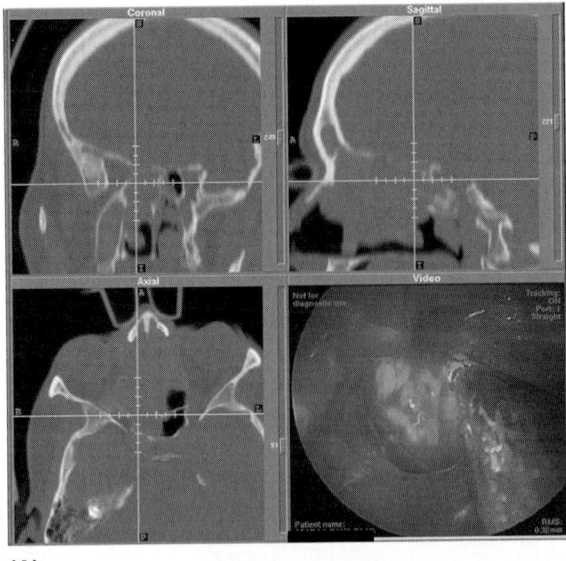

FIGURE 11.1 (A) InstaTrak screen capture shows localization in the posterior ethmoid. The sagittal CT image shows skull base erosion, which was secondary to massive polyposis and allergic fungal sinusitis. (B) InstaTrak screen capture shows localization in the frontal recess. The sagittal CT image shows skull base erosion, which was secondary to massive polyposis and allergic fungal sinusitis.

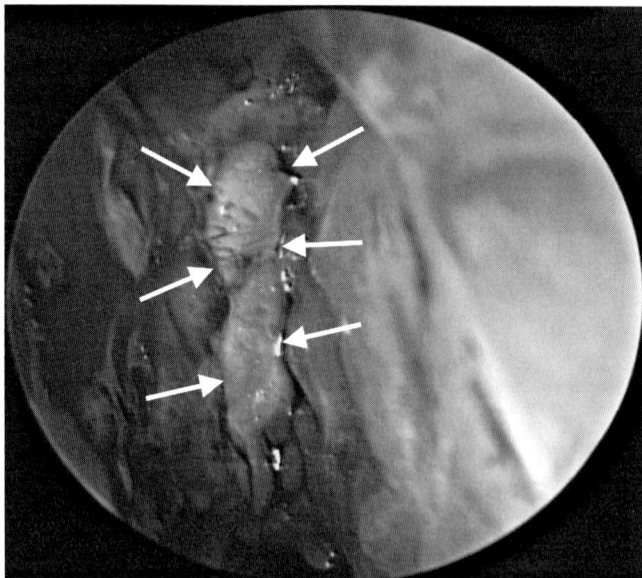

FIGURE 11.2 This endoscopic image shows a 1 × 1.5 cm left ethmoid roof skull base defect due to skull base erosion from a mucocele. Exposed dura (arrows) surrounded by polyps is seen. Intraoperative surgical navigation can help define the bony margins of such defects.

particularly useful in planning the surgical approach to this area. The use of 45- and 70-degree endoscopes, along with a localizing sensor attached to the microdebrider, aids in dissection of this narrow space. Even in FESS cases in which CAS is employed, frontoethmoid mucoceles are opened using the standard endoscopic ethmoidectomy and frontal sinusotomy as described by Kennedy et al. [13,14]. In these cases, CAS can aid in the identification of the usual anatomical landmarks as well as assist in avoiding violation of the orbit or skull base (Figure 11).

Posteriorly, the sphenoid sinus and its surrounding structures also present a difficult and sometimes unpredictable area in which to operate. The carotid canal may be clinically dehiscent in the lateral wall of the sphenoid sinus in up to 22% of specimens, and, significantly less commonly, dehiscences may occur also in the optic canal [15]. In addition to aiding surgical confidence during surgery in this area, CAS is also useful in orbital apex surgery or during optic nerve decompression [11,16]. Additionally, CAS has also been mentioned with respect to the drainage of orbital abscesses [16].

CAS has other potential applications. Surgical navigation can confirm the location of skull base defects for accurate surgery in meningoencephalocele resection and repair of cerebrospinal fluid leaks. The role of CAS in this situation is limited to the precise identification of the bony boundaries of the skull base defect. Because soft tissue is compressible, CAS, which relies upon preoperative imaging data (unless intraoperative MR and/or CT is employed), cannot provide accurate localization along tissue structures in these cases.

When pituitary surgery is performed through a midline approach, it generally carries a low risk of carotid/cavernous injury. However, the potential risk increases when the surgery is performed through either transnasal or transethmoidal approaches because some degree of obliquity is introduced. In this situation, CAS can have significant benefit, reducing the potential for the neurosurgeon to operate through a large tumor towards the opposite carotid artery. Because of the bulk of the self-retaining pituitary retractor, performing transsphenoidal surgery with an electromagnetic-type CAS system can require the use of a special nonferromagnetic retractor.

Many of the advantages of CAS are particularly apparent in cases of neoplasm resection. A number of external and craniofacial approaches can be avoided with the use of endoscopic surgery by the experienced surgeon. Dissection of such mass lesions is supplemented by the application of CAS technology, which reduces the risks of violation of the skull base and dural injury and enhances the safety of removing lesions (such as inverted papilloma) from these areas. Displaced or exposed vital structures including the orbit, optic nerve, and carotid artery can thus be avoided [11]. CAS becomes particularly important for the endoscopic resection of some bony and fibro-osseous sino-nasal tumors. In fact, CAS is essentially a requirement for these cases. Lesions such as ossifying fibroma, osteoma, and fibrous dysplasia frequently need to be removed piecemeal using a drill. It is easy to lose both depth appreciation and landmarks when drilling through a solid tumor. For this reason, the exact site of the tissue on the opposite side of the lesion may be difficult to perceive, especially when the lesion extends intracranially and/or intraorbitally [13].

Localization software has also been applied very successfully in frontal sinus obliteration. However, a system that does not require a headset over the forehead is a requirement for utilization in this manner. In a study of frontal sinus obliteration by Carrau, the accuracy of CAS systems was shown to be greater than the traditional use of a template of the patient's sinus made from a 6-foot Caldwell plain x-ray view [17].

11.4 ADVANTAGES AND DISADVANTAGES
11.4.1 Advantages

In addition to the specific advantages outlined above, the triplanar format provided by the CAS computer significantly aids in surgical planning. The added perspective gained by the sagittal view, coupled with the axial and coronal views, completes a "three-dimensional" picture and significantly helps with anatomical conceptualization for the surgeon [18]. By scrolling sequentially through these three views simultaneously, the surgeon may better comprehend the relevant surgical anatomy. Indeed, in some cases the capacity of CAS to foster the surgeon's understanding of anatomical relationships may be the most important contribution of CAS. In this regard, computer-enabled CT review may be even more helpful than instrument localization.

The orientation afforded by intraoperative surgical navigation does enhance endoscopic sinus surgery and does facilitate a more complete procedure. Potentially, this may lead to improved treatment and reduce the need for revision surgery. Although the use of CAS is not a substitute for experience, it may also facilitate timely dissection for more hesitant and tentative surgeons. Although it is reasonable to believe that computer-guided information might allow for the surgery to be performed with increased safety, this remains to be proven. However, CAS is a perfect teaching tool for residents and those learning functional endoscopic sinus surgery [4,8,18]. CAS can enhance physician education both in the cadaver lab as well as in the operating room. Finally, the database capabilities of the systems also allow for comparison studies that can contribute to research.

11.4.2 Disadvantages

The most significant disadvantage of CAS is added cost. This includes the frequent necessity for a repeat CT scan, capital equipment expenses and disposable instrument costs, additional set-up time and labor, and, possibly, increased intraoperative time. Since fine-cut CTs are required for three-dimensional reconstruction, additional x-ray exposure also occurs to the lens, although this effect may be minimal. As is the case with all complex equipment, learning how to use and troubleshoot it can take considerable time and effort. CAS carries a rather steep learning curve, but this challenge is surmountable. Even surgeons who are well versed in CAS technology may find that troubleshooting these systems is problematic. For practical reasons, calling technical support in the middle of the procedure is not a good option. Alternatively, a CAS technician in the OR may be an ideal solution for this technical challenge, but most institutions do not have the resources for this position.

CAS system complexity can be overwhelming. Obviously, the probability of difficulties and delays related to the system varies directly with the number of steps necessary in the use of the system. Failure of the system can prolong or even lead to cancellation of the surgical procedure if the patient and surgeon were anticipating its use.

Another potential problem associated with CAS systems involves the performance of the preoperative CT scan and its transfer to the CAS workstation.

Endoscopic Sinus Surgery

If the CT scan is not performed in the proper format, the CAS computer may be unable to use the data. Although standards for CT scan data have been established, the data may not be easily transferred between institutions or even between CT scanner computers in one institution. For this reason, CT scans need to be performed according to specific protocols at the institution that houses the CAS system. Of course, this requirement produces added costs for some cases.

The evolution of CAS devices has led to their reported accuracy of within 1–3 mm of the actual anatomy [4,8]. Device inaccuracy beyond this measurement can lead to disorientation and errors that together expose the patient to an increased risk of complications. In addition, surgical navigation accuracy may degrade during the surgical procedure. This may result from an inadvertent shift in the relative positions of the patient and the tracking system. For all practical purposes, this problem in FESS results from movement of the patient or the system headset during the procedure (Figure 11.3). Damaged localizing probes can also produce inaccurate localizations. As a result, the surgeon must maintain awareness of these possibilities throughout the procedure. It should be empha-

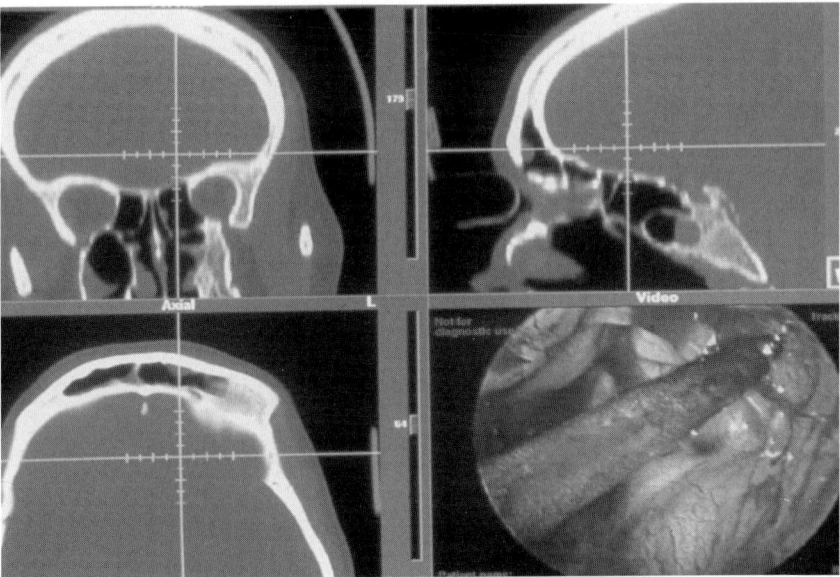

FIGURE 11.3 This InstaTrak screen capture demonstrates loss of system surgical navigation accuracy during surgery. The endoscopic view, which is rotated 45° clockwise, shows probe tip placement in the posterior ethmoid cavity, but the system displays a localization within the intracranial cavity. This discrepancy was due to headset distortion from sterile draping placed for the procedure. (Visualization Technology, Inc., Lawrence, MA.)

sized that small incremental changes in position are often not noticeable. If system accuracy degrades due to these problems, repeat system and/or tool calibration may be necessary, but this alternative disrupts the surgical procedure and increases the operative time. Since failure to recognize the need for recalibration can lead to complications, most CAS systems have built-in functions that require that the surgeon verify system accuracy against defined checkpoints and anatomical landmarks. In addition to these software precautions, it is important that the surgeon use the usual anatomical landmarks throughout the case for repeated comparisons for the confirmation of navigation accuracy.

The surgeon should keep in mind several other precautions with regard to use of CAS stereotactic navigation for endoscopic sinus surgery. There is a significant potential for a false dependence on CAS. CAS should only be used as a guide during surgery; it should not be the major means of orientation and localization. Again, the surgeon should depend on knowledge of paranasal sinus anatomy through study and cadaver dissections. The surgeon should constantly compare actual anatomy with the accuracy of system. A false sense of confidence could lead to more aggressive surgery with its attendant complications. Furthermore, it should be remembered that successful outcomes in sinus surgery do not come just from aggressive surgery; rather comprehensive perioperative medical management, meticulous, mucosal-sparing surgical techniques, and regular postoperative surveillance all contribute to the success of FESS procedures.

Finally, current CAS systems rely on imaging information that is obtained preoperatively. This does not allow for tissue shifts or changes that occur during the course of surgery [11].

11.5 CURRENT SYSTEMS

We currently use both electromagnetic and infrared tracking systems. The current electromagnetic CAS in use at our institution is the InstaTrak System (Visualization Technology, Inc., Lawrence, MA). This system uses low-frequency magnetic fields to detect the relative positions of a probe with ferromagnetic sensors. The InstaTrak software then correlates this information with patient's preoperative CT image data and displays the calculated localization (relative to the preoperative CT scan) on the computer monitor.

The Instrak requires a special preoperative CT scan. During this preoperative CT scan, the patient wears a special headset, which contains fiducial markers. The patient also must wear an identical headset, which is disposable, during the actual surgery. Since the headset can only fit on a patient in one way, the relationship between the fiducial markers and the anatomical region of interest is maintained during the preoperative CT scan and surgery. At the time of surgery, an electromagnetic transmitter is connected to the headset. For surgical navigation, a simple probe calibration is necessary. Registration, or the correlation of points in the operative field and the CT scan volume, is automatic, since the relative position of the headset does not change. The InstaTrak software automatically recognizes the fiducial points in the CT scan. Since the headset remains stationary in relationship to the patient, the patient's head can be moved during the procedure for optimal surgical access.

We find the system straightforward and user-friendly. Little teaching is required in its set-up and use. Use of the system results in few interruptions during the surgical procedure. There have been occasional technical difficulties relating to the transfer of the CT data to the computer, but tending to this task prior to surgery has minimized interruption of surgery.

The InstaTrak does impose restrictions on the surgical procedure. The headset extends across the forehead to the dorsum of the nose and is somewhat uncomfortable to wear for a prolonged periods. The headset also prevents the routine use of the device in open approaches to the frontal sinus. Because the localization is based upon an electromagnetic field, metallic instruments in the operative field may interfere with surgical navigation and localization. Additionally, because the electromagnetic source is connected to the anterior portion of the headset and the headset fiducial markers are all anterior, there is the potential for loss of accuracy in the more posterior anatomical structures.

The other system we use is LandmarX (Medtronic Xomed, Jacksonville, FL). This system uses an optical digitizer, which tracks the positions of LED arrays, known as dynamic reference frames (DRFs), on surgical instruments. In this system, anatomical fiducial landmarks, which must be manually identified in the preoperative CT data set, serve as guides for system calibration. During registration, each of these points is directly correlated to the corresponding point on the patient with the localizing probe. The patient wears a headset that contains a mount for a DRF that tracks patient position. Since this DRF is attached to the patient's head, the head may be moved if necessary.

Before surgery, the LandmarX must reconstruct the sagittal and coronal images as well as a three-dimensional model. In order to minimize delays during the actual surgical procedure, this step may be performed in advance. In comparison with the automatic registration approach of the InstaTrak, LandmarX's landmark-based registration process is more complicated. Registration based on anatomical landmarks requires practice. Adequate registration can be more time-consuming if multiple iterations are necessary. Clinical impressions suggest that the LandmarX offers superior surgical navigation accuracy in the posterior ethmoid and sphenoid regions. This probably reflects the greater dispersion of the fiducial points in three-dimensional space in landmark-based registration. Unfortunately, LandmarX is less intuitive and more labor intensive during routine use.

The commonly used headset for the LandmarX system is rigid and somewhat bulky. As a result, the headset can be intrusive and can limit head positioning. Additionally, the correct degree of tension when applying the headset is not predefined. Its successful application requires skill in order to balance the risk of headset slippage and inadvertent soft tissue erosion at the headset contact points. Recently, a less bulky and simplified head set has been demonstrated. The LandmarX headsets also limit access to the frontal region for open approaches.

The LandmarX's optical tracking system requires that the overhead camera array recognize the signals produced by the DRFs in the operating field. Blocking the line of sight between the cameras and the DRFs will interfere with the system's operation. Careful placement of instrumentation, which can be a significant problem in a crowded operating room, can minimize this problem.

Both the InstaTrak and LandmarX require specific CT scan protocols. In general, an axial CT scan at a slice thickness of 1 mm is performed for either system. As described above, the patient must wear a specialized headset if the scan will be used with the InstaTrak. Data must then be transferred to the computer workstation via a direct network connection or digital media. Data processing and transfer as well as software problems can lead to discrepancies in the reconstructed images and ultimately affect device accuracy. Of course, technical errors at each of the steps necessary for set-up of the system may result in the operating delays and may even prevent the use of either system.

11.6 COST

The expense of new technology is often a deciding factor in its procurement and utilization. The average cost of a CAS system for sinus surgery today is approximately $150,000. Some of the cost could be deferred if other specialties share use of the system. On the other hand, supplementary equipment, such as modified surgical instruments, can add several thousand dollars to the package. An additional CT scan formatted for use by the specific CAS system adds to the total cost of the patient's care. Other additional costs include added operating room time. Equipment problems can create delays that carry even additional expense.

Surgeon reimbursement for CAS in sinus surgery has been problematic. Although current definitions for procedural codes seem to support the use of Current Procedural Terminology (CPT) code 61795 [19], anecdotal evidence would suggest that third-party reimbursement of this code for sinus surgery applications has been minimal. In fact, the 2000 Health Care Financing Administration coding edit effectively prohibited the use of CPT code 61795 with other codes for endoscopic sinus surgery. Later, this coding edit was reversed, but implementation of this change has not yet been verified by common observations.

11.7 THE FUTURE AND ALTERNATIVE CAS SYSTEMS

BrainLab (Munich, Germany) recently introduced a laser-based system for registration. In this approach, the computer correlates calculated surface contour data from the CT scan with the patient's actual facial contour, which is determined by the reflection of light from a hand-held laser. Although this technology holds the promise of significantly simplifying registration, its applicability and accuracy in clinical practice has yet to be verified.

CBYON (Palo Alto, CA) is also introducing a new CAS platform, which uses an optical tracking system. For sinus surgery, the registration is automatic in that a headset with built-in fiducial markers (similar to the IntaTrak headset) is used. In addition, the CBYON system has advanced graphics capabilities based on perspective volume rendering. It also can perform virtual endoscopy of three-dimensional models reconstructed from axial CT scan data. In an application known as image-enhanced endoscopy, this system can register the perspective virtual endoscopy view with the real world endoscopic image.

The use of MR-based CAS in FESS is under investigation. Preliminary reports by Fried et al. using an open surgical magnet show that advanced MR techniques can quickly provide useful, real-time images [20]. This technology, controlled by the surgeon intraoperatively, provides constantly updated information about tissue changes and progress during the surgical procedure. Intraoperative MR is of major benefit where tissue shifting may occur during surgery, such as intracranially or intraabdominally. However, the use of this system has less benefit when working within the bony paranasal sinus confines. Obviously, MR does not image bone well, since bone does not produce a MR signal. Also, significant tissue shift does not occur within the sinuses during standard FESS cases. Some situations where MR guidance has been said to be potentially useful include tumor resection, complex and revision FESS cases, and skull base and orbital surgery.

A number of factors are likely to ensure that intraoperative MR is not widely used for endoscopic sinus surgery in the near future. Magnet use in the operating room requires special construction. All instruments must be entirely nonferromagnetic. The list of specialized equipment includes all instruments, endoscopes, anesthesia equipment, and other ancillary equipment (such as light sources). The costs are considerable. Additionally, the current surgical MR units are cramped and prevent full access to the patient.

Other imaging technologies may be incorporated into the OR. These alternatives include intraoperative ultrasound or portable CT scanners. Either modality may serve to update the preoperative images intraoperatively.

New localization devices are also under development. Tiny electromagnetic devices may be utilized on instrument tips. This technology may improve the flexibility of surgical instruments during CAS-based navigation.

11.8 CONCLUSION

The bony framework of the paranasal sinuses provides an excellent realm for the use of CAS. This tool allows surgeons to accomplish ever more complex procedures while avoiding the necessity for external approaches. When used for selected cases, the benefits of CAS in FESS outweigh its disadvantages. Rhinologic surgeons are encouraged to use CAS as a guide for surgery, rather than as a substitute for surgical judgment, careful study, and cadaveric dissection experiences. Presently it is unknown if CAS can actually reduce FESS complications rates. Additional rapid developments in CAS technology may be anticipated. Surgeons should monitor these advances with significant interest, since they may offer advantages over currently accepted technology.

REFERENCES

1. Zinreich SJ, Dekel D, Leggett B. 3D CT interactive "surgical localizer" for endoscopic sinus surgery and neurosurgery. 76th Annual Meeting of the Radiological Society of North America, Chicago, 1990.
2. Zinreich SJ. Image-guided functional endoscopic sinus surgery. In: Kennedy DW, Bolger WE, Zinreich SJ, eds. Diseases of the Sinuses. Diagnosis and Endoscopic Management. Hamilton, Ontario: B.C. Decker Inc., 357–368, 2000.
3. Anon JB, Lipman SP, Oppenheim D, Halt RA. Computer-assisted endoscopic sinus surgery. Laryngoscope 104:901–905, 1994.
4. Fried MP, Kleefield J, Gopal H, Reardon E, Ho BT, Kuhn FA. Image-guided endoscopic surgery: results of accuracy and performance in a multicenter clinical study using an electromagnetic tracking system. Laryngoscope 107:594–601, 1997.
5. Bolger WE, Kennedy DW. Complications of surgery of the paranasal sinuses. In: Eisele DW, ed. Complications in Head and Neck Surgery. St. Louis: Mosby-Year Book, Inc., 1993, pp. 458–470.
6. Kennedy DW, Shaman P, Han W, Selman H, Deems DA, Lanza DC. Complications of ethmoidectomy: a survey of fellows of the American Academy of Otolaryngology-Head and Neck Surgery. Otolaryngol Head Neck Surg 111:589–599, 1994.
7. May M, Levine HL, Mester SJ, Schaitkin B. Complications of endoscopic sinus surgery: analysis of 2108 patients—incidence and prevention. Laryngoscope 104: 1080–1083, 1994.
8. Anon JB. Computer-aided endoscopic sinus surgery. Laryngoscope 108:949–961, 1998.
9. Roth M, Lanza DC, Zinreich J, Yousem D, Scanlan KA, Kennedy DW. Advantages and disadvantages of three-dimensional computed tomography intraoperative localization for functional endoscopic sinus surgery. Laryngoscope 105:1279–1286, 1995.
10. Watanabe E, Watanabe T, Manaka S, Mayanagi Y, Takakura K. Three-dimensional digitizer (Neuronavigator): new equipment for computed tomography-guided stereotaxic surgery. Surg Neurol 27:543–547, 1987.
11. Senior BA, Lanza DC, Kennedy DW, Weinstein GS. Computer-assisted resection of benign sinonasal tumors with skull base and orbital extension. Arch Otolaryngol Head Neck Surg 123:706–711, 1997.
12. Owens RG, Kuhn FA. Supraorbital ethmoid cell. Otolaryngol Head Neck Surg 116: 254–261, 1997.

13. Kennedy DW, Keogh B, Senior B, Lanza DC. Endoscopic approach to tumors of the anterior skull base and orbit. Oper Tech Otolaryngol Head Neck Surg 7:257–263, 1996.
14. Kennedy DW. Functional endoscopic sinus surgery: Technique. Arch Otolaryngol 111:643–649, 1985.
15. Kennedy DW, Zinreich SJ, Hassab MH. The internal carotid artery as it relates to endonasal sphenoethmoidectomy. Am J Rhinol 4:7–12, 1990.
16. Anon JB, Klimek L, Mosges R, Zinreich SJ. Computer-assisted endoscopic sinus surgery. An international review. Otolaryngol Clin North Am 30:389–401, 1997.
17. Carrau RL, Snyderman CH, Curtin HB, Weissman JL. Computer-assisted frontal sinusotomy. Otolaryngol Head Neck Surg 111:727–732, 1994.
18. Mann W, Klimek L. Indications for computer-assisted surgery in otorhinolaryngology. Computer Aided Surg 3:202–204, 1998.
19. Current Procedural Terminology (CPT 2000). Chicago, IL: American Medical Association, 1999.
20. Fried MP, Topulos G, Hsu L, Jalahej H, Gopal H, Lauretano A, Morrison PR, Jolesz FA. Endoscopic sinus surgery with magnetic resonance imaging guidance: Initial patient experience. Otolaryngol Head Neck Surg 119:374–380, 1998.

12

Image-Guided Functional Endoscopic Sinus Surgery

Martin J. Citardi, M.D., F.A.C.S.
Cleveland Clinic Foundation, Cleveland, Ohio

12.1 INTRODUCTION

Within the domain of otorhinolaryngology–head and neck surgery, computer-aided surgery (CAS) technology has reached its greatest state of development for endoscopic sinus surgery applications. Essentially all of the commercially available CAS systems have an "ENT package" that adapts each CAS platform to sinus surgery. Scientific papers on CAS are increasingly common in the otorhinolaryngological literature each year, and more presentations on this topic are occurring at the specialty's scientific meetings. These papers almost completely focus on the use of CAS in sinus surgery. CAS has attracted attention from general otolaryngologists as community-based hospitals and surgery centers install CAS systems for sinus surgery in their facilities. Obviously, CAS has attracted a significant amount of notice from otorhinolaryngologists. Despite this apparent stature, the exact role of this exciting technology for sinus surgery has not been established. In fact, rhinologists, who are widely recognized as leaders in the field, differ greatly on how CAS should be applied.

Many reports describe the use of CAS for sinus surgery [1–9]. For the most part, the authors of these articles have focused on the technology and its adaptation for sinus surgery. Of course, this emphasis reflects the novelty of the technology.

It is important to remember that the impact of CAS on surgical techniques is very difficult to quantify. In fact, it is difficult even to describe that impact. Even those surgeons who have positive experiences with CAS probably will admit that conveying that experience to other physicians is a challenging task.

At this point, the need for further descriptions of the technology is minimal. Instead, reports should highlight the positive impact of CAS on surgical decision making and execution. This shift is critical, since CAS for otorhinolaryngology is at a critical point. The simple fact is that most sinus surgeons do not use CAS; these individuals will require convincing reports as justification for their adoption of CAS. The vendors and designers of CAS platforms also need additional guidance from surgeons; these engineers know how the systems work on a mechanistic level, but they do not know how surgeons use these systems or how these systems can be improved so that surgeons can use them more effectively. In addition, CAS is expensive technology, and hospital and surgery center administrators are requesting objective evidence of the benefits of CAS. Similarly, managed care companies and governmental regulatory agencies also have begun to ask appropriate questions about the cost-effectiveness of this technology. These demands are significant, and descriptions of an interesting technology will be insufficient for these audiences.

This chapter proposes an approach for the integration of CAS into functional endoscopic sinus surgery. Strategies for the adaptation of CAS for sinus surgery will be presented. Specific cases are presented, and the impact of CAS in these cases is demonstrated. In these discussions, the advantages of CAS should be self-evident. This chapter begins to answer the CAS critics who propose that CAS is an expensive novelty with little clinical use; this chapter also provides information for individuals who are independently trying to reach their own conclusions about CAS. Admittedly, this chapter will probably fall short of its lofty goals. At the very least it will provide a framework for further discussions, and it will engender additional debate in this area.

12.2 RATIONALE FOR CAS IN ENDOSCOPIC SINUS SURGERY

Rhinologic surgeons have expressed interest in CAS technologies because of the unique challenges in rhinology. The paranasal sinuses are a complex, three-dimensional space with close relationships with adjacent structures, including the optic nerve, the medial rectus muscle, the cavernous sinus, the carotid artery, etc. The patterns of paranasal sinus pneumatization can vary greatly among patients and even between sides in the same individual. The bony boundaries separating the intrasinus space from the adjacent structures may be congenitally absent. For instance, the bone of the lateral sphenoid wall may be dehiscent so that the sinus mucosa is draped directly across the optic nerve and/or carotid artery. For these reasons, minimal surgical imprecision can lead to catastrophic results.

The introduction of the rigid nasal telescopes and computed tomography (CT scan) has facilitated greater understanding of this anatomy. The patterns of anatomical relationships are better categorized, and, using nasal endoscopy and CT scans, experienced sinus surgeons can more readily recognize paranasal sinus anatomy in a specific patient. Together nasal endoscopy and CT scans have driven a fundamental shift in the strategy for the evaluation and treatment of inflammatory diseases of the paranasal sinuses; however, it must be remembered that even CT scans and nasal telescopes have inherent limitations.

Of course, CT scans offer tremendous advantages over standard plain films in the evaluation of the paranasal sinuses, since CT scans simply provide additional information in additional images, where as in plain films all of this information is superimposed in a single image. Yet standard CT scans, printed on film and reviewed on a traditional x-ray light box, provide only a finite amount of imaging information. During review of these images, the surgeon must interpret the images and mentally reconstruct "virtual image slices" for those areas that are between each pair of consecutive CT slices. Furthermore, the surgeon then must mentally fashion a three-dimensional model that is used for preoperative assessment and surgical planning. At the time of surgery, the surgeon then extrapolates from this model, which can only be seen in his or her personal "mind's eye," to the intraoperative anatomy. During each step of this process, inadvertent errors can compromise the ultimate precision of the process. Computer-enabled review of high-quality thin-cut CT images can minimize these issues.

The Hopkins rod telescopes provide brilliant illumination, and the resultant image quality is excellent. The slender profile of these instruments provides surgical access that would otherwise be impossible. It must be remembered that the endoscopic image is only a two-dimensional representation of three-dimensional anatomy. Furthermore, the endoscopic image also has a consistent amount of distortion that is intrinsic to the Hopkins rod lens systems; that is, looking through the telescope is simply not the same as looking through a window or through a standard movie camera viewfinder. The use of angled telescopes, which provide a field of view that is displaced 30°, 45°, 70°, or 120° from the main axis of the telescope, compounds this tendency for disorientation. The net result of these factors is that the views provided by the nasal telescopes are often difficult to interpret for even experienced sinus surgeons. CAS surgical navigation provides a potential solution for the problems of the nasal telescopes.

These issues also adversely effect physician education. Rhinologic surgery is fraught with potential catastrophic complications that reflect the position of the paranasal sinuses and adjacent structures as well as their variability. For this reason, physician education is of paramount importance, but learning the techniques of nasal endoscopy and CT scan review is not an easy task. Computer-based systems, to the extent that they simplify anatomical complexity, may facilitate physician education as well.

12.3 IG-FESS PARADIGM

Messerklinger observed mucociliary clearance patterns directly through nasal and sinus endoscopy in live patients [10] as well as through time-lapse photography in fresh cadaveric specimens [11,12]. From these observations, it became apparent that relatively minimal swelling in the narrow mucosa-lined channels of the anterior ethmoid sinuses of the middle meatus can lead to secondary mucosal retention, which in turn leads to bacterial infection. From a clinical standpoint, the precise diagnosis of sinusitis depends on the accurate recognition of these often subtle abnormalities. Standard plain films and anterior rhinoscopy do not provide poor visualization of these critical areas; however, CT scans and nasal endoscopy permit reliable diagnosis of even mild mucosal changes. As rhinologists gained knowledge of normal mucosal mucociliary clearance and abnormal mucociliary dysfunction (i.e., the fundamental issue in the pathogenesis of sinusitis), the aim of sinus surgery shifted from the removal of "irreversibly diseased" tissue to the restoration of mucociliary clearance. Through the early work of Messerklinger [13] and others in Europe as well as rhinologists in Japan, this concept of functional endoscopic sinus surgery (FESS) became popular. In the mid-1980s, Kennedy introduced FESS to the United States [14,15].

The paradigm of *image-guided functional endoscopic sinus surgery* (IG-FESS) attempts to integrate CAS technology into functional endoscopic sinus surgery [16]. Principles of this approach include:

> The goal of sinus surgery that targets medically refractory chronic rhinosinusitis is the restoration of normal mucociliary clearance. The normal patterns of mucociliary clearance are well known, and nasal endoscopy provides direct visualization for diagnosis as well as surgical manipulations. The surgery is finesse-based, rather than destructive. IG-FESS extends these basic concepts of standard FESS.
>
> CAS surgical navigation systems should provide more than simple localization; that is, they should not be used as mere "point-and-hunt" devices. Contemporary sinus surgery is derived from sophisticated principles, and the integration of new technology should be done in a sophisticated manner. Violation of this principle violates the fundamental core of functional endoscopic sinus surgery.
>
> CAS computer workstations provide powerful platforms for the review of preoperative CT data. Through software-enabled review, surgeons can develop a more accurate understanding of three-dimensional anatomical relationships. Similarly surgical planning is facilitated by the use of the computer workstation.
>
> Intraoperatively, the surgeon can relate the preoperative imaging to the intraoperative anatomy. In this way, the surgeon can directly implement his surgical plan.

Image-Guided Functional Endoscopic Sinus Surgery

The CAS surgical navigation system should be used throughout the entire procedure. In order to facilitate this, surgical instruments, including curved aspirators, pointers, forceps, and even microdebriders, should be modified so that their positions can be tracked through surgical navigation. The designs of these modified instruments should facilitate their use. Bulky or otherwise unworkable instruments not only serve to frustrate the operating surgeon; their poor design adversely effects the potential impact of CAS in FESS (Figure 12.1).

Through these principles, IG-FESS moves CAS from a means of confirmation to a critical method for the completion of the surgical procedure.

The term "image-guided functional endoscopic sinus surgery" obviously builds upon the widely accepted term "functional endoscopic sinus surgery." One must not dismiss this as trivial wordplay. First, early reports on surgical navigation for sinus surgery in the United States and Japan, commonly talk about "image-guided surgery" (IGS); in rhinology, the IGS terminology still predomi-

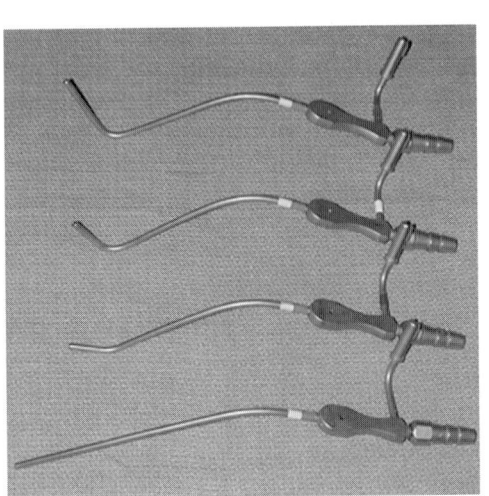

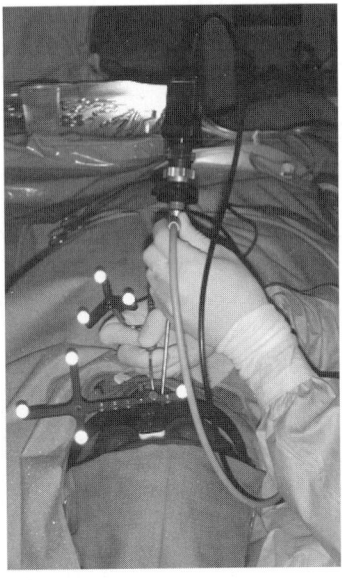

(A)   (B)

FIGURE 12.1 Proper instrument design is critical for the successful integration of CAS instrumentation into routine endoscopic sinus surgery. Optically based surgical navigation requires line-of-sight between the instrument tracking platform and the overhead camera array. A simple post for the tracking platform is inadequate; instead, the post should include an offset (A) so that line of sight can be maintained during surgery (B).

nates, although the term "computer-aided surgery" has gained considerable international exposure through the actions of the International Society of Computer-Aided Surgery (ISCAS) [17]. IG-FESS refers to this heritage of IGS. In addition, the IG-FESS term draws attention to the importance of images—which really guide the surgery. In IG-FESS, these images come from multiple sources. Clearly, the nasal telescopes provide a direct view of the operative field. The CAS system generates images that simulate a virtual world. Both the CAS-generated images and the endoscopic images direct the surgery.

12.4 COMPUTER-AIDED CT IMAGE REVIEW

IG-FESS incorporates not only intraoperative surgical navigation, but also the image review features of CAS systems. CAS software generally include a variety of tools:

- Simultaneous view of the axial, coronal, and sagittal images in the three orthogonal planes through a given point
- Coronal and sagittal image reconstruction
- 3D model reconstruction
- 3D model cut-view reconstruction
- Distance-measurement tools
- CT window and level adjustment

These software tools provide technological means for the review of preoperative images in ways that the standard observation of the CT films on a radiology light box cannot. A standard sinus CT (namely 3 mm coronal slices, printed on regular x-ray film) provides a finite number of images. Anatomical structures between the scanned slices can only be inferred from the information captured on the surrounding slices. In contrast, CT scans for CAS are obtained at much

---

FIGURE 12.2 These series of images serve as example of the importance of CAS workstation review of preoperative CT scans in complex revision sinus surgery cases. (A) The standard coronal image depicts bilateral frontal sinus opacification as well as hazy new bone formation (star) and dehiscence of the right frontal sinus floor (arrow). (B) The midline frontal sinus seems well aerated; the reasons for the superior frontal sinus opacification are unclear. (C) The CT scan images of the three orthogonal planes through a point in the right frontal recess is shown. The sagittal reconstruction image demonstrates that complete dissection of the frontal recess has already been completed and that the inferior frontal sinus and frontal recess are both aerated and healthy; however, new bone formation separates the superior frontal sinus, which is opacified, from the inferior sinus and its normal outflow. (D) The findings on the left side are similar. The images in A and B are partial screen captures from the SAVANT (CBYON, Palo Alto, CA). C and D show screen captures from SAVANT (CBYON, Palo Alto, CA).

Image-Guided Functional Endoscopic Sinus Surgery

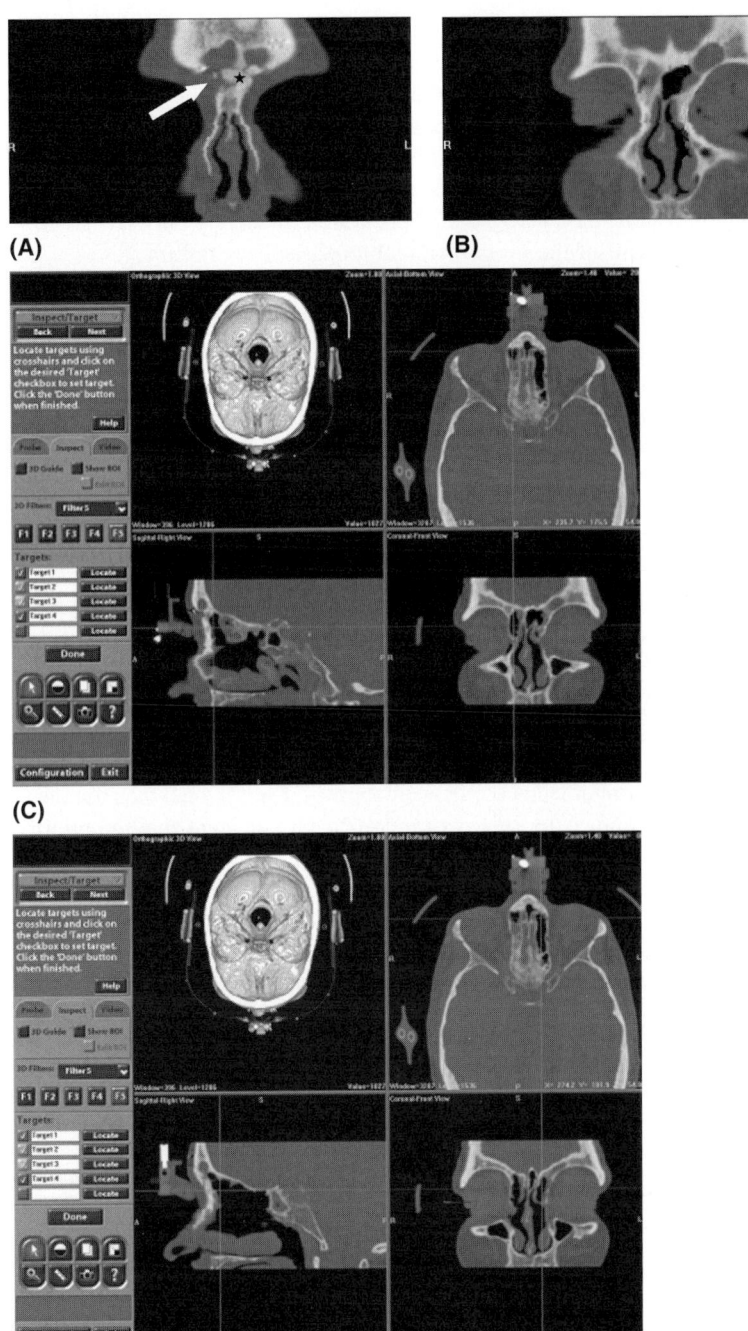

thinner slice thickness (often 1.0–1.5 mm); these scans depict more data. Furthermore, the CAS system reconstructs the axial data into coronal and sagittal images, and the user can scroll through any of these images. Finally, the CAS computer presents axial, coronal, and sagittal images for each orthogonal plane through each point in the scan volume; that is, the axial, coronal, and sagittal images are all arranged 90° to each other. The net result is a complete set of anatomical information that can be easily accessed. This notion of accessibility is also critical. Simply printing all of the 1 mm axial, coronal, and sagittal images to x-ray film cannot be equivalent, since that approach would create an overwhelming morass of visual information. The key point is that CAS provides more information in clinically useful ways.

Computer-enabled review of the preoperative CT scan can directly influence preoperative surgical planning, as shown in Figure 12.2. The patient, a 61-year-old woman who had undergone one previous osteoplastic frontal sinus procedure as well as three endoscopic sinus surgery procedures, presented with persistent frontal headache. Her nasal endoscopic examination showed healthy, relatively thin mucosa in each frontal recess; in fact, on each side, the frontal ostium was well seen and the internal frontal sinus mucosa also seemed healthy. However, the apparent volume of the frontal sinus on each side seemed small, since the endoscopic view did not extend as far superiorly as anticipated. A CT scan was obtained. Two coronal images are shown in Figure 12.2A and B. In Figure 12.2A, the image showed that the frontal sinus was opacified bilaterally, that the right frontal sinus floor was absent/eroded, and bone with a hazy appearance formed most of the frontal sinus floor. In another coronal image (Figure 12.2B), the midline frontal sinus seems well aerated. The CT scan was reviewed on the CAS workstation. After this review, it became apparent that the inferior aspect of each frontal sinus was aerated and draining into the frontal recess, but that the superior aspect of each sinus was opacified and separated from the inferior frontal sinus by reactive new bone formation (Figure 12.2C and D). This new bone formation occurred at the location of the bone cuts for the previous osteoplastic flap. Intraoperative findings confirmed these conclusions.

12.5 SURGICAL NAVIGATION FOR SINUS SURGERY

Through intraoperative surgical navigation, CAS also provides precise localization relative to the preoperative imaging data set. The paranasal sinuses are truly an ideal location for surgical navigation, since they are contained inside a rigid bony space. In this environment, surgical navigation can be performed without concern about soft tissue deformations due to surgical manipulations. Furthermore, as FESS is performed, the relative positions of the adjacent critical soft-tissue structures (namely brain and orbit) are not disturbed unless an inadvertent violation of an adjacent cavity has occurred. As a result, for FESS the navigation

Image-Guided Functional Endoscopic Sinus Surgery

is confined to the space of the paranasal sinuses; the boundaries of this space are relatively inviolate. Therefore, localization is relatively straightforward, especially compared to the challenges of neurosurgery, where soft-tissue deformation (brain shift, etc.) is almost unavoidable.

Other endoscopic techniques (such as endoscopic optic nerve decompression and endoscopic closure of cerebrospinal fluid leaks) differ from standard FESS, since the surgical procedure for these so-called "advanced" techniques deliberately occurs outside the paranasal sinuses, which only serve as a route of access. Even in these circumstances, localization information relative to the known bony anatomy can be helpful. In fact, such information may be of even greater importance for these challenging cases.

Surgical navigation depends upon registration, which is basically a calibration step for surgical navigation. All registration strategies map corresponding points in the preoperative imaging data set and the operating room. Registration may be divided into two categories:

1. In automatic registration, the patient wears a special headset at the time of the preoperative CT scan and surgery (Figure 12.3). The headset contains special fiducial markers that the computer can recognize automatically in the CT data. Since the headset fits the patient in only one way and since the relationship between the tracking device (also known as the dynamic reference frame or DRF) and the headset is predefined, the registration process is complete as soon as the computer has determined the location of the fiducial points in the CT scan. All localizations are relative to these points.
2. If the preoperative CT scan does not contain any information about the position of the DRF relative to the surgical volume; manual registration must be performed. In point-mapping registration, the surgeon must manually correlate corresponding points on the preoperative imaging data set and the surgical field. Anatomic fiducial points (such as the tragus and/or the medial canthus) may serve this purpose. Alternatively, external fiducial markers can be applied prior to the preoperative CT scan; in this case, the markers cannot be moved before surgery. Early CAS systems used bone-anchored fiducial points. Although such markers provide the best registration, they are cumbersome and impractical, and the other alternatives provide satisfactory registration accuracy. Surface contour maps also can support registration. In this approach, the surgeon maps approximately 30–40 points on relatively immobile surface contours, and the computer computes a registration by fitting the curve defined by these points to the surface contour of a three-dimensional model that has been reconstructed from the thin-cut axial CT data. A new system that automates the surface matching process has been developed (Figure 12.4).

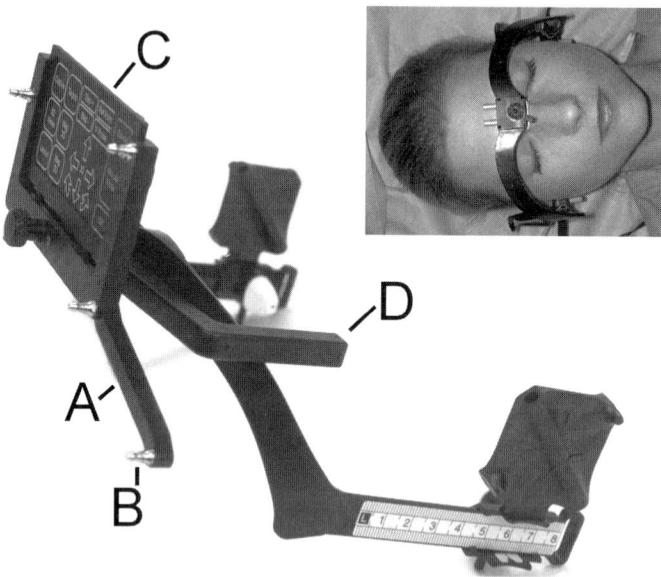

FIGURE 12.3 The CBYON SAVANT ENT headset (Cbyon, Palo Alto, CA) is typical of CAS headsets that support automatic registration for sinus surgery. These headsets rest on the patient's nose and are secured in place at each external auditory canal (inset photo). The headset components include (A) dynamic reference frame (DRF) platform for the tracking system, (B) posts for reflective spheres, which can be recognized by the CAS camera array, (C) virtual mouse pad, and (D) fiducial markers. In the SAVANT headset, a plastic frame houses the metal fiducial markers. The headset for the InstaTrak (Visualization Technology, Inc., Lawrence, MA), which is also designed for automatic registration, is similar; the major difference is that VTI system uses electromagnetic tracking rather than optical tracking. (Original headset photo courtesy of CBYON, Palo Alto, CA.)

During registration, the CAS computer calculates a registration accuracy value, which is actually an arithmetic expression of the average standard deviation of each fiducial point relative to the whole registration. If the registration accuracy is less than a critical value, then the registration is deemed potentially acceptable. The CAS user must manually accept the registration in order to proceed to surgical navigation.

In general, lower registration accuracy values are associated with greater surgical navigation accuracy; however, this may not be so in each specific case. As a result, the surgeon must estimate surgical navigation accuracy manually by localizing to known points in the surgical volume and making a visual estimate of localization accuracy. It is important that the estimates of surgical navigation

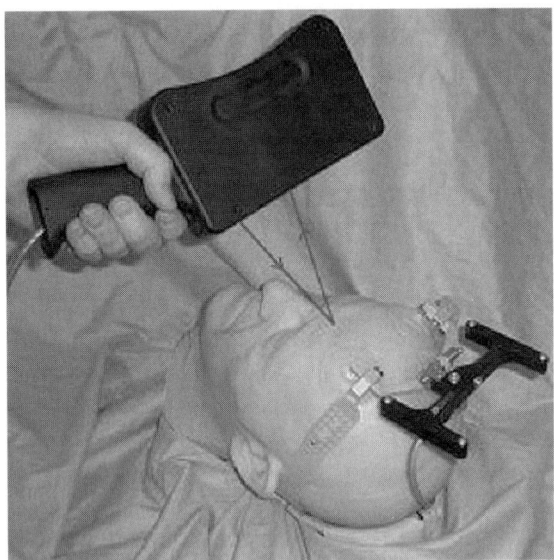

FIGURE 12.4 The Xomed FAZER® (Medtronic Xomed, Jacksonville, FL) automates surface merge registration by performing a surface laser scan; during this scan, the reflected light contains the information about the surface contour. Then registration is calculated through a surface matching algorithm, which relates the surface anatomy information with the CT images that have been reconstructed from the preoperative CT scan. During registration, the CAS system tracks the locations of the headset DRF and the FAZER. (Photo courtesy of Medtronic Xomed, Jacksonville, FL.)

accuracy be completed at several points randomly distributed in the surgical volume, since localization accuracy may vary among points in different parts of the surgical volume. In addition, surgical navigation accuracy should be verified throughout the duration of the procedure, since inadvertent drift may alter accuracy during the case.

Registration accuracy (registration error calculated by the CAS system) and surgical navigation accuracy are not equivalent. Registration accuracy is the error calculated by the CAS system; to a large extent, it reflects the position of the fiducial points on the CT scan. Surgical navigation accuracy is the real-life value that is much more important. Numerous factors—including tracking system precision, registration accuracy, and instrument calibration (i.e., bent vs. "true" instruments)—all influence surgical navigation accuracy. Although surgical navigation accuracy is just a visual estimate of localization accuracy, it is the only way to confirm the precision of surgical navigation and monitor the continued performance of the system during surgery.

Available CAS systems routinely provide a surgical navigation accuracy of 2 mm or better, and in many cases an accuracy of 1 mm or better can be achieved. This level of accuracy must be considered relative to the anticipated dimensions of relevant structures (such as the lamina papyracea, which has a thickness of less than 1 mm). Since the critical dimensions of these structures are less than 1 mm, one may assume that the intraoperative margin of error for surgical navigation should also be less than 1 mm; however, this assumption is inaccurate. The net intraoperative margin of error must be smaller than that critical dimension, but the net margin of error includes surgical navigation accuracy as well as the judgment of the operating surgeon. Information from CAS localization is not used in isolation; rather, CT scan images, the endoscopic view, and surgical navigation are all complementary. The net surgical precision is greater than the estimated accuracy of surgical navigation alone; the net surgical precision with CAS is also greater than endoscopy and CT scans together (in the absence of CAS). The bottom line is that the effective intraoperative accuracy of CAS surgical navigation is greater than the estimated accuracy of isolated localizations provided by CAS surgical navigation.

12.6 THE SPECIFIC UTILITY OF CAS IN FESS

The practical implications of IG-FESS are best explained through a series of examples, which illustrate the impact of CAS on surgical decision making and execution [16]. In this series of examples, the focus is not upon the novelty of CAS. Similarly, the focus is not simply point localization. Rather, the emphasis is on how CAS positively influences surgical planning and the actual procedure.

Case 1: Frontal Sinus

R.V., a 46-year-old man with a long history of sinonasal polyposis, chronic rhinosinusitis, and asthma, presented with complaints of facial pressure, nasal congestion/obstruction, and purulent rhinorrhea. He also described periodic asthma exacerbations that he subjectively related to rhinosinusitis exacerbations. He had undergone surgery at another facility in the recent past. Since his medical treatment had not been maximized, he was first treated with systemic steroids and culture-directed antibiotics, but his symptoms persisted. He then was brought to the operating room for IG-FESS. Initial review of his preoperative CT seemed to reveal a septated frontal sinus; however, careful examination of the images on the CAS workstation showed the presence of a right supraorbital ethmoid cell and a left frontal sinus that had pneumatized across the midline into the right frontal bone (Figure 12.5). Intraoperatively, a right frontal ostium could not be identified.

CAS surgical navigation was used to confirm localization relative to the preoperative CT scan; in doing so, the CAS-enabled assessment of the frontal

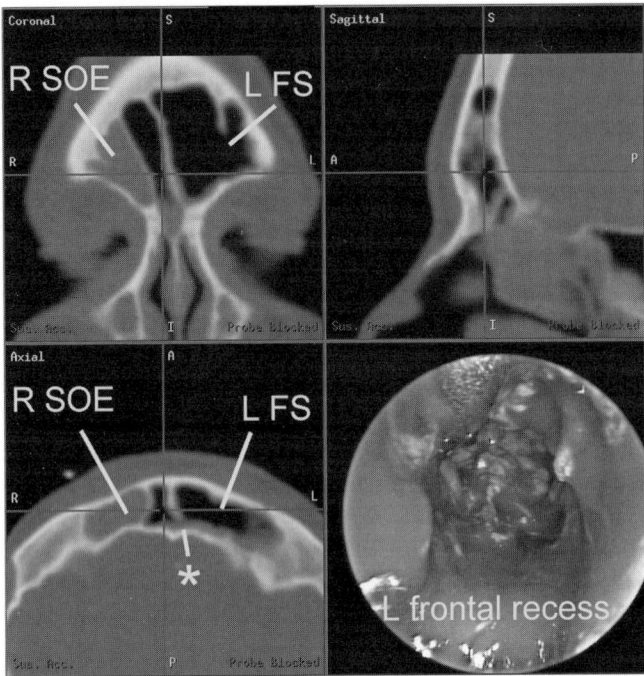

FIGURE 12.5 No right frontal sinus is present, although a cursory review of the coronal CT image suggests the presence of a septated frontal sinus. In this instance, the left frontal sinus has pneumatized across midline. The asterisk shows the connection between the left frontal sinus and its contralateral extension. During surgery, a curved suction probe was passed from the left frontal recess into the contralateral portion of the left frontal sinus. This CAS screen capture shows localization relative to the point of this instrument. The inset endoscopic picture shows this view of the left frontal recess. (LandmarX 2.6.4, Medtronic Xomed, Jacksonville, FL.) (From Ref. 16.)

sinus pneumatization was directly related to the intraoperative surgical field. The complexity of the frontal sinus pneumatization patterns is well known. Since CAS provides a simple way to recognize the specific patterns in a given patient, it can enhance the efficacy and reduce the morbidity of frontal sinus surgery.

Case 2: Sphenoid and Sphenoethmoid Region

M.S., a 44-year-old woman with a history of sinonasal polyposis, described symptoms of facial pain, purulent nasal discharge, and anosmia. Medical management had been effective. She then underwent IG-FESS. Review of the preopera-

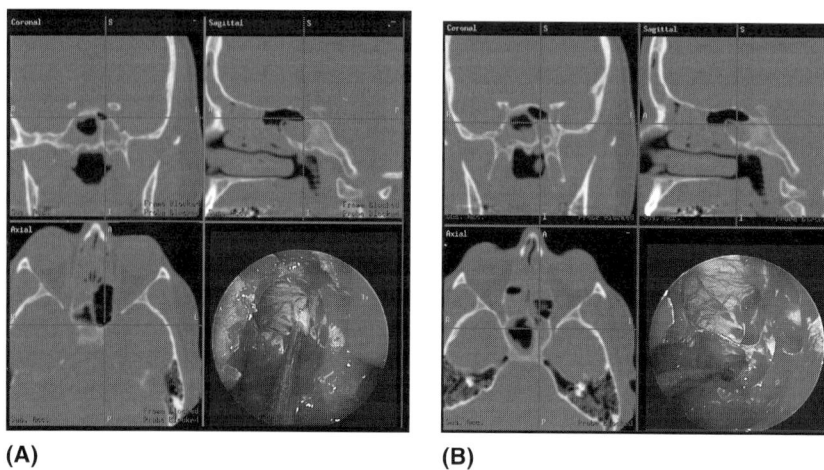

FIGURE 12.6 (A) The sphenoethmoid cell can be clearly identified on the sagittal image. This CAS screen capture shows the endoscopic view of the localizing suction as well as its localization relative to the preoperative CT scan images. In this way, identification of the sphenoethmoid cell is confirmed. (B) The sphenoethmoid cell can be clearly identified on the sagittal image. This CAS screen capture shows the endoscopic view of the localizing suction as well as its localization relative to the preoperative CT scan images. In this way, successful completion of the endoscopic sphenoidotomy is confirmed. (LandmarX 2.6.4, Medtronic Xomed, Jacksonville, FL.) (From Ref. 16.)

tive CT scan demonstrated the presence of left sphenoethmoid cell (Figure 12.6). Intraoperatively, the sphenoidotomy was performed safely and quickly; similarly, the sphenoethmoid cell was opened. Surgical navigation was used to confirm relevant landmarks, including the skull base, the sphenoid face, the sphenoid sinus, and the sphenoethmoid cell.

Neither standard coronal CT images nor intraoperative endoscopic views can conclusively demonstrate the presence or absence of sphenoethmoid cell. CAS can provide relatively straightforward information about this issue. Since the sphenoethmoid cell has a close anatomical relationship to the optic nerve and internal carotid artery, this information can be critically important.

Case 3: Residual Ethmoid Partitions and Sinonasal Polyposis

D.M., a 70-year-old woman with a history of chronic sinusitis, sinonasal polyposis, and asthma, described severe purulent rhinorrhea and secondary cough. She had received systemic corticosteroids and antibiotics, but her symptoms persisted.

She had also undergone a surgical procedure at another institution approximately 7 months earlier. Since her symptoms were persistent, she then underwent IG-FESS. As anticipated, her sinus mucosa had undergone extensive polypoid degeneration. The mucosa was hyperemic and bled easily. As a result, identification of surgical landmarks was difficult. The sagittal CT, which was reviewed on the CAS workstation, provided information about the number and location of residual ethmoid partitions (Figure 12.7). Each partition was sequentially identified and excised with through-cutting forceps. Surgical navigation was used to confirm each partition as well as location relative to the ethmoid roof and the lamina papyracea.

This case illustrates two critical points. In the bloody field, CAS surgical navigation can compensate for suboptimal endoscopic visualization. It should be emphasized that CAS is not a substitute for visualization; rather, CAS provides supplementary guidance. In addition, after previous partial or subtotal ethmoidectomy, CAS surgical navigation can assist the identification of each residual parti-

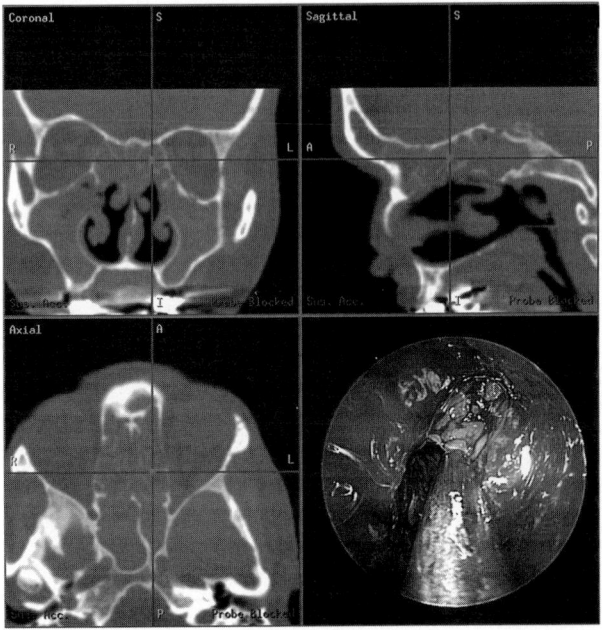

FIGURE 12.7 Residual ethmoid partitions can be easily seen on the sagittal CT scan. Intraoperative surgical navigation can be used to confirm positioning on each of these partitions. A representative localization is shown. (LandmarX 2.6.4, Medtronic Xomed, Jacksonville, FL.) (From Ref. 16.)

tion. Of course, such identification is necessary for the complete removal of each partition.

Case 4: Revision Maxillary Antrostomy

H.J., a 53-year-old woman who had undergone sinus surgery 4 years earlier and again 2 years earlier for chronic rhinosinusitis and sinonasal polyposis, described facial headache and purulent rhinorrhea. Initial treatment included culture-directed antibiotics and systemic corticosteroids, but this approach proved ineffective. She then underwent IG-FESS. Intraoperative findings included previous maxillary antrostomies. On each side, the endoscopic view suggested that residual uncinate process was present; however, the axial CT did not show residual uncinate process. CAS surgical navigation was used to confirm the anterior boundary of each maxillary antrostomy as well as each nasolacrimal system so that revision maxillary antrostomy could be achieved without nasolacrimal duct injury (Figure 12.8). Because of the previous surgery, formal uncinate removal was not neces-

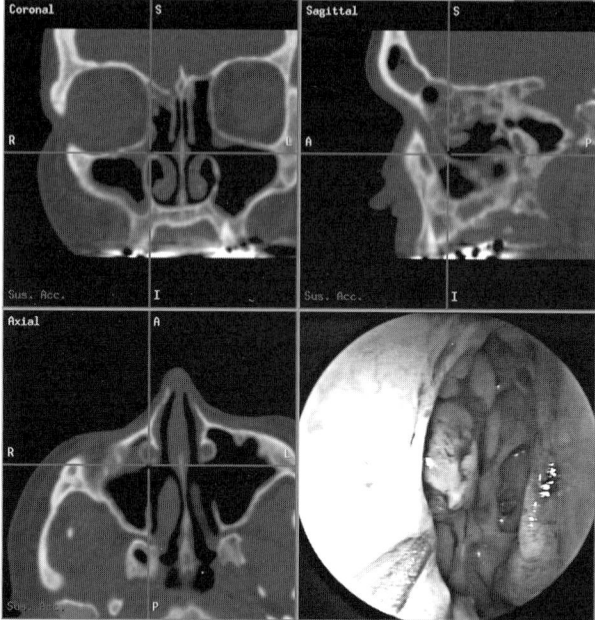

FIGURE 12.8 Localization at the anterior aspect of the previous maxillary antrostomy confirms the location of the nasolacrimal system. This information minimized the risk of inadvertent nasolacrimal system injury. The CAS screen capture shows the CT localization and corresponding endoscopic view. (LandmarX 2.6.4, Medtronic Xomed, Jacksonville, FL.) (From Ref. 16.)

sary; instead, polypoid mucosa and soft-tissue scar was cleared from the previous maxillary antrostomies under endoscopic visualization and CAS surgical navigation.

Although endoscopic maxillary antrostomy is a relatively simple procedure, in certain instances even maxillary antrostomy can be problematic. As a result, CAS guidance can be useful.

Case 5: Skull Base Identification

R.T., a 53-year-old man, whose history included previous surgery for refractory chronic sinusitis, described severe headaches, rhinorrhea, and cough. Since he had failed medical treatment, bilateral IG-FESS was performed. Intraoperative findings include previous middle turbinate resection as well as numerous residual ethmoid cells. The loss of the middle turbinate as a surgical landmark made visual identification of the skull base difficult. Osteitic new bone formation also compounded this problem. CAS surgical navigation was used to directly confirm the location of the ethmoid roof (Figure 12.9).

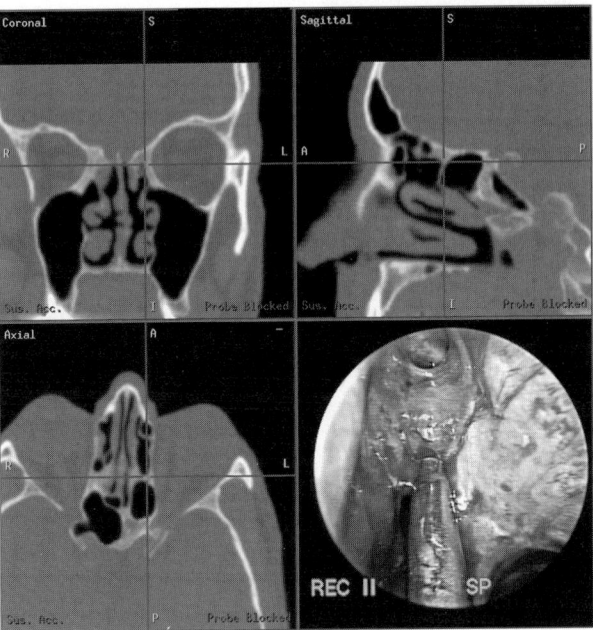

FIGURE 12.9 Localization along osteitic new bone in the posterior ethmoid confirms the skull base boundary location. The CAS screen capture shows the CT localization and corresponding endoscopic view. (LandmarX 2.6.4, Medtronic Xomed, Jacksonville, FL.) (From Ref. 16.)

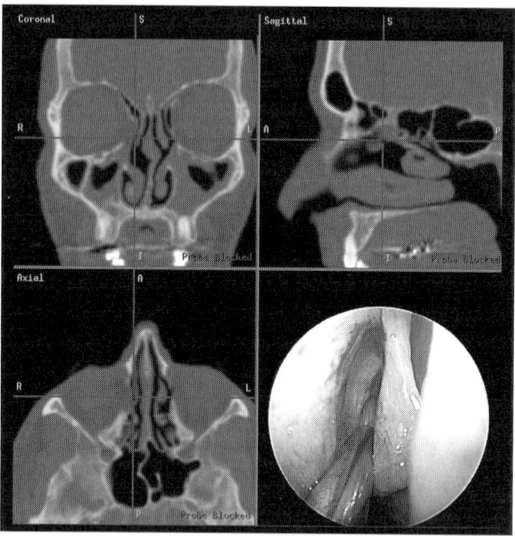

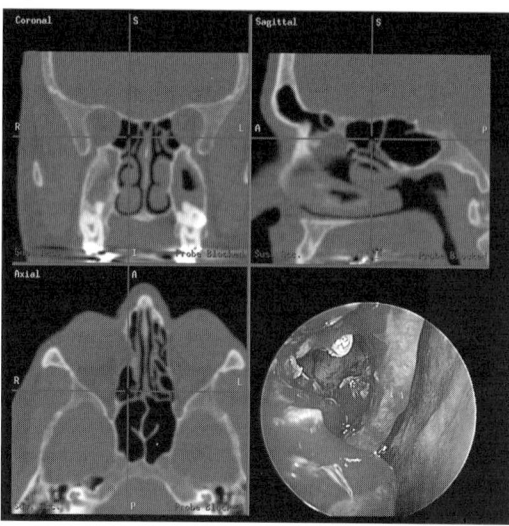

FIGURE 12.10 (A) A dehiscent medial orbital wall is seen on the coronal CT, but the endoscopic view suggests residual uncinate process. Intraoperative localization on the apparent "uncinate process" directly illustrates that the area of the dehiscence. (B) A dehiscent medial orbital wall is seen on the coronal CT, but the endoscopic view suggests residual uncinate process. Dissection around the dehiscence to the posterior ethmoid has been completed. In this CAS screen capture, localization to a posterior ethmoid cell is shown. The endoscopic image is a view into this posterior ethmoid cell. (LandmarX 2.6.4, Medtronic Xomed, Jacksonville, FL.) (From Ref. 16.)

Since the roof of the ethmoid defines the anatomical extent of superior dissection during endoscopic ethmoidectomy, the identification of the skull base is obviously important. Although this is a critical boundary from a surgical perspective, the ethmoid roof often does not have any distinguishing features. Previous surgery can further obscure landmarks, and the inflammatory changes, such as osteitic new bone formation, can further distort the anticipated anatomical relationship. In these instances, CAS surgical navigation can supply critical localization information.

Case 6: Orbital Dehiscence

L.M., a 60-year-old man with a history of chronic rhinosinusitis, sinonasal polyposis, and asthma, described episodic congestion, rhinorrhea, and midfacial pressure. He reported that he had received sinus surgery several years earlier; according to his recollection, the surgery was uneventful. His symptom severity seemed to be worsening, although he received aggressive medical treatment. He then underwent bilateral IG-FESS. Computer-enabled review of the preoperative CT scan revealed that the right medial orbital wall was partially dehiscent. Since he did not have a history of significant trauma, this finding was ascribed to his previous sinus surgery. Endoscopic examination of the right lateral nasal wall suggested residual uncinate process; in reality, the orbital dehiscence was mimicking the appearance of an uncinate process. During surgery, CAS surgical navigation was used to define the limits of the orbital wall dehiscence and to guide dissection around the dehiscence for access to the posterior ethmoid cells (Figure 12.10).

It is important to remember that the endoscopic view can be misleading. In this case, the orbital dehiscence was the critical finding, but the endoscopic view suggested residual uncinate process! CAS defined the extent of the orbital dehiscence and intraoperatively, the boundaries of dehiscence, was mapped by successive localizations. This case also demonstrates another critical point. Previous surgery can disrupt standard anatomy in ways that are difficult to predict. CAS can minimize this complexity if revision surgery proves necessary.

12.7 INDICATIONS FOR CAS IN SINUS SURGERY

Discussions about the indications for CAS in sinus surgery have engendered considerable debate and controversy. Most surgeons will at least admit that CAS has the greatest role in the more complex rhinologic surgeries. Of course, procedural complexity reflects anatomical complexity; as a result, CAS is most useful for surgery of the frontal recess, the sphenoethmoid recess, and the posterior ethmoid region. In addition, certain conditions can obscure anatomical landmarks—making procedures, which would otherwise be simple and straightforward, especially complex and challenging. Therefore, sinonasal polyposis, pansinusitis, and previous surgery can all be considered indications for CAS in sinus surgery.

It is important to consider those instances in which CAS is probably inappropriate. Simple, limited procedures do not require CAS. For instance, endoscopic maxillary antrostomy for isolated chronic maxillary sinusitis in a patient who has failed medical treatment but has not already undergone sinus surgery would not routinely require CAS.

The indications for CAS are relative, not absolute indications. The decision to use CAS is really at the discretion of the rhinologic surgeon, since CAS is merely a tool that the operating surgeon may select for a specific application. CAS is not a substitute for surgical expertise.

12.8 LIMITATIONS

Since IG-FESS depends upon the robustness of CAS technology, surgeons must be cognizant of the limitations of CAS. With such knowledge, the surgeon may recognize CAS technical failures early and thereby avoid potentially catastrophic complications. In addition, the knowledgeable surgeon can better integrate CAS into his surgical decision-making and execution.

The limitations of CAS for sinus surgery can be divided into three categories:

1. Since current CAS platforms rely upon preoperative CT images, intraoperative surgical navigation cannot reflect the anatomical changes caused by the actual procedures. For soft tissue surgery, where intraoperative tissue deformation can be significant, this limitation may be a major problem; however, standard sinus surgery is performed within a bony box, which is the ideal environment for surgical navigation that depends upon preoperative imaging. Intraoperative MR and CT scanners may permit real-time updates for surgical navigation, but they have not been fully integrated with CAS surgical navigation. Furthermore, intraoperative scanners are cumbersome, time-consuming, and expensive. Also, the quality of the images from current intraoperative scanners is also less than the quality of comparable preoperative images, since the intraoperative scanners use faster scan sequences and thicker scan slices. The poorer resolution of these images limits the maximal surgical navigation accuracy that they can support.
2. Accurate surgical navigation depends upon precise registration. If the registration tightly maps imaging data set volume to the surgical field of the real world, then surgical navigation will be optimal. It should be emphasized that all registration protocols are less than perfect. Even registration based upon bone-anchored fiducial markers may be com-

Image-Guided Functional Endoscopic Sinus Surgery

promised by minor deviations in instrument tracking precision. Bent instruments can also degrade registration. Registration protocols also contain adaptations so that the CAS system is more useful in the clinical setting. Bone-anchored fiducial markers clearly provide the best registration accuracy, but they are unacceptable for ambulatory procedures (such as sinus surgery). As a result, alternative approaches for registration—including anatomical fiducial points, surface contour mapping, and DRF headset frames—have been developed. Although these alternatives increase the usability of the system, they all degrade registration accuracy to a certain degree. In general, this trade-off has been considered an acceptable compromise. Since registration is the critical step in intraoperative surgical navigation, all surgeons who use CAS must be able to recognize registration failures and troubleshoot registration problems.

3. Hardware failure and software bugs can compromise all CAS systems. Although these problems are becoming less common, they can occur in all systems. Most CAS platforms include diagnostics, which can help determine the source of a potential system failure. For instance, optically based systems often can display aiming information that depicts the relationship between the overhead camera array and the DRF. Software engineers and designers have modified the CAS software interfaces so that these software diagnostic tools are more helpful. Surgeons should be familiar with these aspects of the software.

Although CAS is an impressive tool for sinus surgery, CAS is not a substitute for surgical expertise. CAS merely provides additional information that can simplify complex procedures. As a result, CAS is an enabling technology. It does not radically change the nature of the surgery; rather CAS facilitates the completion of procedures according to currently accepted surgical principles. CAS does not change the details of the surgery.

12.9 CONCLUSION

The image-guided functional endoscopic sinus surgery paradigm incorporates CAS technology into sinus surgery. CAS provides intraoperative surgical navigation as well as a series of software tools that support computer-enabled review of preoperative CT images. Because of the anatomical complexity of paranasal sinuses, rhinologic surgeons have begun to embrace CAS as a means of improving surgical outcomes and decreasing surgical morbidity. Clinical experiences have shown that CAS is most helpful in the frontal recess, in the sphenoethmoid recess, in the posterior ethmoid and at the roof of the ethmoid. In addition, CAS offers significant advantages in specific situations, including previous sinus surgery, extensive sinonasal polyposis, and other scenarios that are characterized by a loss of surgical landmarks. CAS (namely preoperative computer-based CT review and intraoperative surgical navigation) should be routinely utilized for these more complex cases. This IG-FESS paradigm should serve to decrease surgical morbidity and increase surgical effectiveness.

REFERENCES

1. JB Anon. Computer-aided endoscopic sinus surgery. Laryngoscope 108:949–961., 1998.
2. JB Anon, L Klimek, R Mosges, et al. Computer-assisted endoscopic sinus surgery. An international review. Otolaryngol Clin North Am 30:389–401, 1997.
3. JB Anon, SP Lipman, D Oppenheim, et al. Computer-assisted endoscopic sinus surgery. Laryngoscope 104:901–905, 1994.
4. M Roth, DC Lanza, J Zinreich, et al. Advantages and disadvantages of three-dimensional computed tomography intraoperative localization for functional endoscopic sinus surgery. Laryngoscope 105:1279–1286, 1995.
5. MP Fried, J Kleefield, R Taylor. New armless image-guidance system for endoscopic sinus surgery. Otolaryngol Head Neck Surg 119:528–532, 1998.
6. MP Fried, PR Morrison. Computer-augmented endoscopic sinus surgery. Otolaryngol Clin North Am 31:331–340, 1998.
7. R Metson. Intraoperative image-guidance technology. Arch Otolaryngol Head Neck Surg 125:1278–1279, 1999.
8. R Metson, M Cosenza, RE Gliklich, et al. The role of image-guidance systems for head and neck surgery. Arch Otolaryngol Head Neck Surg 125:1100–1104, 1999.
9. R Metson, RE Gliklich, M Cosenza. A comparison of image guidance systems for sinus surgery. Laryngoscope 108:1164–1170, 1998.
10. Messerklinger W. Über die Drainage der Menschlichen Nasennebenholen unter nomalen und pathologischen Bedingungen: II. Mitteilung die Stirnhohle und ihr Ausfuhrungssystem. Monatsschr Ohrenheilkd 101:313–326, 1967.
11. Messerklinger W. On the drainage of the normal frontal sinus of man. Acta Otolaryngol 63:176–181, 1967.
12. Messerklinger W. Über den Recessus Frontalis und seine Klinik. Larynol Rhinol Otol 61:217–223, 1982.
13. Messerklinger W. Endoscopy of the Nose. Urban & Schwarzenberg, Baltimore, 1978.
14. DW Kennedy, SJ Zinreich, AE Rosenbaum, et al. Functional endoscopic sinus surgery (theory and diagnostic evaluation). Arch Otolaryngol 111:576–582, 1985.
15. DW Kennedy. Functional endoscopic sinus surgery (technique). Arch Otolaryngol Head Neck Surg 111:643–649, 1985.
16. G Olson, MJ Citardi. Image-guided functional endoscopic sinus surgery. Otolaryngol Head Neck Surg 123:188–194, 2000.
17. International Society for Computer-Aided Surgery. Computer-aided surgery: aims and scope. www.iscas.org/aims.html 1999 (abstract).

13

Computer-Aided Revision Sinus Surgery

**Michael J. Sillers, M.D., F.A.C.S., and
Christy R. Buckman, M.D.**
University of Alabama–Birmingham, Birmingham, Alabama

13.1 INTRODUCTION

Functional endoscopic sinus surgery (FESS) has become the standard surgical approach for medically refractory paranasal sinus disease since its introduction in the United States in 1985. It is estimated that over 400,000 sinus surgeries are performed each year. Successful outcomes are realized in 76–97.5% of patients, and approximately 10–15% of surgical patients will require revision surgery [1–11]. Kennedy reported a strong correlation between the extent of disease and eventual surgical outcome [6]. Patients with limited disease were more likely to have resolution of their symptoms when compared to patients with more extensive disease. Independent variables, such as asthma, aspirin sensitivity, prior surgery, and allergy did not influence surgical outcome, but the extent of disease noted on preoperative computed tomography (CT) scans was an important factor.

With an incidence of revision surgery of 10–15 % of patients, a significant number of patients will require revision sinus surgery. Most patients who are considered surgical failures become symptomatic within 2–18 months of primary FESS [1]. Perhaps the most difficult, yet most important, challenge in these patients is determining the cause(s) of failure. Potential etiologies include uncontrolled allergic disease, underlying immunological disorder, ciliary dyskinesia, and osteitis. Incomplete surgery and/or scar tissue formation may interfere with paranasal sinus ventilation and drainage and thus lead to revision surgery. The initial evaluation of postoperative patients with persistent/recurrent sinusitis should focus on potential nonsurgical etiologies. If such an etiology is confirmed, then appropriate treatment can be instituted. If systems persist despite such treatment or the search for such an etiology is inconclusive, then careful comprehensive nasal endoscopy, in conjunction with repeat CT scans, will often identify a disease focus that is amenable to revision surgery [8]. Since the normal landmarks have been altered by the previous surgery and/or persistent inflammatory disease, intraoperative recognition of critical structures by endoscopic criteria alone can be very challenging. Computer-aided surgery (CAS), which incorporates software-enabled review of preoperative images as well as intraoperative surgical navigation and localization, can provide critical supplemental information and thereby improve surgical outcomes.

Functional endoscopic sinus surgery has a reported major complication rate of 0–8% [3,12–18]. Major complications include orbital injuries with significant sequelae such as restricted gaze, altered vision, or even blindness. Penetration of the ethmoid roof may result in cerebrospinal fluid fistula, meningitis, or brain abscess. Death may result from catastrophic injury to the cavernous portion of the internal carotid artery or severe brain injury. Minor complications, including bleeding requiring packing, symptomatic synechia formation, periorbital ecchymosis and/or emphysema, and temporary epiphora occur in up to 21% of patients [3,12–18]. Several authors have reported their results with revision FESS: there does not appear to be a higher incidence of major or minor complications with these procedures (compared with primary FESS cases) [1,19,20]. To the extent that CAS facilitates the surgeon's comprehension of intraoperative anatomy, it may be anticipated that risk of both minor and major complications should decrease.

13.2 PATTERNS OF SURGICAL FAILURES

When performing revision FESS, the most important features to recognize are the alterations of normal anatomical surgical landmarks. Most commonly one finds scar tissue between the middle turbinate and the lateral nasal wall [1–4,19]. This scar tissue will contract with time and result in middle turbinate lateralization (Figure 13.1). Scar tissue may also obscure the maxillary sinus natural ostium as well as make identification of the lamina papyracea and anterior skull base difficult [1,4,6,19,21]. When there has been prior partial or complete middle turbinate resection, the orientation for the revision surgeon is significantly altered (Figure 13.2). The inferior free edge of a shortened middle turbinate remnant will be closer to the ethmoid roof when compared to an intact middle turbinate.

Computer-Aided Revision Sinus Surgery

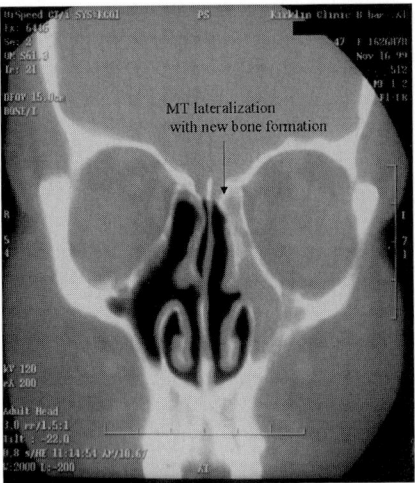

FIGURE 13.1 This coronal CT shows left middle turbinate lateralization with new bone formation in the ethmoid cavity. Soft tissue density, likely scar, obstructs outflow from the maxillary sinus, which is opacified. The inferior border of the preserved middle turbinate lies in the same axial plane as the maxillary sinus infundibulum.

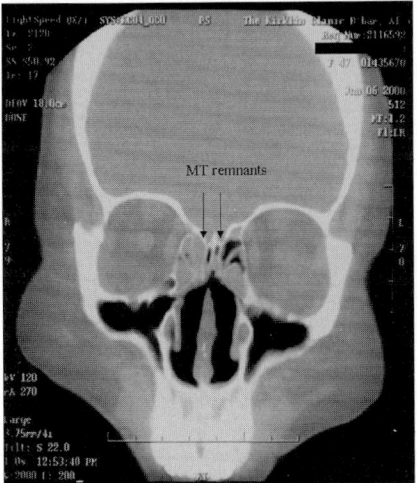

FIGURE 13.2 This coronal CT demonstrate previous inferior, middle, and superior turbinate resection. The ethmoid sinuses are opacified. The inferior border of the middle turbinate remnant sits superior to the maxillary sinus natural ostium in the axial plane. There is residual uncinate process on each side.

Failure to recognize this may lead to an otherwise avoidable injury of the ethmoid roof. Also, the position of the maxillary sinus ostium will appear "lower" in comparison with an intact middle turbinate. Penetration of the lamina papyracea may result if the inferior border of a shortened middle turbinate is used as a landmark during a revision maxillary antrostomy in the presence of a scarred lateral nasal wall

13.3 REPORTS OF CAS IN FESS

The primary goals of surgical navigation are the reduction of complications and the improvement in outcomes as a result of early anatomical landmark recognition and increased surgical precision. With CAS, important anatomical surgical landmarks such as the lamina papyracea, middle turbinate basal lamella, sphenoid face, frontal recess, and posterior skull base can be more easily identified by correlating endoscopic and multiplanar CT images. Although it appears that CAS will allow for increased surgical precision and decreased complications, this has not been proven definitively [22–26].

In a review of the first 107 consecutive patients undergoing endoscopic sinus surgery of the paranasal sinuses and anterior skull base with CAS, Neumann et al. reported no major complications [20]. Minor complications, including persistent symptomatic synechiae (4/107) and postoperative bleeding requiring placement of packing (1/107), occurred in 4.7% of patients. Overall 81 of 107 patients were diagnosed with chronic rhinosinusitis, 78% of whom had undergone prior sinus surgery. Revision surgery was required in 4.7% of patients (5/107). CAS was utilized with an estimated accuracy of better than 3 mm in 97.2% of cases (104/107). In three patients the estimated accuracy was worse than 3 mm. In these cases, CAS was therefore not used. Since this paper was a description of an early experience utilizing new technology, long-term outcomes were not reported.

Caversaccio et al. reported their experience in 25 patients undergoing revision surgery using CAS [26]. Results were compared to a control group of 10 patients undergoing revision FESS without CAS. The reported surgical navigation accuracy was 0.5–2.0 mm. There were no major or minor complications in either group. The author emphasized the improved ability to localize important surgical landmarks with CAS and a subsequent decrease in operator anxiety when compared to patients operated without surgical navigation.

Metson et al. reported 34 surgeons' experience with CAS in 754 patients undergoing sinonasal surgery [27]. Chronic rhinosinusitis was the most common diagnosis. There were no major or minor complications, and outcomes were not reported. In a survey of participating surgeons, 71% responded that they would utilize CAS for revision sinus surgery, while 11% would use surgical navigation in all cases.

Complete description of the numerous reports devoted to CAS in sinus surgery is beyond the scope of this brief discussion. Other authors have presented similar experiences and have described similar conclusions.

13.4 DESCRIPTION OF TECHNIQUE

After the diagnosis of refractory rhinosinusitis, which has persisted despite aggressive medical treatment and previous surgery, has been confirmed, revision FESS may be necessary. Informed consent for the procedure should include an explicit discussion of the surgical risks, including bleeding, scar tissue formation, persistent or new infection, blurred vision, double vision, blindness, cerebrospinal fluid leak, meningitis, brain abscess, brain injury, and death. In addition, the use of CAS should also be discussed with the patient. Since CAS is a new and exciting technology, there is some tendency to overstate its potential benefits. Care should be taken to avoid this problem.

Before surgery, an appropriate CT scan should be obtained. For CAS, direct axial images, from which the CAS workstation can reconstruct coronal and sagittal images and three-dimensional models, are necessary. Preoperative image data may be transferred to the CAS workstation via local networks or on digital media (such as optical disks). In general, the quality of the reconstructed images will be better with thinner axial slice thickness. Software algorithms within the CAS workstation help avoid the stair-stepped appearance of the reconstructed images. One must realize, however, that these reconstructed coronal and sagittal images contain computer-generated data and may not accurately represent the patient's anatomy.

It is helpful to study the multiplanar images (axial, coronal, and sagittal) as part of presurgical planning. Residual ethmoid air cell walls and/or areas of new bone formation can be seen, and their relationships to the ethmoid roof, lamina papyracea, and sphenoid sinus can be appreciated. Structures such as the optic nerve and the cavernous sinus portion of the internal carotid artery can be followed by "scrolling" through images in one plane while following them in the other two planes. This maneuver can provide invaluable information as to areas at risk for catastrophic complications. With current CAS workstations, utilizing a variety of headsets, reference frames, and registration techniques, there is virtually no need to obtain additional CT's immediately prior to performing CAS; that is, the CT scan may be completed days, weeks, or even months prior to the surgery. Of course, long delays between the CT scan and actual surgery are not advisable for other reasons, but at least the newer systems avoid the need for CT scans on the day of surgery.

Computer-aided revision sinus surgery can be performed under local anesthesia with intravenous sedation or general anesthesia. The choice of anesthetic may be based on the surgeon's preference. The specific details of the set-up of the CAS equipment reflects the design and technology of the CAS platform chosen for the procedure. For sinus surgery, essentially all systems employ a headset that provides a reference frame for surgical navigation. Before surgical navigation can be used, registration, a calibration process through which the computer correlates corresponding points in the surgical volume and CT scan data set volume, must be completed. Each CAS system has its own registration protocol. (For a complete discussion of these issues, please refer to Chapters 3, 4, 11, and 12). Then the CAS surgical instruments, which may include straight and curved aspirators, the microdebrider, and through-biting forceps, may be calibrated.

After registration is completed, the accuracy of surgical navigation should be confirmed. An estimate of accuracy is made by comparing known endoscopic anatomical landmarks with the corresponding CAS localizations displayed on the computer monitor. It is helpful to utilize anatomical structures that are not likely to be altered during the revision surgical procedure. Such landmarks include the posterior choana, the vomer of the nasal septum, and the maxillary crest. These anatomical verification points must be utilized throughout the surgical procedure whenever a question regarding localization accuracy arises. Confidence in the reliability of the localization during the surgical procedure is enhanced if the initial correlation between anatomical landmarks and corresponding localizations is estimated to be within 1–2 mm.

After the surgery has begun, it is important to reassess the accuracy of the system against known points. If surgical navigation accuracy does not appear to correlate well with these anatomical landmarks, the initial anatomical verification points—which had indicated acceptable accuracy at the beginning of the case—should be reexamined with the localizing probe. Any inaccuracies should be reconciled. The reference frame position and/or headset should be inspected for proper placement. Repeat registration should be performed if necessary. If the inaccuracies cannot be reconciled, the CAS workstation should not be utilized during the procedure.

After an acceptable registration has been achieved, diagnostic nasal endoscopy is performed with a CAS localizing probe, such as a straight aspirator. This allows the surgeon to correlate endoscopic images and the preoperative CT scan data as a step in the revision sinus operation. In particular, determining the relationship of the middle turbinate or its remnant to the lateral nasal wall provides reliable orientation early in the revision surgical procedure. If the middle and superior turbinates have been completely resected, identification of the sphenoid face and posterior ethmoid roof are early goals. Finally, if the maxillary sinus natural ostium or an accessory ostium can be found, the posterior maxillary sinus wall and its roof can be visualized with an angled telescope. By correlating these maxillary sinus landmarks with its medial wall, the lamina papyracea can be located and established as the lateral boundary of the ethmoid dissection. Any of the above-mentioned techniques can be used, depending on the specific clinical situation.

Computer-Aided Revision Sinus Surgery

The goal of revision ethmoid surgery is the wide marsupialization of the ethmoid labyrinth. This involves removal of all remaining ethmoid air cell walls by dissecting along the lamina papyracea and ethmoid roof while preserving surgical landmarks, such as the middle turbinate basal lamella and its anterior vertical attachment. Of course, maximum mucosal preservation should be attempted. Through-biting instruments are helpful when removing bone from the ethmoid roof and lamina papyracea since they reduce the torque placed on these bony cell wall remnants when compared with curettes and standard grasping forceps.

13.5 SPECIFIC SURGICAL SCENARIOS

One of the most common diagnoses of patients undergoing revision endoscopic sinus surgery is sinonasal polyposis. It is also common for these patients to have had more extensive surgery than nonpolyposis patients. Frequently the middle and superior turbinates have been partially resected. Figure 13.3 depicts a coronal CT image of a patient with recurrent symptomatic nasal polyposis, refractory to medical therapy. Partial resection of inferior, middle, and superior turbinates had

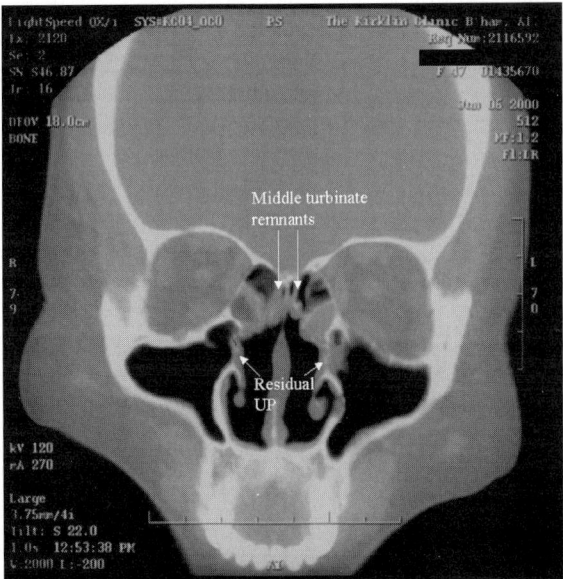

FIGURE 13.3 This coronal CT depicts prior middle turbinate resection and associated ethmoid sinus opacification. The left posterior ethmoid cavity is aerated and represents a key early landmark in this patient's revision ethmoid surgery. The uncinate process is intact bilaterally.

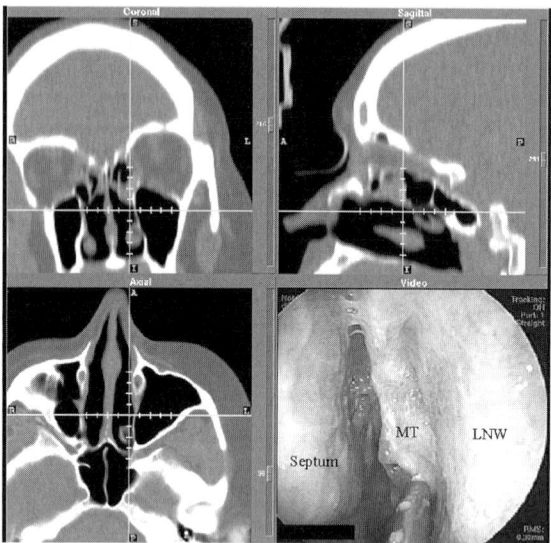

FIGURE 13.4 At the beginning of a revision FESS procedure, diagnostic nasal endoscopy coupled with CAS defines the relevant anatomy. In addition, the accuracy of surgical navigation can be confirmed. In this example, the endoscopic image shows the position of the localizing aspirator. The multiplanar CT images (namely the coronal, sagittal, and axial images in the orthogonal planes through a specific point) show the calculated position of the instrument tip. The middle turbinate is lateralized and there is polypoid mucosa in the middle meatus. The lateral nasal wall (LNW) can be seen. In this way, navigation accuracy is confirmed and key structures may be appropriately localized.

been performed during the patient's initial surgery. A superior nasal septal perforation is present, and both uncinate processes are intact.

During the revision CAS procedure, the first step is to establish the accuracy of surgical navigation by localizing to a known landmark. In Figure 13.4, the multiplanar CT images shows a representative localization that confirms system accuracy; that is, the tip of the probe is seen at the inferior portion of the middle turbinate basal lamella. The sagittal image depicts this information well. Figure 13.4 also demonstrates that the left middle turbinate remnant is scarred to the lateral nasal wall and the mucosa is polypoid. Penetration of the basal lamella allowed the surgeon to enter the posterior ethmoid cavity and readily identify the posterior ethmoid skull base. This can be seen in the next set of multiplanar CT and endoscopic images (Figure 13.5).

Figure 13.6 shows the right nasal cavity in the same patient. The middle turbinate has been partially resected. The multiplanar CT and endoscopic images

Computer-Aided Revision Sinus Surgery

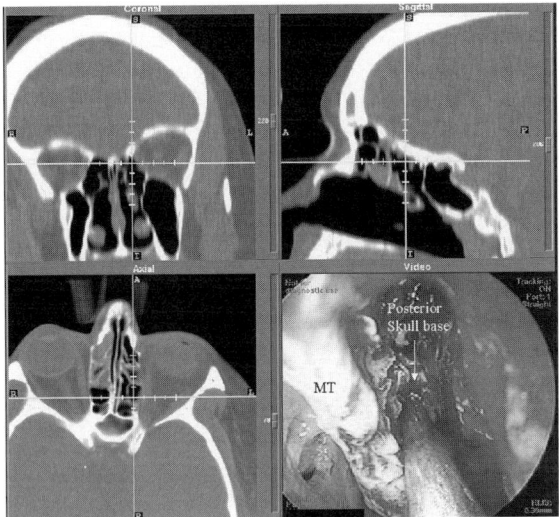

FIGURE 13.5 After penetration of the left middle turbinate basal lamella, the position of the ethmoid roof must be determined. In this instance, the skull base is clearly seen, and the CT scan images obtained via surgical navigation confirm this landmark.

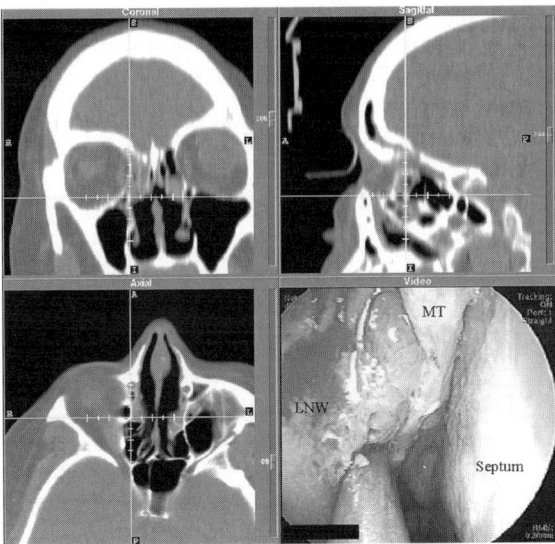

FIGURE 13.6 This intraoperative CAS screen capture shows the precise location of the localizing aspirator in the anterior middle meatus. The right middle turbinate (MT) has been partially resected, and its inferior border is superior to the maxillary sinus natural ostium in the axial plane.

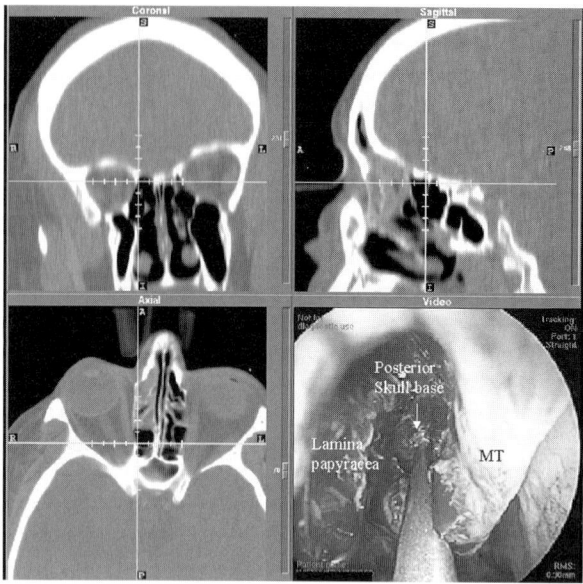

FIGURE 13.7 Another intraoperative CAS screen capture depicts localization through a point in the right posterior ethmoid. The right middle turbinate basal lamella has been penetrated for access to the posterior ethmoid, and the skull base has been identified in the posterior ethmoid cavity. The probe tip is at the junction of the lateral skull base and the superior aspect of the lamina papyracea. The optic nerve is not at immediate risk, as seen on the axial image.

depict the inferomedial boundary of the lamina papyracea and the inferior edge of the middle turbinate remnant. In this anatomical situation, the inferior border of the middle turbinate can mislead the surgeon in regard to the proper location of the maxillary sinus natural ostium. If a "blind" maxillary antrostomy were created in this location, the orbit could be easily penetrated. Instead, careful search for the uncinate process and its complete removal resulted in the proper and safe identification of the natural ostium of the maxillary sinus. Then the middle turbinate basal lamella was penetrated under CAS guidance, and the posterior skull base position was verified (Figure 13.7). After precise identification of the lamina papyracea and the skull base in the posterior ethmoid cavity, the ethmoid cavity was then marsupialized by removing cell wall remnants. In this situation, through-biting forceps are helpful by reducing unnecessary torque and aiding in mucosal preservation (Figures 13.8 and 13.9).

Identification of the anterior vertical attachment of the middle turbinate can be a helpful landmark in the presence of residual and/or recurrent anterior eth-

Computer-Aided Revision Sinus Surgery

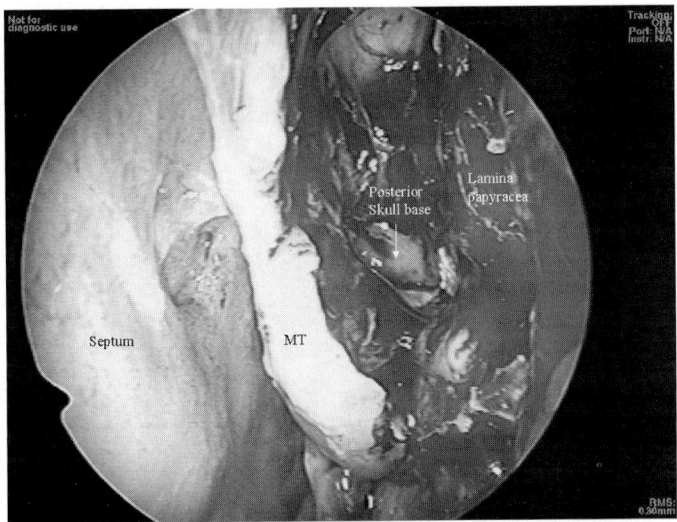

FIGURE 13.8 This endoscopic image shows the appearance of the left nasal cavity at the completion of computer-aided revision FESS. The middle turbinate remnant has been preserved and remaining ethmoid cell walls have been removed.

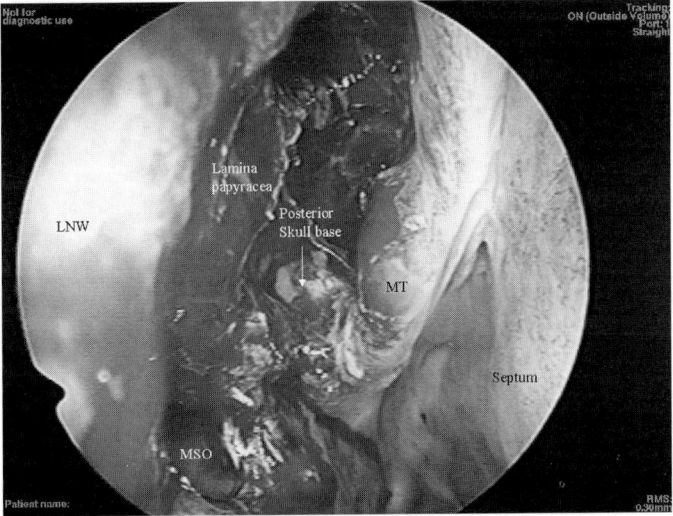

FIGURE 13.9 This endoscopic image shows the appearance of the right nasal cavity at the completion of computer-aided revision FESS. The middle turbinate remnant has been preserved and the natural ostium of the maxillary sinus can be seen. Ethmoid cell wall remnants have been removed from the skull base and lamina papyracea.

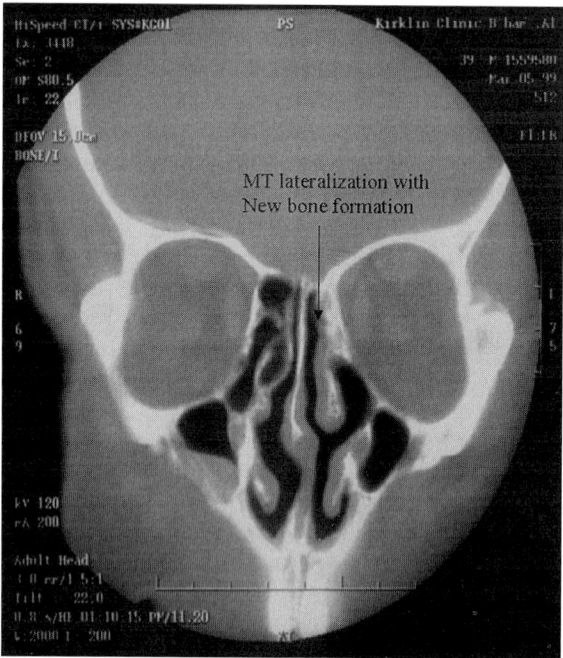

FIGURE 13.10 This coronal CT image demonstrates left middle turbinate lateralization that mimics the endoscopic appearance of a shortened ethmoid.

moid and frontal recess disease; however, in revision FESS cases, careful examination of the preoperative CT may show that this endoscopic landmark has become distorted. In a primary case, ethmoid air cells are located posterior and lateral to the vertical attachment of the middle turbinate. In a revision case, the vertical attachment of the middle turbinate may become lateralized and scarred to the lamina papyracea, resulting in an anterior ethmoid sinus mucocele (Figures 13.10 and 13.11). This creates a misrepresentation of the position of the anterior ethmoid roof and residual ethmoid cell wall remnants from a purely endoscopic viewpoint. Endoscopic dissection in this scarred middle meatus may lead to an inadvertent orbital injury and/or unsuccessful drainage of the mucocele. Appropriate marsupialization of the mucocele in this situation should be performed anterior to the middle turbinate vertical attachment. Increased confidence in choosing the proper location for drainage is improved with CAS by correlating these structures endoscopically with the multiplanar CT images.

Patients who have undergone orbital decompression for Graves' ophthalmopathy may develop symptoms of chronic rhinosinusitis. This is likely to be

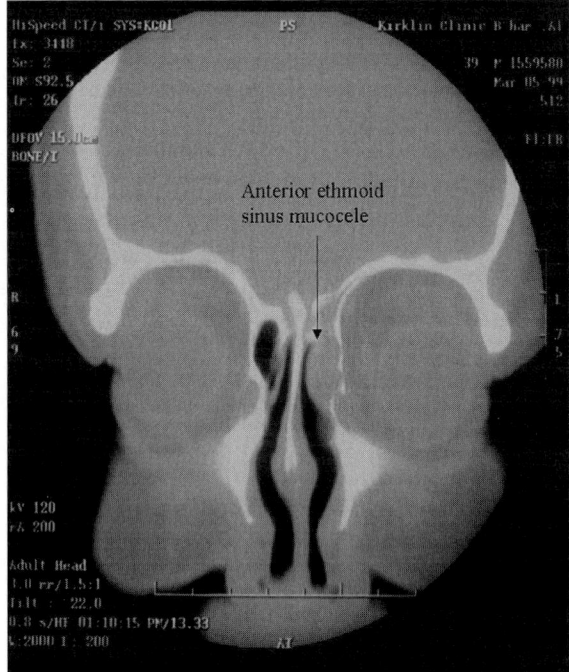

FIGURE 13.11 This coronal CT image is slightly anterior to the image in Figure 13.10. An anterior ethmoid sinus mucocele, resulting from middle turbinate lateralization, is seen.

worse in patients who have undergone prior radiotherapy, which may lead to secondary damage of mucociliary clearance mechanisms. Surprisingly, Mann found that in his series of 23 patients no patient required revision sinus surgery and rather aggressive medical therapy and extended follow-up were sufficient [28]. Of course, some Graves' patients may have concomitant paranasal sinus disease and require eventual surgery. Figure 13.12 depicts anterior ethmoid opacification in a patient who has already received orbital decompression. Under CAS guidance, the inferior and superior margins of lamina papyracea resection could be identified as well as intact lamina papyracea posteriorly. A plane between the orbital fat and the anterior ethmoid polyps was identified by endoscopic criteria; in this way, the careful removal of the polyps proceeded without injury to the orbital contents (Figure 13.13). A similar situation may occur in patients who have undergone a previous external ethmoidectomy approach. In the absence of a true bony wall separating the ethmoid sinus from orbital contents, powered instrumentation should be used with extreme caution. Orbital fat and/or the me-

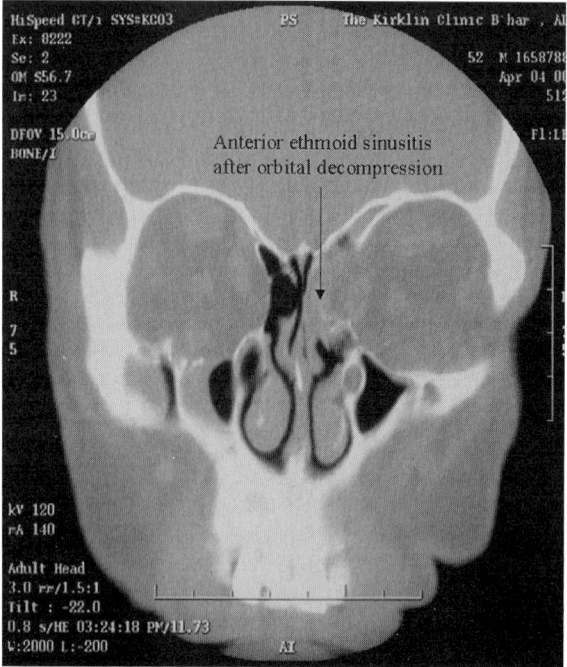

FIGURE 13.12 This coronal CT image shows left anterior ethmoid sinus opacification after prior external orbital decompression. Note the absence of the lamina papyracea.

dial rectus muscle can be pulled into the oscillating blade, which can injure soft tissues quickly and easily.

In extreme cases of prior surgical alteration of landmarks, CAS is invaluable in identifying even the most basic landmarks. Figure 13.14 depicts a patient in whom both traditional surgical approaches (namely Caldwell-Luc procedures) and intranasal endoscopic techniques have been utilized for the treatment of nasal polyposis. One can appreciate the absence of reliable landmarks. In these patients, CAS perhaps offers the most assistance. In this case, the left posterior ethmoid roof and lamina papyracea was identified endoscopically and verified through surgical navigation early during the surgical procedure. Similarly, the right posterior ethmoid roof and lamina papyracea was identified after penetration of the remnant of the middle turbinate basal lamella.

In patients with diffuse sinonasal polyposis, which may be associated with tissue hyperemia and significant intraoperative blood loss, CAS is a useful adjunct. Patients with extensive disease are likely to have more bleeding when compared to patients with less extensive disease. While this blood loss is not

Computer-Aided Revision Sinus Surgery

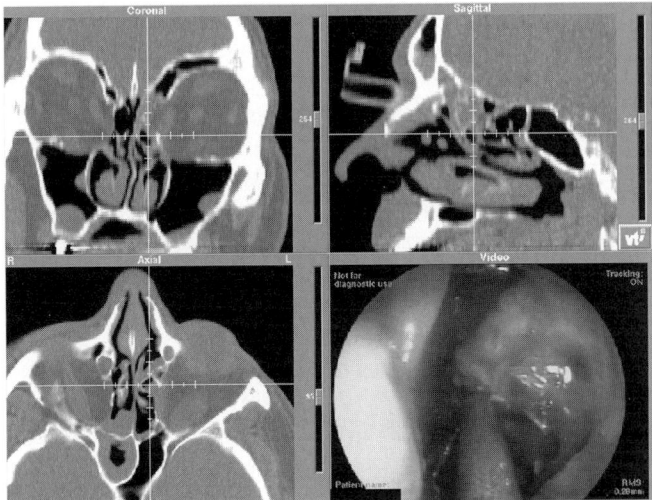

FIGURE 13.13 This intraoperative CAS screen capture was obtained during computer-aided FESS in a patient who had previously undergone orbital decompression. In the endoscopic image, anterior ethmoid sinus polyps are seen adjacent to orbital fat. The relative position of the instrument tip is shown by the crosshairs on the CT images.

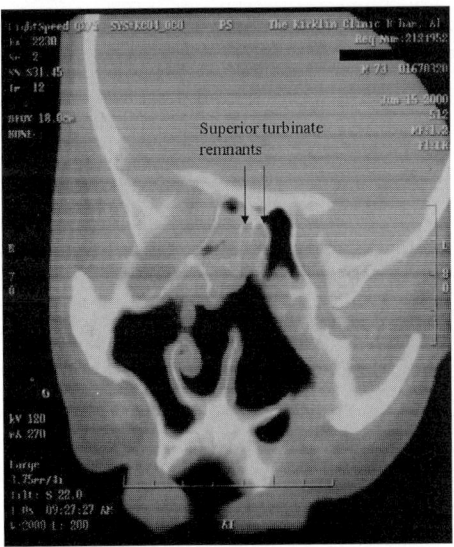

FIGURE 13.14 This coronal CT image depicts the absence of surgical landmarks as well as a large nasal septal perforation in patient who had previously undergone a Caldwell-Luc procedure as well as extensive transnasal endoscopic surgery. The left posterior ethmoid sinus is aerated and provides a reliable landmark early in the revision surgery.

likely to be physiologically significant, it may obscure visualization, making the surgical procedure more difficult. It is important to remember that if visualization is poor and reasonable hemostasis cannot be achieved, the procedure should be terminated. FESS is largely performed on an elective basis for benign inflammatory disease, and major complications are difficult to justify.

In patients with allergic fungal sinusitis with diffuse polyposis, landmarks are difficult to identify because of the fungal debris, allergic mucin, and polypoid mucosa (Figure 13.15). With CAS, the surgeon can more readily localize the lamina papyracea and the skull base.

In some cases, revision ethmoid surgery is performed in the presence of new bone formation. Typically osteoneogenesis occurs adjacent to areas of inflammation. New bone may form to the extent of causing obstruction of outflow from the paranasal sinuses. Figure 13.16 shows new bone formation along the ethmoid roof bilaterally. Previously, the patient had undergone drainage of a right frontal sinus mucocele with an acute orbital abscess. After resolution of the acute inflammatory process, follow-up CT scanning showed bilateral frontal sinus opacification with anterior ethmoid sinus opacification. Using CAS, the new bone formation in the anterior ethmoid sinus and frontal recess was reduced

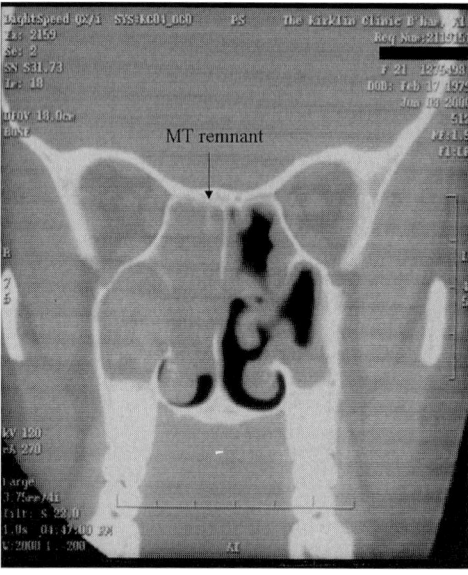

FIGURE 13.15 This coronal CT image shows many of the common features seen in allergic fungal sinusitis. Differing densities are notable in the right maxillary sinus. The ethmoid sinus is filled with soft tissue density, but no bony remnants are visible.

Computer-Aided Revision Sinus Surgery

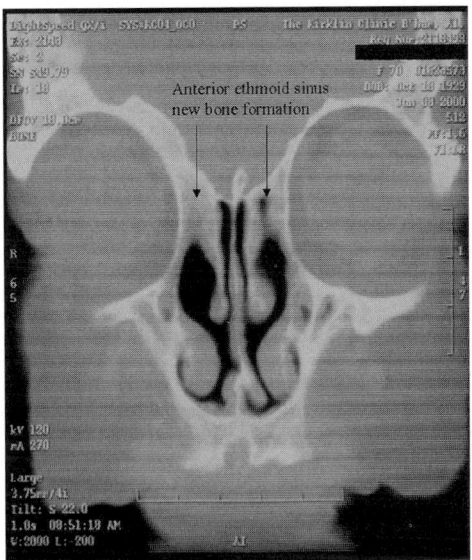

FIGURE 13.16 This coronal CT image demonstrates osteoneogenesis (new bone formation) along the ethmoid roof bilaterally.

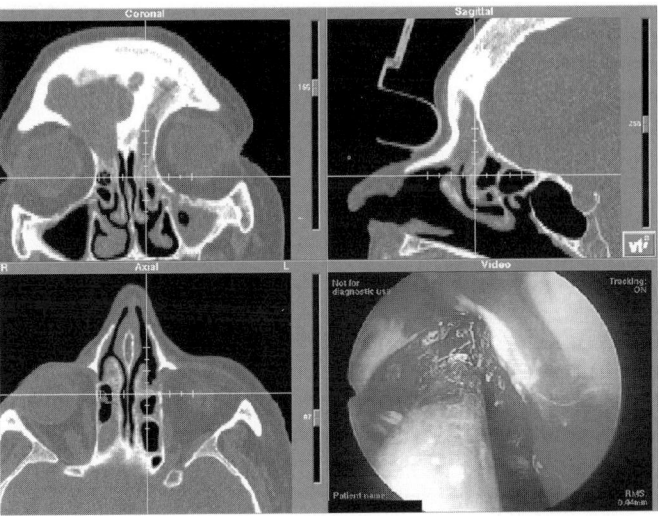

FIGURE 13.17 In this case, new bone formation has obstructed the left frontal sinus, causing a mucopyocele. The microdebrider was used to reduce new bone formation along the anterior ethmoid sinus roof as a means of decompressing the mucopyocele. The microdebrider tip's position is indicated by the crosshairs on the CT images.

and a large frontal sinus mucopyocele was decompressed on each side (Figure 13.17).

13.6 CAS PITFALLS

Current CAS workstations do not provide real-time data that reflect changes that take place during the surgical procedure. This may not be problematic in a fixed, bony environment, such as the paranasal sinuses. However, as CAS indications broaden, significant limitations would exist when current technology is adapted for the resection of soft tissue tumors of the cranial base. In these procedures, simply exposing the posterior or lateral skull base and achieving initial vascular control would significantly alter the size and position of the tumor, making CAS navigation inaccurate. Fried et al. [29] published preliminary reports of performing cadaveric sinus surgery in an open MRI unit. The highly sophisticated operating suite and specialized surgical instrumentation required are currently cost-prohibitive, but it is conceivable that modifications will be made to enable real-time surgery using both CT and MRI.

Perhaps the most significant concern with CAS is that the technology tends to decrease the tendency for the surgeon to be a good anatomist. It is easy to have the expectation that the technology alone will prevent complications. Of course, such an attitude is false, since CAS is simply a guide. While this technology may enhance operator confidence, it is still incumbent upon the physician to become an expert surgical anatomist through multiple cadaver dissection and experience [20,22,23,27,30,31].

The use of CAS has been associated with an increase in operative time as reported by Metson et al. [27]. This increase in operative time was most notable during the surgeon's early use of this new technology (15–30 min) and was found to improve with experience (5–15 min). Most new technologies are associated with a ''learning curve'' during which period an increase in surgery length is anticipated. However, as the surgeon and operating room personnel become more familiar with the new technology, the increase in operative time should decrease. Further, with improved anatomical localization and surgical precision available with CAS, an eventual overall decrease in surgery length may be achieved.

13.7 CONCLUSION

Computer-aided revision functional endoscopic sinus surgery can be performed safely and effectively. Since CAS provides confirmatory localization of potentially obscured surgical landmarks, areas of recurrent or residual disease may be appropriately treated. At the same time, CAS assists in the identification of the ethmoid roof and lamina papyracea. In this way, CAS may reduce surgical morbidity and improve the surgical outcomes of revision FESS.

REFERENCES

1. JM King, DD Caldarelli, JB Pigato. A review of revision functional endoscopic sinus surgery. Laryngoscope 104:404–408, 1994.
2. DH Rice. Endoscopic sinus surgery: results at 2-year follow-up. Otolaryngol Head Neck Surg 101:476–479, 1989.
3. HL Levine. Functional endoscopic sinus surgery: evaluation, surgery, and follow-up of 250 patients. Laryngoscope 100:79–84, 1990.
4. M May, SJ Mester. Endoscopic Endonasal Sinus Surgery: Factors contributing to Failure. Presented at the First International Symposium on Contemporary Sinus Surgery, Pittsburgh, November 4–6, 1990.
5. BL Matthews, LE Smith, R Jones, et al. Endoscopic sinus surgery: outcome in 155 cases. Otolaryngol Head Neck Surg 104:244–246, 1991.
6. DW Kennedy. Prognostic factors, outcomes and staging in ethmoid sinus surgery. Laryngoscope 102 (suppl57):1–18, 1992.
7. JP Corey, RM Bumsted. Revision endoscopic ethmoidectomy for chronic rhinosinusitis. Otolaryngol Clin North Am 22:801–808, 1989.
8. GP Katsantonis, WH Friedman, MC Sivore. The role of computed tomography in revision sinus surgery. Laryngoscope 100:811–816, 1990.
9. WH Friedman, GP Katsantonis, BN Rosenblum, et al. Sphenoethmoidectomy: the case for ethmoid marsupialization. Laryngoscope 96:473–479,
10. VL Schramm, MZ Effron. Nasal polyps in children. Laryngoscope 90:1488–1495, 1980.
11. LF Smith, PC Brindley. Indications, evaluation, complications, and results of functional endoscopic sinus surgery in 200 patients. Otolaryngol Head Neck Surg 108(6): 688–696, 1993.
12. JA Stankiewicz. Complications of endoscopic intranasal ethmoidectomy. Laryngoscope 97:1270–1273, 1987.
13. JA Stankiewicz. Complications in endoscopic intranasal ethmoidectomy: an update. Laryngoscope 99:686–690, 1989.
14. M May, HL Levine, SJ Mester, B Schaitkin. Complications of Endoscopic sinus surgery: analysis of 2108 patients—incidence and prevention. Laryngoscope 104: 1080–1083, 1994.
15. AJ Maniglia. Fatal and other major complications of endoscopic sinus surgery. Laryngoscope 101:349–354, 1991.
16. SD Schaefer, S Manning, LG Close. Endoscopic paranasal sinus surgery: indications and considerations. Laryngoscope 99:1–5, 1989.
17. H Stammberger. Endoscopic endonasal surgery: concepts in treatment of recurring rhinosinusitis. Part I Anatomic and pathophysiologic considerations. Otolaryngol Head Neck Surg 94:143–146, 1986.
18. H Stammberger. Endoscopic endonasal surgery: concepts in treatment of recurring

rhinosinusitis. Part II Surgical technique. Otolaryngol Head Neck Surg 94:147–156, 1986.
19. RH Lazar, RT Younis, TE Long, et al. Revision functional endonasal sinus surgery. Ear Nose Throat J 71:131–133, 1992.
20. AM Neumann Jr., K Pasquale-Niebles, T Bhuta, MJ Sillers. Image-guided transnasal endoscopic surgery of the paranasal sinuses and anterior skull base. Am J Rhinol 13(6):449–454, 1999.
21. DW Kennedy, SJ Zinreich, H Shaalan, et al. Endoscopic middle meatal antrostomy: theory, technique, and patency. Laryngoscope 97(43):1–9, 1987.
22. JB Anon, SP Lipman, D Oppenheim, RA Halt. Computer-assisted endoscopic sinus surgery. Laryngoscope 104:901–905, 1994.
23. J Claes, E Koekelkoren, L van den Hauwe, PH Van de Heyning. Computer assisted E. N. T. surgery, a preliminary report. Acta Oto-Rhino-Laryngol Belg 53:117–123, 1999.
24. MP Freid, J Kleefield, R Taylor. Drug/Device capsules. Otolaryngol Head Neck Surg 119(5):526–532, 1998.
25. R Mosges, L Klimek. Computer-assisted surgery of the paranasal sinuses. J Otolaryngol 22(2):69–71, 1993.
26. M Caversaccio, R Bächler, K L Lädrach, G Schroth, L-P Nolte, R Häusler. Frameless computer-aided surgery system for revision endoscopic sinus surgery. Otolaryngol Head Neck Surg 122(6):808–813, 2000.
27. RB Metson, MJ Cosenza, MJ Cunningham, GW Randolph. Physician experience with an optical image guidance system for sinus surgery. Laryngoscope 110:972–976, 2000.
28. WJ Mann, G Kahaly, W Lieb, RG Amedee. Orbital decompression for endocrine ophthalmopathy: the endonasal approach. Am J Rhinol 8(3): 123–127, 1994.
29. MP Fried, L Hsu, GP Topulos, FA Jolesz. Image-guided surgery in a new magnetic resonance suite: preclinical considerations. Laryngoscope 106:411–417, 1996.
30. MP Fried, J Kleefield, H Gopal, E Reardon, BT Ho, FA Kuhn. Image-guided endoscopic surgery: results of accuracy and performance in a multicenter clinical study using an electromagnetic tracking system. Laryngoscope 107:594–601, 1997.
31. M Roth, D Lanza, et al. Advantages and disadvantages of three-dimensional computer tomography intraoperative localization for functional endoscopic sinus surgery. Laryngoscope 105:1279–1286, 1995.

14

Computer-Aided Frontal Sinus Surgery

Frederick A. Kuhn, M.D., F.A.C.S.
Georgia Nasal & Sinus Institute, Savannah, Georgia

James N. Palmer, M.D.
University of Pennsylvania Health System, Philadelphia, Pennsylvania

14.1 INTRODUCTION

Chronic frontal sinusitis resistant to medical management has long posed a difficult problem for the otolaryngologist. Multiple surgical approaches for chronic frontal sinusitis have been advocated over the past century, suggesting that no single procedure yielded good reproducible results from patient to patient and from surgeon to surgeon. What has been needed is an organized, integrated approach to frontal sinus surgery (as outlined in this chapter).

Intranasal procedures were first proposed in the 1890s, and by 1917 multiple articles discussing the use of intranasal frontal sinusotomy in chronic disease had been published [1–3]. However, these procedures fell from favor and were replaced by a group of external procedures. We suspect that a high failure rate or complication rate associated with intranasal procedures caused them to disappear from the scene. Interestingly, the original articles, as well as the later works of Van Alyea and Mosher, pointed out the importance of the frontal recess in frontal sinus disease [4–7]. This concept of frontal recess disease as the cause of frontal sinusitis was apparently lost with the advent of external procedures and frontal sinus obliteration. Today, however, meticulous attention to endoscopic frontal recess dissection and removal of frontal recess disease in endoscopic sinus surgery has become the hallmark of successful frontal sinus treatment (8).

Endoscopic sinus surgery has been a major advance in the surgical treatment of sinusitis and has brought with it a widespread increase in the understanding of nasal and sinus anatomy. However, even with our improved visualization and increased anatomical knowledge, we commonly have difficulty determining where we are in the sinuses. Stereotactic computer-assisted surgical navigation, or image-guided surgery, is another major advance that has greatly enhanced the ease and completeness of sinus surgery, particularly the endoscopic approach to frontal sinus and frontal recess surgery. Computer-aided surgery (CAS) allows the surgeon to understand the complex frontal recess anatomy and to treat more advanced frontal sinus disease, such as osteoma, mucocele, polyps, and tumor. Because of noticeable improvements in safety and completeness of the procedure, endoscopic frontal recess dissection combined with CAS is the procedure of choice for treatment of chronic frontal sinus disease.

In the first part of this chapter, we will cover frontal sinus mucociliary clearance, frontal recess anatomy, and several anatomical variants, which must be understood in order to perform frontal recess dissection successfully. The use of CAS clarifies these anatomical structures and improves frontal recess dissection. The second portion of the chapter will highlight the utility of CAS in more advanced endoscopic procedures, including treatment of lateral frontal sinus lesions, osteomas of the frontal sinus, mucoceles and even an osteoplastic frontal sinus obliteration. Taken as a group, the procedures outlined comprise an integrated approach to the frontal sinus that CAS can enhance. It is important to emphasize that these procedures (Table 14.1) are used with the least invasive first; progression to the more invasive techniques occurs in a graduated stepwise approach only as the patient's disease dictates. Due to the added dimension of CAS, the least invasive procedures are often successfully applied in more advanced cases; in this way, CAS reduces the patients' exposure to more invasive surgery and lessens the risks of complications associated with these more aggressive procedures.

TABLE 14.1 The Integrated Approach for Frontal Sinus Surgery

1. Endoscopic frontal sinusotomy
2. Above and below approach (endoscopic & trephine)
3. Frontal sinus rescue (FSR)
4. Modified endoscopic Lothrop (Draf drill out)
5. Above and below approach (endoscopic and osteoplastic)
6. Frontal sinus obliteration

14.2 FRONTAL SINUS PHYSIOLOGY AND ANATOMY

14.2.1 Frontal Sinus Mucociliary Clearance

Mucus transport in the frontal sinus is governed by its mucosal ciliary beat patterns. This pattern is up the interfrontal sinus septum, then laterally across the frontal sinus roof, and finally medially along the frontal sinus floor (orbital roof) to the ostium. Approximately, 40–60% of the mucus recirculates up the interfrontal sinus septum and around the sinus again, while the other 60–40% is swept out the ostium and down the medial orbital wall. The recirculating mucus loop may actually extend down into the frontal recess, where it could possibly pick up bacteria or fungus, transporting them into the frontal sinus. The frontal recess cilia play a very active role in frontal sinus health; therefore, this mucosa and its attendant cilia must be carefully preserved. Since Moriyama et al. [9] demonstrated that cilia do not regenerate if mucosa is stripped from bone, it is obvious that drilling or leaving exposed bone in the frontal recess is counterphysiologic.

14.2.2 Frontal Recess Dissection

The express goal of endoscopic frontal recess dissection is to open the drainage pathway from the frontal sinus into the middle meatus by removing all air cells and attendant bony lamella from the boundaries of the frontal recess. The frontal recess boundaries are (1) posterior—skull base; (2) anterior—anterior wall of the agger nasi cell or the middle meatus; (3) lateral—lamina papyracea/superior medial orbital wall; and (4) medial—vertical attachment of middle turbinate to skull base. The frontal recess is a potential space frequently filled by air cells, known as frontal recess cells. Removal of these cells in frontal recess dissection will clear the frontal recess, "removing the cork from the bottle," and thereby open the frontal sinus drainage pathway. The various frontal recess cells will be described and techniques will be suggested for their removal using image guidance.

Figure 14.1 is an endoscopic picture of a patient's left frontal recess following endoscopic surgery, which resulted in frontal ostium stenosis. This photograph, combined with Figure 14.2, demonstrates the utility of CAS in endoscopic frontal recess dissection. The three depressions, from medial to lateral, are (1) a blind depression, (2) the stenosed frontal ostium, and (3) a supraorbital ethmoid cell. Using CAS and frontal recess dissection techniques, the frontal sinus was identified and opened, the mucocele drained from the frontal sinus, and the recurrent frontal sinus disease resolved. It should be mentioned that meticulous postoperative care is also required to achieve long-term successful results.

Knowledge of the individual patient's frontal sinus drainage pathway is best determined preoperatively using the CAS computer to review the images sequentially. Once the drainage pathway is established and understood, resection of cell

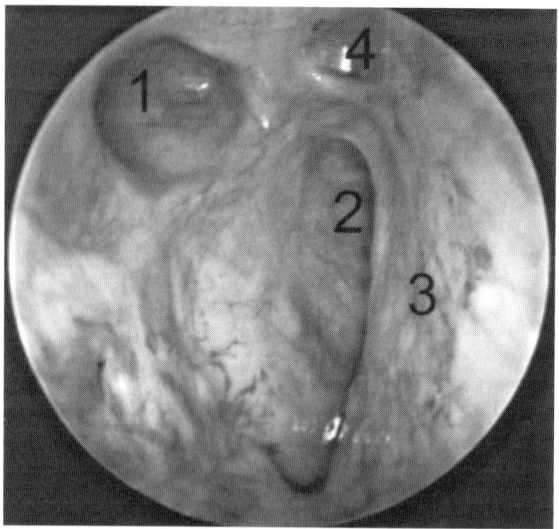

FIGURE 14.1 This endoscopic view of the left frontal recess shows with interfrontal sinus septal cell (1), supraorbital ethmoid cell (2), medial orbital wall (3), and scarred over frontal sinus ostium (4). No obvious frontal sinus drainage pathway is apparent.

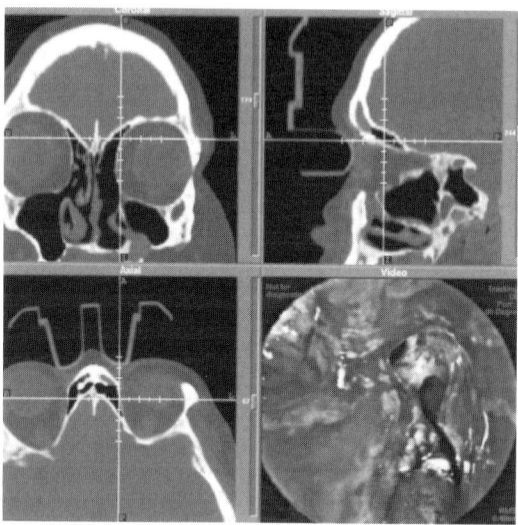

FIGURE 14.2 This intraoperative CAS screen capture (InstaTrak, Visualization Technology, Lawrence, MA) shows that the left frontal sinus and supraorbital ethmoid cells have been opened into the left frontal recess. The localizing pointer is on the medial orbital wall in the supraorbital ethmoid cell. The preoperative view is shown in Figure 14.1.

Computer-Aided Frontal Sinus Surgery

walls can be planned. Removal of the uncinate process and cell walls from the frontal recess is best accomplished using a combination of frontal sinus seekers and curettes to fracture the cell walls and through cutting punches, giraffe forceps, or gentle application of curved powered dissection to remove redundant mucosa and bone. Meticulous attention is required to preserve mucosa in all quadrants of the frontal sinus drainage pathway. The object is to clear the frontal recess, restore physiological mucociliary clearance, and allow frontal sinus disease to resolve.

14.2.3 Agger Nasi Cells

Agger nasi, translated from Latin, means nasal mound. When this region, which is located slightly above and anterior to the middle turbinate, is pneumatized, it contains the most anterior ethmoid cell and the most consistent cell of the frontal recess. The agger nasi cell develops from the first embryological frontal pit or furrow as described by Schaeffer [10] and Kaspar [11], whereas the frontal sinus itself develops from the second frontal pit. These frontal pits or furrows are at the upper end of the first and perhaps second embryological ethmoturbinal groove.

The agger nasi cell commonly fills most of the frontal recess, as it pneumatizes the lateral and anterior frontal recess walls. The frontal sinus drains over the posterior and medial walls of its cap or dome. Since the posterior and medial walls are the only two walls that are not part of the skull, these two partitions can be removed. Disturbance of natural mucociliary flow across the agger nasi cell roof is the most common cause of frontal recess obstruction. Multiple mechanisms for frontal sinus disease involve the agger nasi dome if it is not removed. Edema at its posterior or medial portion may occlude the drainage pathway in the patient who has not had surgery. A remnant agger nasi cap or dome left behind during surgery may scar to the posterior frontal recess, to the ethmoid bulla lamella, or to the vertical middle turbinate attachment to skull base, closing off the drainage pathways [10]. Sagittal computed tomography CT scan reconstructions and CAS allow precise location of the agger nasi cap and guide the surgeon to its careful removal.

To remove the agger nasi cap, one must identify the cell boundaries on the CAS sagittal CT view. Once open inferiorly, only the medial and posterior walls of the cell can be removed, as the other walls are common with the skull. To achieve this objective, the 90-degree frontal sinus curette is slid between the skull base and the posterior agger nasi cell wall and then pulled anteriorly and slightly inferiorly. This maneuver breaks the cell wall anteriorly. Next the remaining medial agger nasi wall may be removed by sliding the curette between this cell wall and the middle turbinate. Gentle traction laterally and somewhat inferiorly will break free the medial agger nasi wall. Meticulous attention to both mucosal preservation and turbinate stability is of paramount importance. After the curettes have broken the medial and posterior agger nasi wall, the loose bony fragments may be removed with 45-degree and 90-degree side-toside and front-to-back grasping frontal giraffe forceps. Bone fragments, which have been inadvertently pushed up into the frontal sinus, may be pulled down into the frontal recess with frontal sinus seekers. They may then be removed with giraffe forceps for removal. The frontal recess mucosa should not be grasped with forceps, as it may strip out of the frontal recess. Mucosal loss will result in scarring and possibly osteoneogenesis. Redundant pieces of mucosa may be removed with through-cutting forceps or the gentle application of curved powered dissection blades. At this point, the ostium should be open and a suction canula may be gently passed into the frontal sinus to aspirate debris for microbiological and pathological examination as well as for frontal sinus irrigation. Irrigation of the sinus can be particularly helpful to clear a bloody field, reduce edema, and allow direct visualization of bony fragments and mucosal edges. If the suction canula is also a CAS surgical navigation probe, it will demonstrate that the frontal sinus ostium is open.

Figure 14.3 demonstrates an agger nasi cell cap that is obstructing the frontal recess in a patient with recurrent frontal recess disease. The suction probe is in the obstructing cell, while the true passageway to the frontal sinus is medial to the probe. The frontal ostium is above the agger nasi cell cap, and the frontal

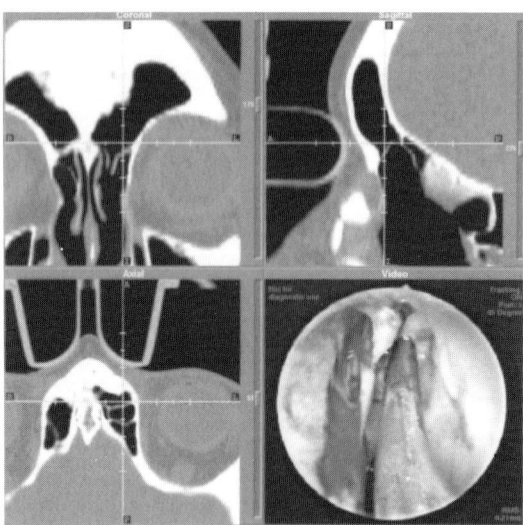

FIGURE 14.3 This intraoperative CAS screen capture (InstaTrak, Visualization Technology, Lawrence, MA) shows that the remnant agger nasi cap has scarred to ethmoid bulla remnant posteriorly (sagittal view). In addition, remnant cells are seen medially (coronal CT and endoscopic view). In the endoscopic view, the probe has displacing the agger nasi cell cap superiorly; this causes the crosshairs to appear in frontal sinus.

Computer-Aided Frontal Sinus Surgery

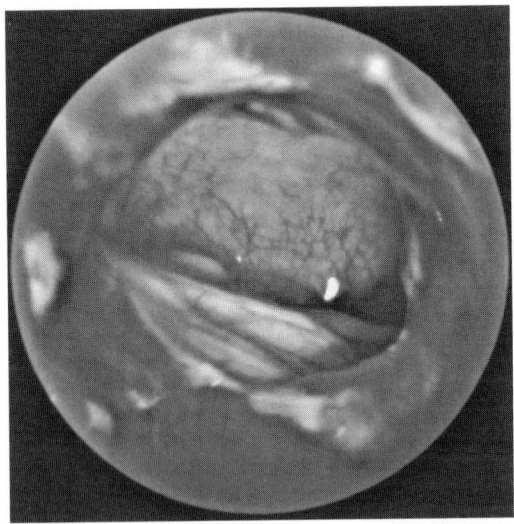

FIGURE 14.4 This endoscopic image shows the left frontal ostium after removal of remnant agger nasi cap. The intraoperative views are shown in Figure 14.3.

sinus must drain over and medial to it. Figure 14.4 is the postdissection image, with the frontal ostium open. This approach is preferable to the drill-out procedure, since the surgical goal of an open frontal ostium is obtained and the functional mucosa lining the ostium and the frontal recess is preserved.

14.2.4 Frontal Cells

Frontal cells also originate as anterior ethmoid cells and pneumatize the frontal recess and frontal sinus in four distinct types. Frontal cells are the second most anterior of the ethmoid cells. The origins for these cells are located posterior to the agger nasi cell. Frontal cells then pneumatize superior to the agger nasi cell into the frontal recess or even up into the frontal sinus, where they may cause frontal recess obstruction. A type I frontal cell is defined as a single cell occurring in the frontal recess above the agger nasi cell. A type II frontal cell is part of a tier of two or more cells above the agger nasi cell in a tier extending up into the frontal recess or even into the frontal sinus. A type III is a single massive cell that extends from the middle meatus, pneumatizing above the agger nasi cell up into the frontal sinus. Before CT image reconstruction CAS, type IV cells initially seemed to be isolated cells in the frontal sinus without any obvious connection to the anterior ethmoid region [13]. Sagittal CT reconstruction, with CAS, shows that the connection between a type IV frontal cell and the anterior ethmoid region may be found posteriorly in the middle meatus. In contrast, a type III cell opens into the anterior middle meatus just behind the agger nasi cell. Frontal recess obstruction from frontal cells can occur in a similar fashion to that of the agger nasi cell; that is, edema in very small, tight drainage pathways, or iatrogenic scar may close the frontal recess [13].

The CAS computer is particularly valuable for surgical planning when these cells are present. The sagittal reconstruction will demonstrate the labyrinth of bony lamella creating various drainage pathways, while coronal and axial scans primarily demonstrate the location of the pathology. Without all three CT planes, location and removal of the cell walls is very difficult.

Frontal cell dissection is performed in the manner described for agger nasi cells. First, the cell walls that can be removed must be identified. Then, the frontal sinus curettes or through-cutting instruments are used to break down the walls. Finally, the loose bony fragments are removed with giraffe forceps. Of course, mucosal preservation must be achieved. Types II–IV frontal cells may be too far superior or lateral to be removed completely by frontal recess dissection. In those instances, the frontal recess dissection should be performed first and then a frontal sinus trephine or osteoplastic flap may be added to improve access from above.

Figure 14.5 demonstrates a type I frontal cell above an agger nasi cell on the medial orbital wall. The probe or suction tip is medial and anterior to the

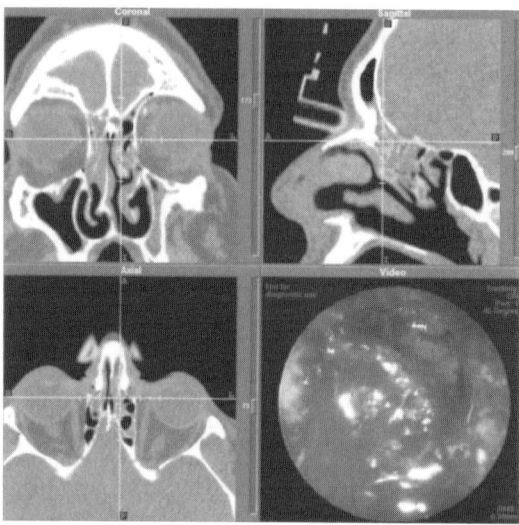

FIGURE 14.5 This intraoperative CAS screen capture (InstaTrak, Visualization Technology, Lawrence, MA) shows a left type I frontal cell. The pointer is at the medial wall of frontal cell. The endoscopic image demonstrates open frontal cell.

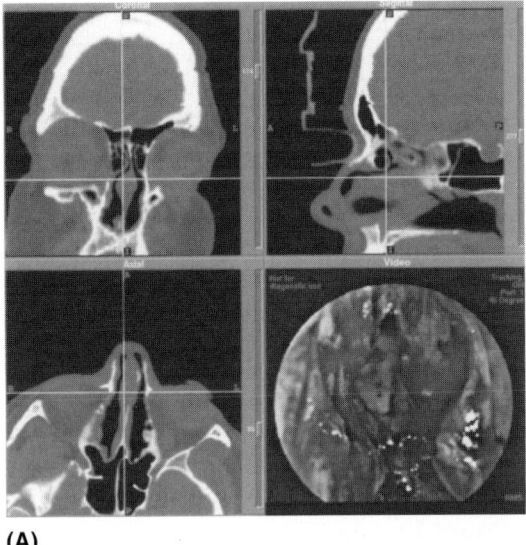

(A)

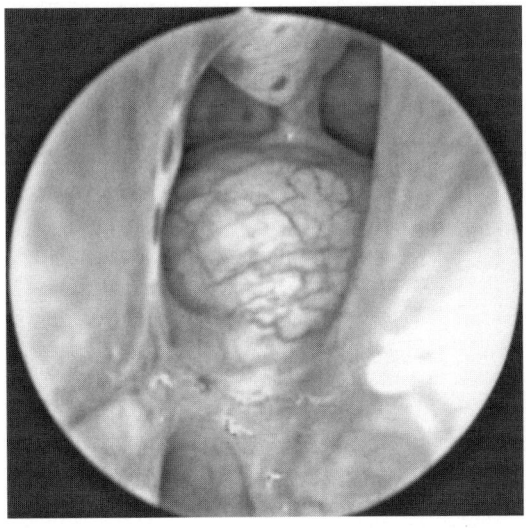

(B)

FIGURE 14.6 (A) This intraoperative CAS screen capture (InstaTrak, Visualization Technology, Lawrence, MA) shows type II frontal cells on the preoperative CT scan as well as the patent frontal ostium after frontal recess dissection. The pointer is below the area of removed agger nasi cell and type II frontal cells. A patent frontal ostium can be seen. (B) This postoperative image, obtained approximately 3 months after surgery, show a healed, patent frontal ostium.

cell. This correlates with the endoscopic image, which demonstrates the open obstructing cap of the cell. The pathway to the frontal sinus is medial to this cell (namely, between the medial cell wall and the middle turbinate attachment to skull base. In Figure 14.6A the CT demonstrates a type II frontal cell. The sagittal CT image depicts this type II frontal cell well. It could be argued that this cell is perhaps a suprabullar cell; however, the CT demonstrates two cells that are stacked in tier configuration. The corresponding endoscopic picture is the frontal recess after the cells have been dissected and the frontal ostium has been open. Note that the probe is actually below the frontal recess so that the endoscopic picture is not obscured. Figure 14.6B is the 3-month postoperative healed right frontal recess in this patient. Figure 14.7 is an excellent example of a type III frontal cell. The sagittal view demonstrates that the drainage pathway for the cell is actually back into the anterior ethmoid, behind the agger nasi cell. The probe is at the posterior skull base so that a clear view of the type III cell pneumatized above a small agger nasi cell into the frontal sinus may be obtained.

14.2.5 Supraorbital Ethmoid Cells

The supraorbital ethmoid cell or cells develop posterior to the agger nasi cell from the third frontal pit or groove of Schaeffer [10]. They occur along the skull base

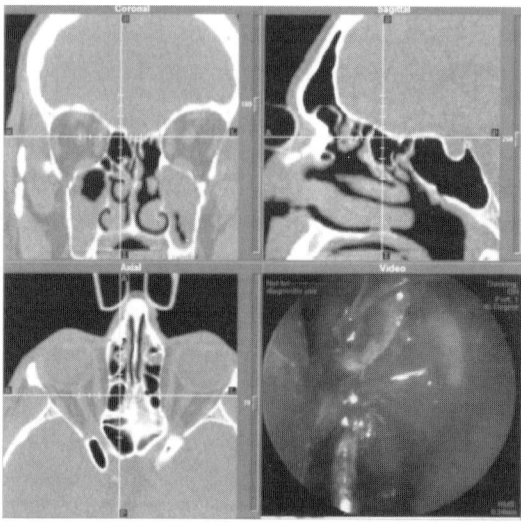

FIGURE 14.7 This intraoperative CAS screen capture (InstaTrak, Visualization Technology, Lawrence, MA) shows a type III frontal cell, which can be best seen on the saggital CT image. The pointer is located in the posterior ethmoid.

in the frontal recess behind the frontal sinus. They may be multiple, may occur anterior or posterior to the anterior ethmoid artery, and usually are separated from the frontal sinus by the ethmoid bulla lamella. They may extend back to or even past the middle turbinate basal lamella . The important common feature of these cells is that they pneumatize laterally out over the orbit. They may also pneumatize forward from their lateral position and appear to be part of a septated frontal sinus. Understanding the spatial relationship of supraorbital ethmoid cells to the frontal sinus, orbit, and skull base is an important key to frontal recess dissection [14].

Axial scans as well as sagittal CT reconstructions are important in delineating the drainage pathway of a supraorbital ethmoid cell. It will usually drain just posterior to the frontal sinus ostium. Due to its proximity to the frontal ostium, the entrance to an extensively pneumatized supraorbital ethmoid cell can be easily confused with it, leaving the internal frontal ostium obstructed at the end of the procedure. This is especially true when viewing the area endoscopically in a bloody field. CAS CT review (particularly the sagittal view) and intraoperative CAS surgical navigation make this differentiation much easier. The CAS probe will distinguish between the supraorbital ethmoid cell opening and the frontal sinus; in doing so, the CAS system demonstrates whether additional dissection is needed.

It is important to remove the common wall between the supraorbital ethmoid cell and the internal frontal ostium as far superiorly as possible, preferably to the skull base. This will prevent recirculation of mucus at either cell ostium. When cell walls are only partially removed, mucociliary clearance may be disrupted, leading to recirculation and trapping of mucus in the frontal recess. CAS facilitates the identification and removal of this septation. Completely opening the supraorbital ethmoid cells creates a much larger common drainage pathway for the two cells. It is much less likely that this pathway will be less likely to become obstructed by edema. Figure 14.2 demonstrates an optimal intraoperative result.

It should also be noted that extensive pneumatization of a supraorbital ethmoid cell can doom frontal sinus obliteration to long-term failure. If the anterior lateral portion of a supraorbital ethmoid cell is confused with a septated frontal sinus, frontal sinus obliteration will be very difficult. Mucous membrane removal in the most lateral or posterior recesses of the cell over or behind the orbit is often impossible and will create a situation of almost certain mucocele development. Therefore, the CT scans obtained in preparation for CAS are very important in presurgical planning, since they will demonstrate a laterally pneumatized supraorbital ethmoid cell, which is a contraindication to frontal sinus obliteration.

14.2.6 Interfrontal Sinus Septal Cell

The interfrontal sinus septal cell appears less frequently than the agger nasi and supraorbital ethmoid cells. It develops in the septum between the two frontal sinuses. This cell may pneumatize to different degrees, varying from just the lower septum all the way to the frontal sinus apex or into a pneumatized crista galli. This cell empties into one frontal recess, usually medial and anterior to the internal frontal ostium. It may also empty into one frontal sinus (rather than directly into the frontal recess). Disease in this cell can cause frontal sinus disease by creating edema and narrowing the total drainage pathway of the frontal recess. Either edema from residual interfrontal sinus septal cell disease or iatrogenic scarring can contribute to frontal recess obstruction and therefore frontal sinus disease in the previously operated patient [15].

CAS is important for intraoperative identification of this cell. Thin-cut coronal scans usually identify its position and contribution to pathology. The interfrontal sinus septal cell's opening and its common wall with the larger frontal recess are difficult to identify. They are best identified by using the 30- and 70-degree telescopes after frontal recess dissection in combination with the CAS probe. Once the frontal recess has been cleared, the common wall between the interfrontal sinus septal cell and the frontal sinus should be removed as far superiorly as possible. One method is to place a frontal sinus 90-degree curette into the interfrontal sinus septal cell and break the intervening wall laterally. However, it is more important to recognize the existence of an interfrontal sinus septal cell and open it inferiorly than it is to remove the entire common wall. Once the cell

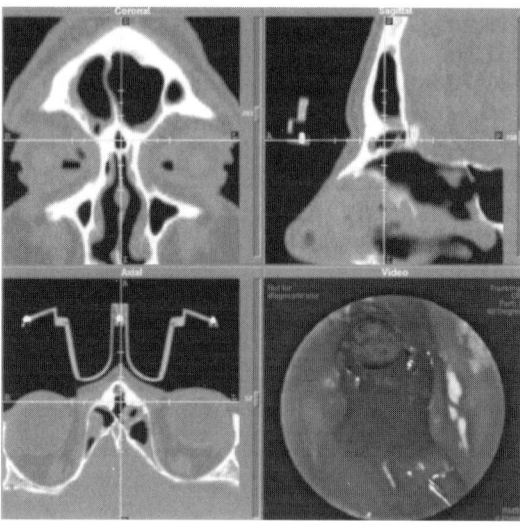

FIGURE 14.8. This intraoperative CAS screen capture (InstaTrak, Visualization Technology, Lawrence, MA) shows an interfrontal sinus septal cell and a left supraorbital ethmoid cell.

is open and draining into a large and disease-free frontal recess, rarely will it play a role in recurrent frontal sinus disease.

The coronal view in Figure 14.8 demonstrates an interfrontal septal cell that has pneumatized into the lower interfrontal sinus septum. The suction probe is at the most anterior part of the endoscopic image, which demonstrates the open frontal ostium. Its tip is in the cell between the frontal sinuses. The coronal view from the same patient (Figure 14.9) demonstrates that the interfrontal sinus septal cell opens into the left frontal recess. The supraorbital ethmoid cell is also extensively pneumatized. The endoscopic images in Figures 14.8 and 14.9 demonstrate a complete frontal recess dissection, including an open supraorbital ethmoid cell laterally. The common partition between the supraorbital ethmoid cell and the frontal sinus has been resected as close to the skull base as possible.

14.2.7 Suprabullar Cell

The suprabullar cell is found above the ethmoid bulla. This cell occurs in the ethmoid bulla lamella or pneumatizes forward through it. This is the only ethmoid cell, which closes the frontal recess from posterior. The suprabullar cell is well visualized only on sagittal CT [14]. CAS is necessary to remove it. Without

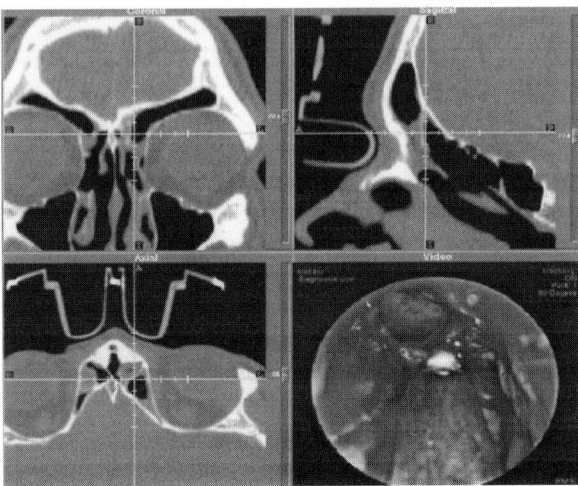

FIGURE 14.9 This intraoperative CAS screen capture (InstaTrak, Visualization Technology, Lawrence, MA) shows that the left frontal ostium and supraorbital ethmoid cell open into frontal recess. The common partition has been resected to skull base in the endoscopic view. The frontal ostium is anterior and the supraorbital ethmoid cell is posterior to the suction tip.

CAS, it is impossible to differentiate the walls of the cell from the skull base endoscopically. Due to its position along the skull base, delicate dissection using the frontal sinus seekers, curettes, and CAS suction tips are required to first break the cap of the cell from anterior to posterior and then remove it. Once the cell walls are broken, they are best meticulously removed in a similar fashion to agger nasi cell caps.

Figure 14.10 demonstrates a right supraorbital ethmoid cell that has pneumatized out over the orbit and a suprabullar cell medially at the skull base.

14.2.8 Recessus Terminalis

If the uncinate process inserts on the medial orbital wall, the ethmoid infundibulum will end in a blind pocket. This blind pocket is called the recessus terminalis. This anatomical variation forces the frontal sinus drainage pathway down the medial surface of the uncinate and thereby directly into the middle meatus. This variant occurs more commonly than often thought (as much as 50%) [7]. The recessus terminalis is important in the surgical approach to the frontal sinus. Complete uncinate removal at its medial orbital wall attachment is the goal when dealing with a recessus terminalis.

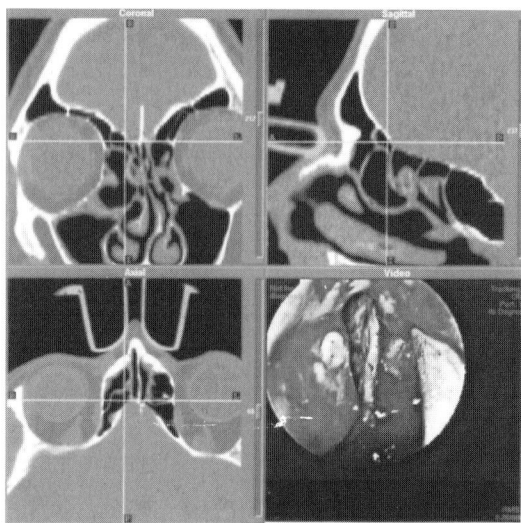

FIGURE 14.10 This intraoperative CAS screen capture (InstaTrak, Visualization Technology, Lawrence, MA) demonstrates a suprabullar cell. In the endoscopic view, the probe tip is within the suprabullar cell. Intraoperative surgical navigation was necessary to differentiate this cell from the skull base.

14.3 SPECIFIC CAS APPLICATIONS

14.3.1 Frontal Sinus Mucocele

Frontal sinus mucoceles occur secondary to frontal recess obstruction that most commonly may be attributed to injury to the frontal recess. As mucoceles develop, they tend to be asymptomatic. The frontal recess insult that leads to mucocele formation may be iatrogenic; that is, endoscopic or external frontoethmoid sinus surgery may cause scarring in the frontal recess. Similarly, frontoethmoidal fractures and frontal sinus fractures also may injure the frontal recess.

In these cases the first and preferred approach should be frontal recess dissection to drain the mucocele into the nasal cavity [17]. If this approach fails, then more aggressive alternatives may be necessary. CAS may be of paramount importance to enable safe frontal recess dissection and mucocele drainage, as illustrated in Figure 10.11. Note that the frontal sinus posterior table is missing; in this situation, inadvertent intracranial penetration during intranasal surgery is much more likely. Intraoperative surgical navigation was critical for the determination of the correct area for deliberate penetration of the mucocele.

Occasionally, anatomical variations (due to trauma) and very hard bony lamellae (due to osteoneogenesis) will be encountered in the course of frontal recess dissection. CAS provides to the surgeon additional comfort when working

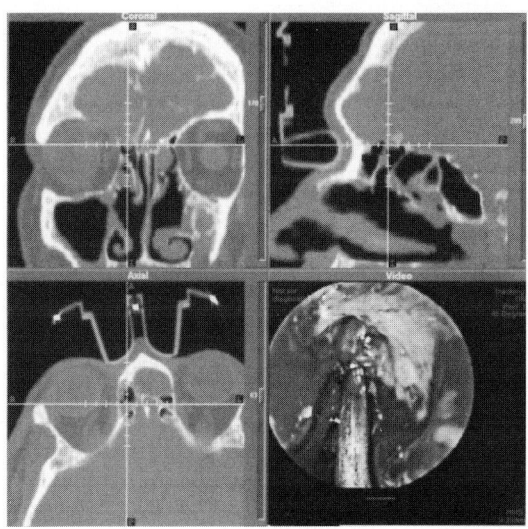

FIGURE 14.11 This intraoperative CAS screen capture (InstaTrak, Visualization Technology, Lawrence, MA) demonstrates a massive bilateral frontal sinus mucocele with erosion of the entire posterior frontal sinus table and anterior skull base.

through these areas of greater bone density; in this way, CAS increases the safety of intranasal mucocele drainage. During these procedures, the surgeon should follow the skull base upward from the posterior portion of the frontal recess. The posterior frontal recess table can be penetrated easily creating a CSF leak, especially in the context of an altered surgical field. Consequently the direction of dissection must always be from posterior to anterior—never from anterior to posterior (Figure 14.12). After the frontal sinus is open, vigorous irrigation of the sinus will help remove inspissated mucus and debris (Figure 14.13). If the mucosal lining be damaged severely during this process, placement of a stent to hold the frontal ostium open may be important. Neel and Lake, in a series containing animal studies and clinical experience, suggest thin soft silastic sheeting loosely rolled in a funnel shape [18,19]. Our current recommendations include use of thin silastic sheeting cut into a truncated triangle with a T wing of silastic at the apex (Figure 14.14). The triangular part of the stent is rolled, grasped with a 45- or 90-degree frontal sinus side biting forceps, and the wings of the T are pushed up into the frontal sinus and allowed to unfurl. The stent is pulled back down into the frontal recess, leaving the wings to anchor it in the frontal sinus, and the body of the stent is partially unrolled in the frontal recess. This allows

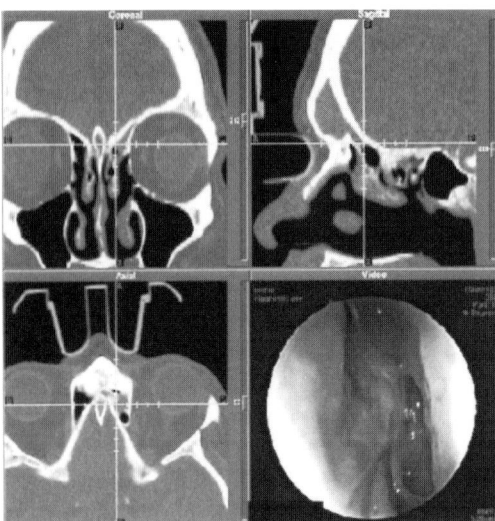

FIGURE 14.12 This intraoperative CAS screen capture (InstaTrak, Visualization Technology, Lawrence, MA) demonstrates a frontal sinus mucocele that occurred previous endoscopic surgery. The frontal sinus is completely closed by remnants of the agger nasi cell anteriorly and a supra bullar cell posteriorly. The endoscopic view is undissected frontal recess.

Computer-Aided Frontal Sinus Surgery

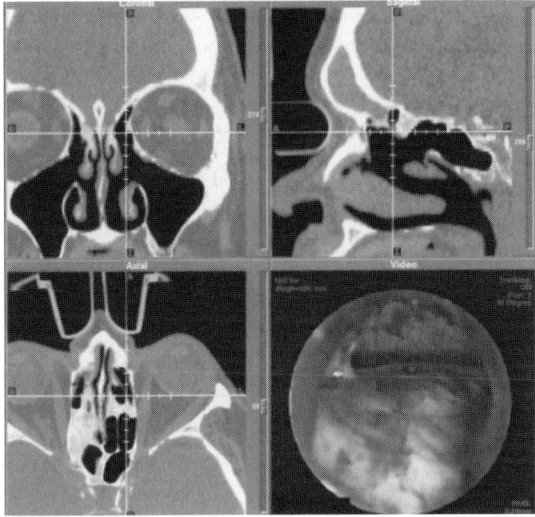

FIGURE 14.13 This intraoperative CAS screen capture (InstaTrak, Visualization Technology, Lawrence, MA) demonstrates a left frontal sinus mucocele, which developed after previous endoscopic ethmoidectomy. The sagittal view demonstrates that the mucocele is bounded posteriorly by suprabullar cell and osteitic bone at skull base. Endoscopic view demonstrates widely patent frontal ostium after succesful endoscopic frontal recess dissection for removal mucocele.

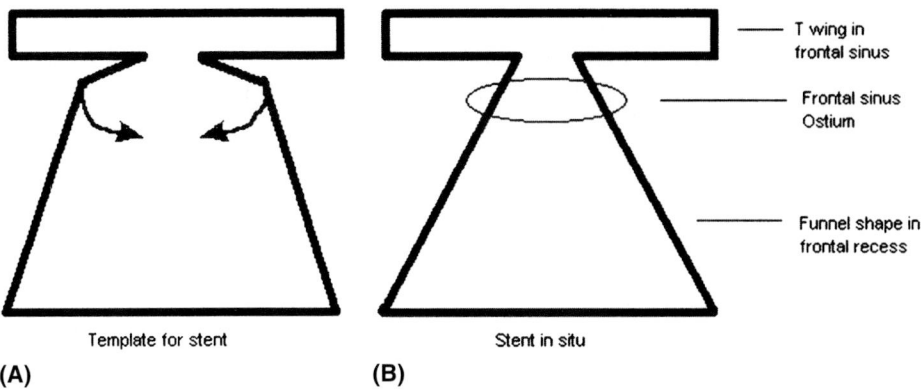

FIGURE 14.14 This schematic illustration shows the basic design (A) and placement (B) of a simple but efficacious frontal sinus stent.

the stent to cover a larger part of the mucosa and prevents the tightly rolled stent from acting like a tube. It is important to remember that tube-like frontal stents tend to cause circumferential scarring down to the diameter of the stent.

The stent is left in for at least 6 months, and the patient is followed with serial office endoscopic examinations to check stent placement and to treat any bacterial infections that might arise. Occasionally the stents become infected with a mucoid phase bacterial infection such as *Pseudomonas*. When this occurs, the infection should be managed with culture-directed antibiotics. Unfortunately, the infection may not clear up until the stent is removed.

Figure 14.13 demonstrates a marsupialised frontal sinus mucocele and open supraorbital ethmoid cell posteriorly—this mucocele was created by scar tissue from previous surgeries. Figure 14.14 depicts the ideal end result after the frontal sinus is irrigated with debris and mucus removed.

14.3.2 Lateral Frontal Sinus Lesions

When a lesion is located laterally in the frontal sinus, endoscopic frontal recess dissection should be performed first. At that point, if the lesion cannot be grasped and brought down into the nasal cavity and removed endoscopically, an external approach may be required to remove the lesion completely [18]. Examples of these lesions are laterally positioned cells with chronic sinusitis, frontal sinus osteomas, foreign bodies, or small mucoceles. Most CAS headsets for ENT surgery are positioned directly over the frontal sinus. Repositioning of the headsets from the standard placement often will provide access for external frontal sinus approaches. Alternatively, the tracking system can be moved from the headset so that it is directly attached to the patient's skull, or a Mayfield head-holder, which tightly secures the patient's head and mounts the tracking system, may also be used. This latter arrangement is the typical arrangement for neurosurgical procedures. When using these modifications of the standard ENT set-up, it is important that the registration for surgical navigation be completed very carefully. Most systems will require registration based upon anatomical fiducial landmarks or traditional external fiducial markers.

After the CAS system has been prepared for external frontal sinus work, it can guide the placement of a trephination. The CAS probe will add another dimension to the utility of this "above and below" approach. In many cases, the trephine combined with the endoscopic approach will be sufficient to remove any lesions in the frontal sinus.

14.3.3 Osteoplastic Flaps

If the necessary exposure is greater than that provided by a standard trephine, an osteoplastic flap can also be performed. Intraoperative surgical navigation can be especially useful in planning the bone cuts. Drill holes can be designed to ensure the safety of the bone cuts and increase their precision. Again, caution must be exercised for correct registration of the CAS system. Since surgical navigation provides greater precision than that afforded by the traditional 6-foot Caldwell plain film, the bone flap may be made larger. The result is better access to the internal frontal sinus. This access will facilitate complete removal of the frontal sinus mucosa if frontal sinus obliteration is planned.

14.4 CONCLUSIONS

CAS technology is extremely beneficial in frontal sinus surgery for many reasons. CAS has the capacity to illustrate anatomical abnormalities in the frontal recess; this knowledge can guide more complete frontal recess dissection. The sagittal CT views provided by CAS increase safety when working in the frontal recess and along the skull base. Intraoperative surgical navigation provides confirmation of complete frontal recess dissection. CAS also can be used for placement of external incisions and trephines.

REFERENCES

1. Anderson CM. Some observations on the intranasal operation for frontal sinusitis. Minn Med 1935; 18:744–747.
2. Wright J. A History of Laryngology and Rhinology. 2nd ed. Philadelphia: Lea and Febiger, 1914:271.
3. Ingals EF. Intranasal drainage of the frontal sinus. Ann Otol Rhinol Laryngol 1917; 26:656–668.
4. Mosher HP. The applied anatomy and the intra-nasal surgery of the ethmoid labyrinth. Trans Am Laryngol Assoc 1912; 34:25–39.
5. Van Alyea OE. Ethmoid labyrinth: anatomic study with consideration of the clinical significance of its structural characteristics. Arch Otolaryngol 1939; 29:881–901.
6. Van Alyea OE. Frontal cells. Arch Otolaryngol 1941; 34:11–23.
7. Van Alyea OE. Frontal sinus drainage. Ann Otol Rhinol Laryngol 1946; 55:267–278.
8. Kuhn FA. Chronic frontal sinusitis: "the endoscopic frontal recess approach." Oper Tech Otolaryngol Head Neck Surg 1996; 7:222–229.
9. Moriyama H, Yanagi K, Ohtori N, et al. Healing process of sinus mucosa after endoscopic sinus surgery. Am J Rhinol 1996; 10:61–66.
10. Schaeffer JP. The genesis, development and adult anatomy of the nasofrontal region in man. Am J Anat 1916; 20:125–145.
11. Kaspar KA. Nasofrontal connections: a study based on one hundred consecutive dissections. Arch Otolaryngol 1936; 23:322–343.
12. Kuhn FA, Bolger WE, Tisdal RG. The agger nasi cell in frontal recess obstruction: an anatomic, radiologic, and clinical correlation. Oper Tech Otolaryngol Head Neck Surg 1991; 2:226–231.

13. Bent J, Kuhn FA, Cuilty C. The frontal cell in frontal recess obstruction. Am J Rhinol 1994; 8:185–191.
14. Owen G, Kuhn FA. The supraorbital ethmoid cell. Otolaryngol Head Neck Surg 1997; 116:254–261.
15. Merritt R, Kuhn FA. The interfrontal sinus septal cell. Am J Rhinol 1996; 10:299–301.
16. Sillers MJ, Kuhn FA, Vickery CL. Radiation exposure in paranasal sinus imaging. Otolaryngol Head Neck Surg 1995; 112:248–251.
17. Kennedy DW, Josephson JS, Zinreich SJ, et al. Endoscopic sinus surgery for mucoceles: a viable alternative. Laryngoscope 1989; 99(9):885–895.
18. Neel HB, Whicker JH, Lake CF. Thin rubber sheeting in frontal sinus surgery: animal and clinical studies. Laryngoscope 1976; 86:524–536.
19. Neel HB, McDonald TJ, Facer GW. Modified Lynch procedure for chronic frontal sinus disease: rationale, technique and long term results. Laryngoscope 1987; 97:1274–1279.
20. Bent JP, Spears RA, Kuhn FA, Stewart SM. Combined endoscopic intranasal and external frontal sinusotomy (the above and below approach to chronic frontal sinusitis: alternatives to obliteration). Am J Rhinol 1997; 11:349–354.

15

Computer-Aided Transsphenoidal Hypophysectomy

Winston C. Vaughan, M.D.
Stanford University, Stanford, California

15.1 INTRODUCTION

The biopsy and removal of pituitary pathology is usually a joint procedure performed by the otorhinolaryngology and neurosurgery services. The transsphenoidal route to the pituitary fossa has become the preferred approach, since it has been shown to offer faster recovery and fewer complications when compared to traditional craniotomies. However, significant complications remain, which usually relate to the close proximity of critical structures. The removal of sellar pathology without injury to the adjacent structures is the main aim of transphenoidal surgery.

Computer-aided surgery (CAS) technology has been implemented in many centers in these procedures, since it offers improved surgical precision and potentially improved surgical outcomes.

15.2 HISTORICAL PERSPECTIVE

The early history of pituitary surgery is filled with renowned surgeons from multiple specialties and countries. It is interesting to consider that these early procedures occurred at a time when antibiotics were not available, microscopes were new devices, and the C-arm image intensifier was considered a major advance in surgical navigation.

Schloffer [1] and Kanavel [2] described an intranasal route that used a subnasal and lateral rhinotomy incision. Halstead introduced the sublabial transnasal route [3]. Cushing followed with the sublabial transeptal approach [4]. He operated on over 240 pituitary masses from 1910 to 1929. This approach lost favor for several years and was replaced by intracranial approaches. Guiot and Thebaul in France, followed by Hardy in Montreal in the 1960s, reintroduced the sublabial, transeptal transsphenoidal route, using the operating microscope and intraoperative fluoroscopy [5–7]. Approximately 40 years later, the sublabial, transseptal, transsphenoidal route to the sella remains the preferred approach for most neurosurgeons.

Over the last decade, otorhinolaryngologists have begun to use endoscopic techniques extensively. More recently, neurosurgeons have started to adopt these techniques. Several joint otorhinolaryngology and neurosurgery teams have published their experiences with these minimally invasive endoscopic applications [8–14].

Endoscopic approaches in the management of sinus inflammatory disease are now some of the most common procedures performed by otorhinolaryngologists. Implementation of CAS surgical navigation during these difficult dissections has improved the safety and efficacy of these procedures.

15.3 COMPUTER-AIDED SINUS SURGERY OVERVIEW

CAS involves the use of an imaging data set for the confirmation of anatomical location during surgical dissection. CAS-based surgical navigation is usually considered a purely semiconductor-based technology; however, use of intraoperative fluoroscopy for localization of instrument positions really is a primitive form of surgical navigation. In this regard, the first real application of this approach involved the use of the C-arm image intensifier to localize the skull base position during sinus dissections. Today computed tomography (CT) scans and magnetic resonance imaging (MRI), coupled with sophisticated tracking systems, are now used.

In early CAS systems, articulated arms provided positional information for the computer system. More sophisticated CAS systems incorporate electromagnetic or optical emitters and sensors for the tracking of instrument positions. Real-time intraoperative imaging is also possible using portable CT scanners [15]. Standard operating rooms have been adapted to accommodate a modified open MRI scanner so that surgical dissection can occur under MRI guidance [16]. (These systems are described in other chapters throughout this book.)

The main indication for CAS in sinus surgery that targets refractory inflammatory rhinosinusitis includes dissection in areas surrounded by vital structures. Furthermore, CAS also offers advantages in the situation where the usual surgical landmarks have become distorted. In a similar fashion, CAS may be useful in transsphenoidal hypophysectomy, since the close proximity of vital structures (namely, the internal carotid arteries, the cavernous sinus and its contents, the brain, and the optic nerve) leads to a very small surgical margin of error. Complications related to inadvertent injury to these structures can be devastating. The guidance provided by CAS cannot substitute for knowledge of anatomy or careful dissection, since CAS is not an infallible technology.

15.4 DEVELOPMENT OF COMPUTER-AIDED TRANSSPHENOIDAL HYPOPHYSECTOMY

In 1969 Hardy published an excellent description of his transsphenoidal technique, which included the use of the operating microscope and televised radiofluoroscopy [7]. In this article he details the benefit of real-time fluoroscopy for identification of surrounding anatomical landmarks. By the time of its publication in 1969, he had performed over 200 cases using fluoroscopic guidance. His work represents the birth of surgical navigation for pituitary surgeons.

Recent advances have included the use of preoperative radiology, along with computer software, to create a navigational data set, which can be used during the surgery. This is usually performed with CT or MRI scans. Specialized software programs also support the simultaneous use of multiple imaging data sets. Ideally, imaging for hypophysectomy should include a CT scan of the bone boundaries, an angiogram of the surrounding vessels and a MRI of the sellar region. For this reason, the use of multiple preoperative images offers significant appeal.

MRI scans obtained before and after transsphenoidal hypophysectomies have demonstrated a fair amount of residual disease. Kremer et al. studied 22 patients with macroadenomas and found 11 cases with residual pituitary tissue [17]. Such residual tissue suggests that more thorough dissection in the sella may reduce disease persistence or progression. CAS has been shown to provide for more thorough dissection in sinus surgery and may prove to do the same in pituitary surgery.

Most CAS systems use a preoperative data set. Recently, both MRI and CT technology have been used for real-time scanning and surgical guidance during hypophysectomies [15,16]. MRI scans, which are a familiar imaging modality for neurosurgeons, offers the advantage of better soft tissue enhancement. MRI also avoids radiation exposure for both patient and staff. Unfortunately, intraoperative MRI systems require special, nonferromagnetic instrumentation, because the MRI scanner generates strong magnetic fields. In contrast with MRI, CT offers better bone margin enhancement. Standard surgical instruments and anesthesia are more easily utilized with an intraoperative CT scanner, but special accommodations for the CT scanner still must be made.

Schwarz et al. utilized intraoperative MRI guidance in 200 intracranial cases [16]. They found that MRI guidance using an open-bore system provided continuous visual feedback and did not affect the complication rate or time of surgery. This series included five cases of transsphenoidal pituitary resections. (For more information about intraoperative MRI, see Chapter 5.)

Real-time CT guidance has also been reported during hypophysectomy. Kitazawa et al. described nine cases in which a mobile CT scanner was used [18]. They felt that the system provided "accurate information about the location and volume of residual tumor as well as . . . surrounding deeper structures." Mattox and Mirvis used real-time CT scanning during sinus surgeries [15]. They stated that in selected cases, the added radiation exposure was justified due to the improved surgical safety for the patient.

Most CAS systems rely upon a preoperative CT or MRI scan. Since these scans are obtained in advance of surgery, surgeons can readily review the images for surgical planning and patient counseling. These systems are also less cumbersome in the operating room, since they do not require the significant modifications that intraoperative MRI scanners and CT scanners require.

CAS in transsphenoidal hypophysectomy carries an important caveat. Since hypophysectomy involves soft tissue manipulation and removal, intraoperative findings that reflect these soft tissue changes cannot be demonstrated on a preoperative imaging data set. For this reason, the incorporation of intraoperative imaging into standard CAS systems would be very helpful.

15.5 SURGICAL TECHNIQUE FOR TRANSSPHENOIDAL HYPOPHYSECTOMY

The otorhinolaryngologist usually provides access and closure during transsphenoidal hypophysectomy. The amount of dissection performed for such access depends on the anatomy and surgeon preferences [19]. Different approaches, including sublabial, open rhinoplasty, transethmoidal, transseptal, and direct transnasal routes, may be performed under the visualization afforded by the operating microscope and/or surgical telescope [20]. Even headlight illumination may be used. The common element in all of these techniques is access to the sphenoid sinus. For this reason, the sphenoid sinuses themselves and the anatomical structures that surround the sphenoid sinus should be carefully reviewed in coronal, axial, and sagittal CT images before surgery. Knowledge of the anatomy in this area provides the otorhinolaryngologist with the information necessary for the choice of the appropriate approach or combination of approaches [21–23].

During the surgical approach to the pituitary fossa, the otorhinolaryngologist must avoid the sphenopalatine artery (Figure 15.1), the internal carotid artery (Figure 15.2), and the optic nerve (Figure 15.3). Furthermore, the bone of the lateral wall of sphenoid sinus may be dehiscent (Figure 15.4). In addition, sphe-

Computer-Aided Transsphenoidal Hypophysectomy

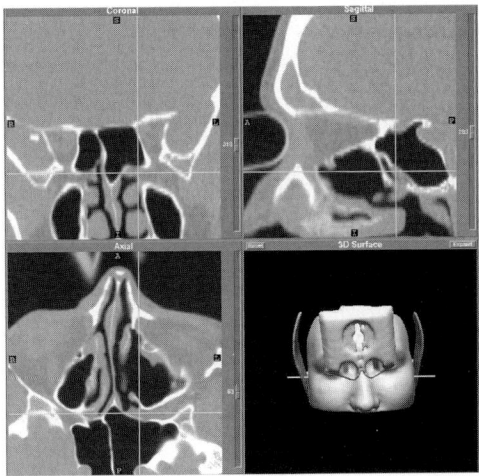

FIGURE 15.1. The crosshairs in this CAS screen capture are on the sphenopalatine neurovascular bundle at a point just medial to the sphenopalatine foramen. The branches of the sphenopalatine artery cross the anterior face of the sphenoid sinus.

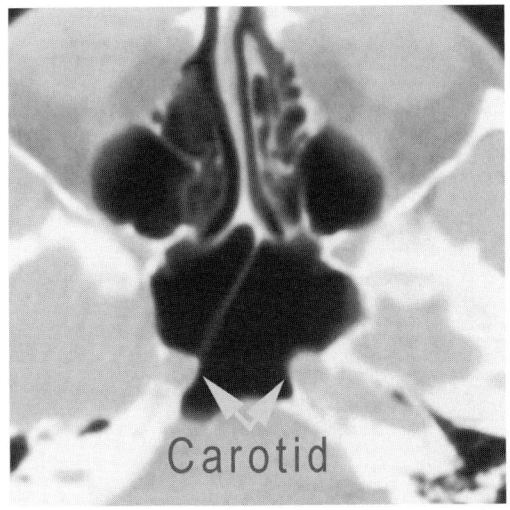

FIGURE 15.2. The internal carotid artery lies in close relationship to the lateral wall of the sphenoid sinus. Often, internal carotid artery will appear as a bulge on the interior aspect of the sphenoid sinus. The extent of sphenoid sinus pneumatization will influence the size of this bulge. Occasionally, the lateral sphenoid sinus wall may be dehiscent; if so, the sphenoid mucosa may lie directly upon the internal carotid artery. In this axial CT, each internal carotid artery clearly protrudes into the sphenoid sinus. Also, the sphenoid internsinus septum inserts directly upon the bone over the right internal carotid artery.

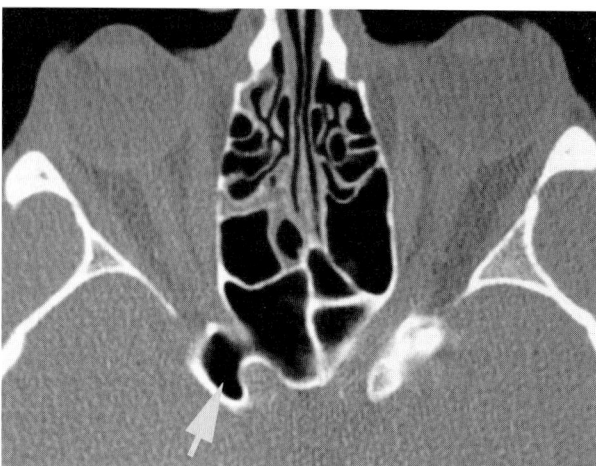

FIGURE 15.3. The optic nerve also may lie in close relationship to the lateral wall of the sphenoid sinus. In fact, the sphenoid sinus may pneumatize around the optic nerve as shown in this axial CT image. It is important to remember that the bone over the optic nerve may be dehiscent.

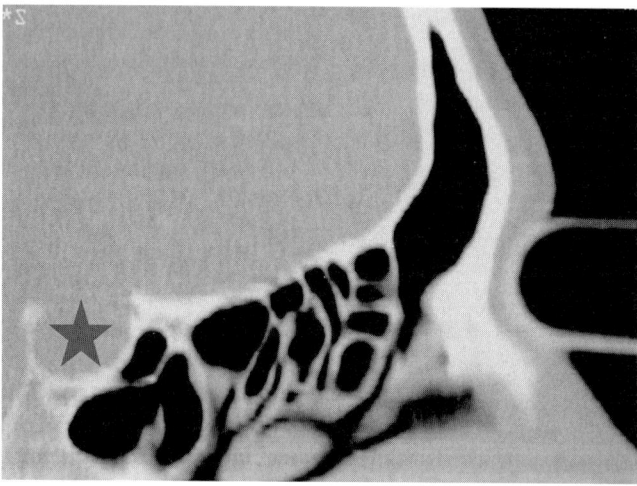

FIGURE 15.4. This sagittal CT reconstruction shows the slope of the skull base and its relationship to the sphenoid sinus and pituitary fossa (star).

Computer-Aided Transsphenoidal Hypophysectomy

noid pneumatization may be asymmetric, and the intersinus septum may directly attach to the bone over the internal carotid artery. The CAS computer workstation provides a platform for the review of the preoperative CT and/or MRI. The location of the adjacent structures as well as the pattern of sinus pneumatization should be reviewed on the preoperative images. Complications due to hypophysectomy are often due to inadvertent violation of these structures themselves or the tissues in immediate proximity to these structures [25–28].

CAS systems provide an excellent medium for presurgical planning and resident education. CAS software tools provide a means for the manipulation of the CT (or MR) images (Figure 15.5). Some systems support the reconstruction of three-dimensional models based on the preoperative image data set. Other systems allow the surgeon to overlap different data sets from MRI and CT. During preoperative planning, the original axial images, as well as the reconstructed sagittal and coronal images, are carefully reviewed on the CAS computer. The coronal images are used to orient transnasal dissection; they also provide information about the septal contour. The axial images depict the relative positions of the sphenoid lateral walls with respect to the optic nerves and the internal carotid arteries. Areas of bony dehiscence may also be identified.

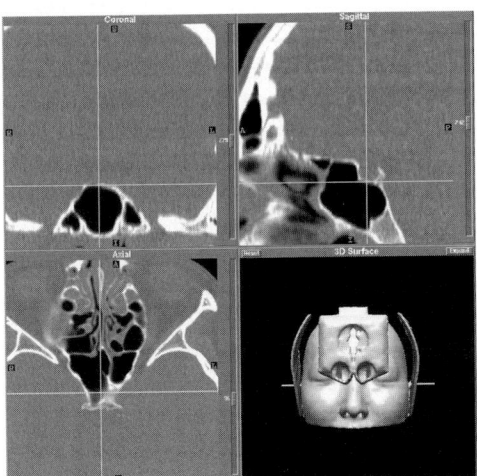

FIGURE 15.5 Software-enabled review of the preoperative CT scan facilitates the surgeon's understanding of complex sphenoid anatomy. By scrolling through the images at the computer workstation, the surgeon can develop a more precise mental model of sphenoid pneumatization. This CAS screen capture shows the standard triplanar CT image layout used for CT scan review. Note that the crosshairs are on the floor of the sella, which is bordered anteriorly and inferiorly by the posterior sphenoid sinus wall.

It should be emphasized that direct midline approaches to the sella (i.e., transseptal routes) provide direct access and afford less perceptual distortion. For this reason, they represent the preferred alternative, although other modifications (such as an endoscopic transnasal route) may also be used. If the route is off of the nasal midline, the potential for inaccurate recognition of relevant landmarks becomes greater. In these instances, CAS may have an even greater role.

After induction of general anesthesia and CAS system calibration and registration, the actual surgery is started. The septum may be used as the direct dissection plane to the sphenoid rostrum in any of the transseptal approaches. Cartilage, mucosa, and the sphenoid keel are removed to open into both sphenoid sinuses. Anterior-to-posterior septal flap elevation at the sphenoid rostrum may be avoided by creating a posteriorly based perforation approximately 1 cm anterior to the rostrum. At this point, a midline sphenoidotomy has been created via the transseptal route.

After completion of the midline sphenoidotomy, the anterior wall of each sphenoid sinus is removed from medial to lateral. During this removal, care should be taken to avoid injury to branches of the sphenopalatine artery, which cross the anterior sphenoid wall (Figure 15.2). The lateral and superior extent of dissection at the sphenoid sinus anterior wall may be guided by CAS surgical navigation.

After removal of the anterior sphenoid walls, the interior surface of the sphenoid sinus should be carefully inspected. The sphenoid intersinus septum may insert on the sella or the internal carotid artery (Figure 15.3). The internal carotid artery and the optic nerve may indent or actually pass through the sphenoid sinus. These anatomical variations, if present, should be identified. Direct visualization (via the operating microscope or nasal telescope), coupled with CAS surgical navigation, serves to accomplish this objective. The angled telescopes (namely, 30°, 45° and 70° telescopes) allow the surgeon to look "around the corner" prior to dissection. This may be very useful for dissection at the most lateral aspects of the sphenoid sinus. Other instruments used during this dissection may also include nasal specula, suction bipolars, suction curettes, sickle knives, and hooks. Suction sphenoid mushroom punches are also available.

The pituitary gland is located in the sella, which is just deep to the posterosuperior wall of the sphenoid sinuses (Figure 15.1). The posterior sphenoid wall may vary in thickness and orientation with respect to the pituitary. Hardy described three types of sphenoid sinus variants with respect to the pituitary [7]. The most common variant (86%) is the sellar type, in which a thin posterior sphenoid wall surrounds the pituitary gland. In the presellar type (11%), the anterior boundary of the sella is the thin posterior sphenoid sinus wall, and the sella's inferior boundary is thick bone. In this anatomical arrangement, sphenoid pneumatization does not extend beyond the vertical plane defined by the anterior sella wall. In the concha type (3%), the sella is surrounded by thick bone, and sphenoid pneumatization is minimal. The last variant may require usage of a drill for removal of thick bone for access to the sellar contents. Some CAS systems support the tracking of drill tip position; obviously, this may be helpful in the dissection of the conchal variant. The sphenoid posterior wall position can be determined by review of the preoperative sagittal CT images, which are reconstructed from the axial CT data on the CAS computer.

After a suitable opening into the sphenoid sinuses has been created, the sella itself must be opened. The mucosa from the posterior sphenoid sinus wall is carefully elevated and preserved. Then the thin bone that defines the boundary between the sella and the sphenoid sinuses is removed. A bipolar cautery is used to gently cauterize the underlying dura. Next the dura is incised for access to the pituitary fossa. Standard microdissection permits removal of the pituitary pathology. Violation of the sellar boundaries must be performed to minimize risk to the adjacent parasellar structures. The neurosurgeon usually performs the intrasellar dissection after the otorhinolaryngologist has provided the surgical access.

After completion of the pituitary dissection, surgical closure of the sellar defect is necessary. Autografts of fat, muscle, and/or fascia may be placed in the sella, but if the adjacent parasellar structures prolapse into the sellar space, the sella may not require packing with autografts. In fact, the avoidance of sellar packing may permit for clearer postoperative imaging for the early detection of recurrence. The posterior sphenoid wall (i.e., the sellar anterior wall) should be repaired to decrease the risk of cerebrospinal fluid leak, encephalocele, pneumocephalus, or meningitis [25–27]. Often the otolaryngologist completes this portion of the surgery. Otologic microinstruments may be helpful during the repair of the sellar wall. A layered reconstruction of the sellar wall is desirable. Temporalis fascia or other autogenous fascia may be placed on the intracranial side of the sellar defect in an "underlay" technique (which is similar to fascial graft placement in tympanoplasty). Acellular dermal allograft (AlloDerm, LifeCell Corporation, Branchburg, NJ) may be substituted for the fascial autografts [28]. Obviously, the use of allografts avoids the potential issues associated with the surgical harvest of autografts. The second layer consists of the positioning a piece of septal bone and/or cartilage (or an autogenous bone graft from the sphenoid anterior wall) so that this graft is wedged into position just deep to the posterior sphenoid wall. Sphenoid mucosa can then be redraped over the anterior sella wall defect. Alternatively, a free mucosal graft from the inferior or superior turbinate may be used for this purpose. Fibrin glue or Tisseel surgical sealant (Baxter Healthcare Corporation, Glendale, CA) may be applied over the reconstruction. Finally, dissolvable hemostatic packing (such as Avitene [MedChem Products, Inc., Woburn, MA], Merogel [Medtronic Xomed, Jacksonville, FL] and/or Surgicel [Johnson & Johnson, New Brunswick, NJ]) is then placed in the sphenoid. Anterior sellar wall reconstruction avoids the need for formal sphenoid sinus obliteration, which is now reserved for selected cases only.

Several variations in the traditional sublabial, transseptal, transsphenoidal approach have been introduced. The introduction of endoscopic visualization now minimizes the risk of septal perforations, which are quite common with the use of the operating microscope. Inadvertent septal trauma is minimized if the telescope is passed between the septal flaps, since the porthole necessary for the telescope is much smaller than the corresponding access needed for the self-retaining nasal speculum and the nasal telescope. Alternatively, the septum may also be left completely undissected; instead the posterior wall of the sphenoid sinus may be exposed via a direct endoscopic unilateral sphenoidotomy. Bilateral endoscopic sphenoidotomies without septoplasty can also be used. Badie et al. [14] studied two groups of patients who underwent standard transseptal transsphenoidal hypophysectomy ($n = 21$) and direct endoscopic transsphenoidal hypophysectomy ($n = 20$). They found that the exposure was equivalent. The endoscopic approach was associated with less facial pain, shorter operative time, and shorter hospitalization. The sublabial technique may be associated with a significant postoperative pain wound infection and nasal deformity. Koren et al. [13] compared the endoscopic transnasal and the sublabial approaches. The endoscopic technique had shorter operative time, shorter hospital stay, and lower incidence of nasal complications.

Today, most otorhinolaryngologists prefer the surgical nasal telescope for visualization during sinonasal procedures, since this instrument offers excellent illumination, visualization, and magnification. Some neurosurgeons have also adopted the telescope for hypophysectomy. The telescope may also supplement the operating microscope during sellar dissections. In particular, the telescope may be used during suprasellar dissections, since the angled telescopes affords visualization that the operating microscope cannot offer. It may be anticipated that the telescope may supplant the operating microscope as more experience with the telescope in pituitary procedures is acquired.

Sethi et al. [21] have developed an entirely endoscopic approach using cadavers. They have utilized this technique in over 40 hypophysectomies and state that it is the preferred technique at their tertiary referral hospital [9]. Carrau and Jho have also instituted a program for similar minimally invasive, endoscopic hypophysectomy at their university-based hospital [10–12]. Both groups believe that actual sella dissection with the 0° and 30° endoscopes permits more thorough dissection since the differences between normal and pathological tissues may be seen more clearly and easily. In addition, the 45° and 70° angled telescopes may also be used to further the extent of dissection in the suprasellar region. A variety of telescope holders and irrigation devices have been introduced; these products allow easier handling of the telescopes and may even permit bimanual dissection.

Vaughan et al. examined the differences among the choices of instruments by three different neurosurgeons who worked in conjunction with a single otolaryngologist [24]. One neurosurgeon preferred the microscope and C-arm, the second neurosurgeon used the operating microscope with CAS surgical navigation, and the third neurosurgeon had chosen the nasal telescope and CAS surgical navigation. Complications, operative times, blood loss, and length of hospital stay were similar in all patients, regardless of the intraoperative preferences of the operating neurosurgeon.

15.6 FUTURE DEVELOPMENTS

Transsphenoidal hypophysectomy has established itself as an effective and well-tolerated approach for pituitary surgery. With additional refinements of endoscopic techniques as well as their greater adoption by both neurosurgeons and otorhinolaryngologists, transsphenoidal hypophysectomy will grow to reflect the trend to minimally invasive surgery.

CAS software modifications will drive additional advances in pituitary surgery. Ideally, the next generation of CAS will support better radiology data set management. Furthermore, modified registration protocols may permit greater surgical navigation accuracy but offer simpler strategies for their routine use. CAS surgical planning modules also need additional revision. In particular, surgical planning should include virtual preoperative dissections, which would facilitate the identification of critical structures. In theory, intraoperative surgical navigation could be integrated with preoperative planning so that the CAS computer becomes a surgical warning system. This future CAS system would warn the surgeon of the close proximity of a critical structure (such as the internal carotid artery or the optic nerve) as the surgeon's instruments approached the structure. Furthermore, robotic instruments, which may be programmed with both preoperative and intraoperative data, may also be developed for hypophysectomies.

15.7 CONCLUSION

Many years ago transsphenoidal hypophysectomy emerged as the preferred approach for pituitary gland surgery. All of the various techniques share the common theme of access to the sella through the sphenoid sinus. Anatomical variability and the close proximity of critical structures represent the key surgical challenges during these procedures. To the extent that CAS facilitates the surgeon's three-dimensional understanding of this anatomy (both through preoperative planning and intraoperative localization), CAS may greatly reduce the potential morbidity and enhance the surgical results of transsphenoidal hypophysectomy.

REFERENCES

1. Schloffer H. Zur Frage der Operationen an der Hypophyse. Beitr Klin Chir 1906; 50:767–817.

2. Kanavel A. The removal of tumor of pituitary body by an intranasal route. JAMA 1909; 53:1701–1704.
3. Halstead A. Remarks on the operative treatment of tumors of the hypohysis. Surg Gynecol Obstet 1910; 10:494–502.
4. Cushing H. Surgical experiences with pituitary disorders. JAMA 1914; 63:1515–25.
5. Guiot G, Thebaul B. L'extirpation des adenomes hypophysaires par voie trans-sphenoidale. Neurochirurgie 1959; 1:133.
6. Hardy J. L'exerese des adenomes hypophysaires par voie trans-sphenoidale. Union Med Can 1962; 91:933.
7. Hardy J. Transphenoidal microsurgery of the normal and pathological pituitary. Clin Neurosurg 1969; 16:185–217.
8. Gamea A, Fathi M, el-Guindy A. The use of the rigid endoscope in trans-sphenoidal pituitary surgery. J Laryngol Otol 1994; 108:19–22.
9. Sethi D, Pillay P. Endoscopic management of lesions of the sella turcica. J Laryngol Otol 1995; 109:956–962.
10. Carrau R, Jho H, Ko Y. Transnasal-transsphenoidal endoscopic surgery of the pituitary gland. Laryngosope 1996; 106:914–918.
11. Jho H, Carrau R. Endoscopic endonasal transsphenoidal surgery: experience with 50 patients. J Neurosurg 1997; 87:44–51.
12. Jho H, Carrau R, Ko Y, Daly M. Endoscopic pituitary surgery: an early experience. Surg Neurol 1997; 47:213–222.
13. Koren I, Hadar T, Rappaport Z, Yaniv E. Endoscopic transnasal transsphenoidal microsurgery versus the sublabial approach for the treatment of pituitary tumors: endonasal complications. Laryngosope 1999; 109:1838–1840.
14. Badie B, Nguyen P, Preston J. Endoscopic-guided direct endonasal approach for pituitary surgery. Surg Neurol 2000; 53:168–172.
15. Mattox D, Mirvis S. Intraoperative portable computed tomography scanning: an adjunct to sinus and skull base surgery. Otolaryngol Head Neck Surg 1999; 121:776–780.
16. Schwarz B, et al. Intraoperative MR imaging guidance for intracranial neurosurgery: experience with the first 200 cases. Radiology 1999; 211:477–488.
17. Kremer P, Forsting M, Hamer J, Sartor K. MR imaging of residual tumor tissue after transsphenoidal surgery of hormone-inactive pituitary macroadenomas: a prospective study. Acta Neurochir Suppl (Wien) 1996; 65:27–30.
18. Kitazawa K, et al. CT guided transsphenoidal surgery: report of nine cases. No Shinkei Geka 1993; 21:147–152.
19. Dew L, Haller J, Major S. Transnasal transsphenoidal hypophysectomy: choice of approach for the otolaryngologist. Otolaryngol Head Neck Surg 1999; 120:824–827.
20. Spencer W et al. Approaches to the sellar and parasellar region: A retrospective comparison of the endonasal-transsphenoidal and sublabial-transsphenoidal approaches. Otolaryngol Head Neck Surg 2000; 122:367–369.
21. Sethi D, Stanley R, Pillay P. Endoscopic anatomy of the sphenoid sinus and sella turcica. J Laryngol Otol 1995; 109:951–955.
22. Chong V et al. Imaging the sphenoid sinus: pictorial essay. Australas Radiol 2000; 44:143–154.

23. Bolger W, Keyes A, Lanza D. Use of the superior meatus and superior turbinate in the endoscopic approach to the sphenoid sinus. Otolaryngol Head Neck Surg 1999; 120:308–13.
24. Vaughan W, Citardi M, Kuhn F. Surgical navigation in pituitary surgery. ERS and ISIAN Meeting '98, Vienna, Austria, July 28–August 1, 1998.
25. Haran R, Chandy M. Symptomatic pneumocephalus after transsphenoidal surgery. Surg Neurol 1997; 48:575–578.
26. Black P, Zervas N, Candia G. Incidence and management of complications of transsphenoidal operation for pituitary adenomas. Neurosurgery 1987; 20:920–924.
27. Ciric I, Ragin A, Baumgertner C, Pierce D. Complications of transsphenoidal surgery: results of a national survey, review of the literature, and personal experience. Neurosurgery 1997; 40:225–36.
28. Citardi MJ, Cox AJ, , Bucholz R. Acellular dermal allograft for sellar reconstruction after transsphenoidal hypophysectomy. Am J Rhinol. 2000; 14:69 73.

16

Computer-Aided Surgery Applications for Sinonasal Tumors and Anterior Cranial Base Surgery

Roy R. Casiano, M.D., F.A.C.S.
University of Miami School of Medicine, Miami, Florida

Ricardo L. Carrau, M.D., F.A.C.S.
University of Pittsburgh Medical Center, Pittsburgh, Pennsylvania

16.1 CHALLENGES

Over the past decade there has been a natural evolution in the capabilities of endoscopic sinus surgeons. Surgeons have continued to fine-tune their endoscopic surgical skills and improve their knowledge of complex orbital and skull base anatomy. The improved ability to successfully endoscopically repair even large skull base defects, combined with the illumination and magnification afforded by rigid telescopes, which provide improved visualization in anatomical recesses, has facilitated removal of a wide variety of nasal and paranasal sinus lesions.

The immediate reaction of those who do not perform endoscopic resection of neoplasms of the nose and paranasal sinuses and those who have not yet mastered this technique is one of skepticism. As with any new surgical approach, questions arise regarding the procedure's safety, morbidity, efficacy, reliability, and cost-effectiveness compared to the accepted "standard of care." Surgeons who are unfamiliar with endoscopic techniques cannot understand how these endoscopic techniques can incorporate fundamental oncological principles so that the endoscopic techniques achieve precision and tissue removal comparable with the more widely accepted, traditional external approaches. Advocates of external approaches are fast to note that facial, cranial, and/or gingival incisions are justifiable in order to attain good exposure and visualization of the surgical field; in this view, such exposure allows for more complete resections. Some surgeons even consider endoscopic treatments to be no more than piecemeal tumor resections. However, for experienced endoscopic surgeons, external incisions are not necessary to attain exposure and visualization. In fact, the visualization of the endoscopic alternative may be even greater than the standard external approaches. In general, most head and neck surgeons who are experienced with endoscopic approaches find few differences between the endoscopic and external procedures for selected lesions in regard to the degree of tissue removal and adequacy of visualization.

Initially advocated for inflammatory disease, endoscopic approaches are increasingly being used for the definitive treatment of nasal and paranasal sinus neoplasms, which previously were resected through more traditional (transfacial or craniofacial) approaches. In the hands of experienced and skilled surgeons, complete endoscopic resection is now attainable in many cases. Endoscopic resection of inverted papillomas, meningoencephaloceles, and a variety of select benign and malignant neoplasms has been advocated as a reasonable alternative to traditional approaches with equivalent efficacy [1–24]. However, large tumor size and uncertainty about the localization of critical neurovascular structures and extranasal tumor margins still limit the use of this approach for a number of other lesions. Today, with the introduction of computer-aided surgery (CAS) and other technological advancements, there are new and exciting surgical possibilities as endoscopic surgeons progressively challenge even these barriers.

16.2 APPLICATIONS

CAS devices complement good clinical judgment, thorough preoperative surgical planning, a solid understanding of the endoscopic anatomy, and sound surgical technique, but CAS can never be a substitute for any of these aspects of surgical care. This observation is especially important when performing endoscopic resection of nasal and paranasal sinus neoplasms. When used appropriately, CAS may be useful for preoperative surgical planning, including the identification of critical anatomical landmarks that may be obscured by inflammation, tumor, congenital anomalies, previous surgery, or neoplasms, and for maxillofacial reconstruction.

CAS devices serve as an excellent teaching tool that bears resemblance to an in-flight simulator, which may provide information for the benefit of operating

Anterior Cranial Base Surgery

surgeons and surgeons-in-training. The correlation of preoperative imaging and intraoperativesurgical anatomy can accelerate the learning curve of inexperienced surgeons and assist them with more difficult cases [25]. Experienced surgeons can also benefit from the use of these devices in complex cases where there is alteration of anatomical landmarks [26].

16.2.1 Preoperative Surgical Planning

The software for most CAS devices provides three-dimensional (3D) reconstructions of the digital data obtained from a fine-cut axial CT scan. This 3D model may be manipulated preoperatively or intraoperatively to simulate a particular surgical approach. CAS enhances the surgeon's ability to perform preoperative surgical planning by simulating the proposed surgical approach through the manipulation of the 3D CT images. Before the surgical procedure, the surgeon may review the 3D reconstructions and identify and delineate the structures of interest. Surgical approaches are then simulated (Figures 16.1 and 16.2). Surgical plans may be discussed with other surgeons and members of the surgical team. The surgical plans may also be reviewed with patients so that patients have a better understanding of their proposed surgical procedures.

16.2.2 Identification of Critical Anatomical Landmarks

In patients with neoplasms of the skull base and paranasal sinuses, tumor or intraoperative bleeding may obscure or even obliterate critical anatomical landmarks. As a result, the endoscopic surgeon may encounter difficulty in the identi-

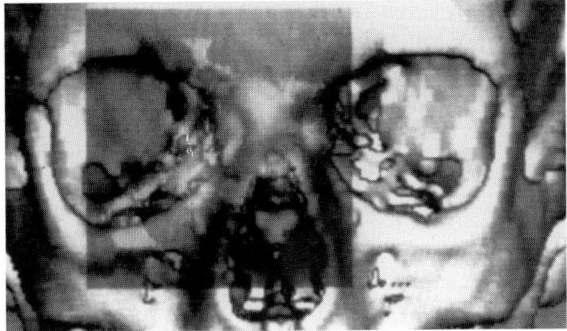

FIGURE 16.1 This three-dimensional CT reconstruction of a right ethmoid neoplasm demonstrates the location of the neoplasm with regard to nasofrontal region and the orbital apex. The lesion required a multidisciplinary approach for resection and reconstruction.

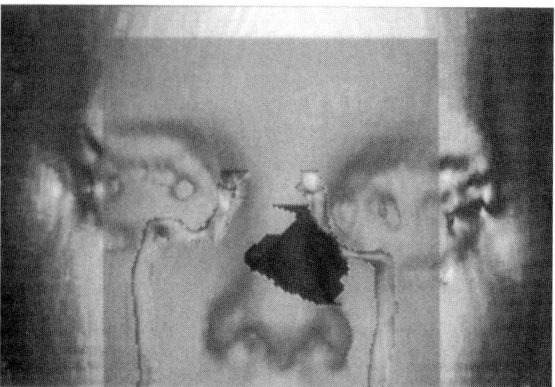

FIGURE 16.2 This three-dimensional CT reconstruction of a left nasoethmoid neoplasm demonstrates its location relative to the midface craniofacial skeleton.

fication of critical anatomical structures and tumor margins. CAS can be a useful adjunct for the identification of these critical structures. During the surgical procedure, the surgeon can reliably identify and preserve critical structures that are in close proximity to the tumor even if they have been displaced, obscured, or destroyed by the tumor. CAS gives the surgeon the most efficient access to the tumor for endoscopic resections, external resections, and even external resections with endoscopic assistance. Furthermore, CAS also increases the surgeon's level of confidence and thereby avoids the need for extensive dissection for the sole purpose of identifying a particular structure. This enhanced margin of safety allows experienced surgeons to consider the use of minimal access approaches. With CAS, the extent of surgical exposure may be more limited, since dissection for the confirmation of neurovascular structures may be minimized. Thus, CAS may expedite the entire surgical procedure. Although this observation has not been objectively confirmed, CAS may decrease surgical morbidity during complex surgeries of the maxillofacial skeleton, orbit, and skull base, while facilitating complete tumor resection.

CAS is most accurate and practical when used to identify fixed bony landmarks such as the paranasal sinuses and neurovascular foramina. It is useful to identify and/or preserve an anatomical barrier (such as the ethmoid sinus roof or orbital wall), a vital vessel (such as the internal carotid artery at its petrous portion), and/or an important cranial nerve (such as the optic or vidian nerve at its foramen or canal). CAS may also serve to plan the margins of tumor resection or to plan a craniotomy or sinusotomy (Figures 16.3 and 16.4). The boundaries of resection during medial maxillectomy may be easily identified with CAS. Similarly, the critical landmarks for endoscopic orbital decompression (namely the

Anterior Cranial Base Surgery

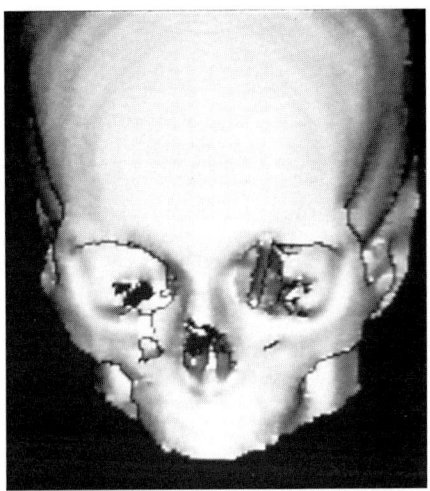

FIGURE 16.3 Another three-dimensional CT reconstruction of a left nasoethmoid neoplasm shows involvement of the medial wall of the orbit as well as the orbital apex.

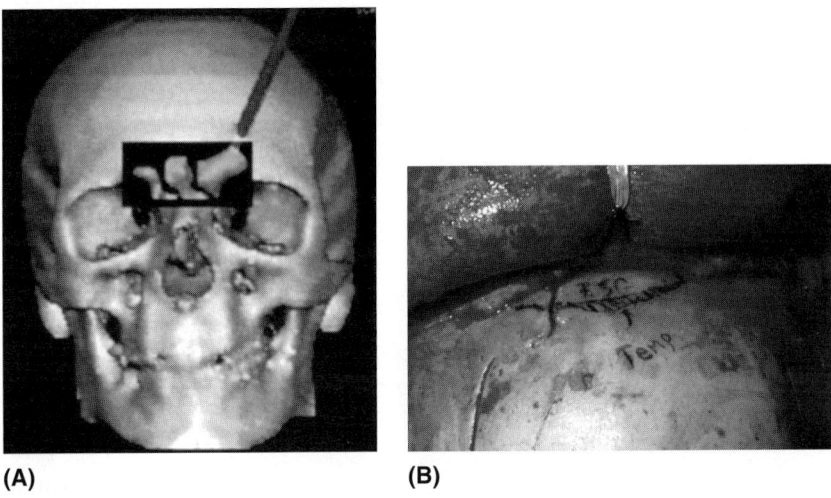

(A)   **(B)**

FIGURE 16.4 (A) This three-dimensional CT model shows the volume of the frontal sinus as well as its relative position. With this information, it is possible to plan the location of the bone cuts for elevation of the anterior table of the frontal sinus. (B) This intraoperative photo shows the outline of frontal sinus pneumatization as determined by a traditional 6-foot Caldwell plain film template (temp) and intraoperative surgical navigation (ISG). CAS provided a more accurate estimation of the size of the frontal sinus; therefore, CAS serves as a better guide for the placement of the bone cuts for osteoplastic sinusotomy.

medial and/or inferior orbital wall) and dacryocystorhinostomy (namely the lacrimal sac and duct) can be recognized. CAS can also be useful for identification of the optic canal or foramen when decompressing the nerve as part of a tumor resection or for posttraumatic neuropathy, especially in the absence of the traditional landmarks. Although CAS cannot provide information about soft-tissue composition and position intraoperatively (since surgery will alter those soft tissues), CAS can identify bony landmarks, which in turn provide important cues about the adjacent soft tissues. For example, intraorbital dissection of the orbital soft tissue during resection of the periorbita as part of an en bloc resection is greatly facilitated by identifying the frontoethmoidal suture and the ethmoidal and/or optic neurovascular foramina. These structures are not as readily visible as when dissecting in a subperiorbital plane, since the periorbita covers the frontoethmoid suture and neurovascular foramina.

16.2.3 Maxillofacial Reconstruction

CAS may facilitate the reconstruction of maxillofacial skeleton after the oncological resection is complete. At the CAS workstation, the surgeon can create a virtual mirror image reconstruction to achieve a symmetrical reconstruction by using the image of the contralateral side as a guide (Figure 16.5). Alternatively, the preoperative image can be used as a virtual moulage or mold to recreate the

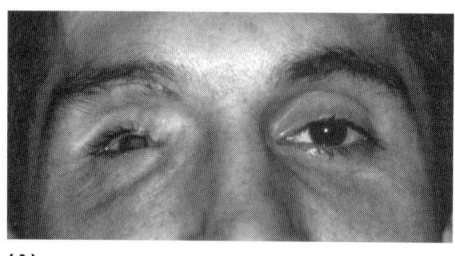
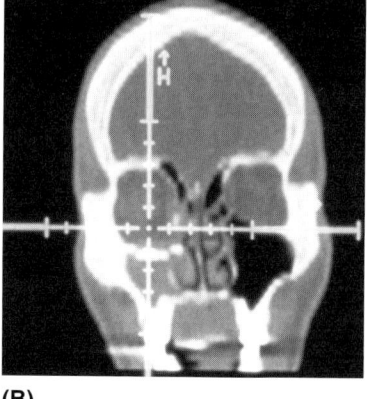

(A)   (B)

FIGURE 16.5 (A) This patient had right enophthalmos after an orbital trauma. Formal orbital reconstruction was necessary. (B) Preoperative CAS-based surgical planning and intraoperative CAS surgical navigation was used to determine the appropriate level of the orbital floor relative to the contralateral side. The crosshairs indicate the desired relative height for the orbital floor reconstruction.

Anterior Cranial Base Surgery

TABLE 16.1 The Ideal Computer-Aided Surgery Device

Good correlation between actual surgical anatomy and CAS images (including reconstructions)
Surgical navigation accuracy of 2 mm or better to minimize the risk of complications
Dynamic registration (which compensates for inadvertent head movement)
Specialized CAS CT or MRI not required
Minimal training for it use
Cost-effective alternative
Easy user interface which does not require the presence of a technician
Real-time update of imaging (compensation for intraoperative tissue manipulation/ distortion)
---

preoperative image. Of course, this option may only be useful if the disease process has not altered that contour. Thus, the surgeon can reconstruct a supraorbital bar, frontal bone, or orbital floor using titanium mesh or other material of preference and then CAS may confirm the adequacy of the profile using CAS.

16.3 ADVANTAGES AND DISADVANTAGES

Table 16.1 outlines the desired qualities of the ideal CAS system. Current CAS devices have inherent properties that may be an advantage or disadvantage, depending on its user (Tables 16.2 and 16.3).

The need for adequate experience, training, and clinical judgment to use these devices effectively and safely cannot be overemphasized. CAS has a learning curve that initially lengthens—rather than shortens—the length of surgery. On the other hand, the learning curve also dictates that with experience, the time associated with CAS set-up decreases. In fact, CAS may even reduce the time required for surgery. Experienced surgeons, who are endoscopically resecting sinonasal neoplasms, may actually find that CAS may reduce or even eliminate

TABLE 16.2 CAS Advantages

Accelerates the learning curve
Facilitates minimal access approaches
Identifies neurovascular foramina
Identifies altered anatomy
Localizes precise osteotomy/craniotomy/sinusotomy
Reduces operative time
Reduces morbidity

TABLE 16.3 CAS Disadvantages

Limited accuracy
No real-time update of intraoperative tissue manipulations
Limits access to the surgical field
Costly:
   The device
   Additional CT or MRI imaging
   Technician
Time necessary for registration
False sense of confidence

the time required for the identification of important structures by minimizing the need for extensive dissection throughout the surgery.

The accuracy of intraoperative CAS surgical navigation must be monitored throughout the procedure. Even in the CAS systems that support dynamic registration (so that the system compensates for inadvertent movement of the patient's head by tracking the head's position), reference frames can slip. When this occurs, the accuracy of surgical navigation will be compromised. Surgical navigation accuracy can be checked by localizing recognizable fixed structures; then the surgeon can compare the calculated position shown by the CAS computer with the known position in the operating field volume. It should be remembered that under the best circumstances, CAS surgical navigation accuracy is still 1–2 mm; therefore, knowledge of anatomy is still critical.

In addition, soft tissue shifts caused by surgical dissection or tumor removal cannot be tracked by any of the currently available CAS devices. The intraoperative monitor display is based on the patient's preoperative CT scan data set. This limitation is particularly important if the surgeon plans to operate beyond the bony confines of the paranasal sinuses. For instance, during endoscopic resection of skull base or orbital lesions, surgically induced distortion of the intracranial, skull base, or orbital soft tissues is a possibility. Intraoperative MRI, CT, or ultrasound have been advocated to circumvent this problem, but these devices are even more costly, are time-consuming, require special surgical instrumentation and operative suites, and/or are not currently widely available.

There are also some limitations with the 3D reconstruction. To truly simulate a surgical procedure in the 3D reconstruction requires intense work in order to delineate every structure that will be encountered in the proposed surgical procedure. In other words, to simulate an infratemporal fossa approach, the surgeon, radiologist, or radiology technician has to delineate the boundaries of the structures that will be manipulated (e.g., temporalis muscle, masseter muscle, parotid, scalp, orbitozygomatic complex, and any structures of interest within the infratemporal fossa). This requires a thorough knowledge of CT or MR anatomy. New CAS software may facilitate these simulations, but these upgrades have not been introduced. In the near future there should be anatomical recognition programs for neural structures to facilitate these tasks.

One of the greatest limitations of CAS devices is their cost. The devices range from $150,000 to $400,000, depending on their capabilities and applications. Adding to the cost is the need for a fine-cut CT scan or MRI, which provides the raw data for the CAS system. Most patients will have already undergone a scan for diagnostic purposes; therefore, the CT or MRI scan for CAS is an additional added cost. Often the device requires a dedicated technician or nurse during the registration process or even throughout the entire surgery. These costs can be amortized by sharing the CAS devices among different surgical services and using fine-cut imaging protocols when the need for CAS is anticipated. Nonetheless, the costs are still considerable and will be passed to the patient or third-party payers and/or absorbed by the buying institution.

16.4 ENDOSCOPIC RESECTION OF SPECIFIC NEOPLASMS AND EROSIVE LESIONS

When compared to other neoplasms of the head and neck, tumors originating in the nose or the paranasal sinuses present with a relatively low incidence in the general population. The most common of the malignant neoplasms is squamous cell carcinoma, occurring in less than 1 in 200,000 inhabitants per year [27]. Benign neoplasms are found even more infrequently. The most frequent benign tumors arising from this region are inverted papillomas, osteomas, hemangiomas, and juvenile nasopharyngeal angiofibroma (JNA). Although they are not true neoplasms, sinus mucoceles, meningoceles, and encephaloceles may present as intranasal or sinus masses and can be equally destructive to neighboring orbital and skull base structures. Three-dimensional reconstruction utilizing CAS can be utilized to guide the limits of resection by outlining the margins of the tumor resection margin or point of entry during a mucocele decompression.

Many lesions of the skull base are not easily accessible for biopsy. Frequently a seemingly minor biopsy requires a fairly extensive surgical approach to obtain an adequate specimen. This is especially true for lesions in the pterygopalatine, clival, and parasellar regions. The use of endoscopic approaches, assisted by CAS, can avoid the morbidity of a transfacial or transbasilar approach (Figures 16.6).

Some patients may have unresectable lesions threatening vital structures such as the optic nerve and other orbital structures. In these cases, tumor debulking and decompression of vital structures may be indicated. Benign lesions, such as fibrous dysplasia, can safely be debulked. In these procedures, the optic nerve, orbit, or secondary mucoceles in the dependent sinuses can be decompressed

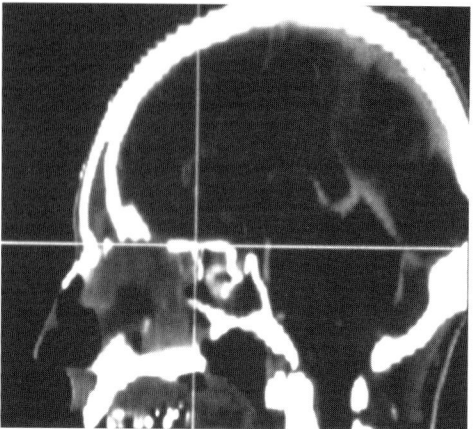

FIGURE 16.6 The crosshairs on this sagittal CT reconstruction show posterior tumor boundary, which guided planning for an intracranial osteotomy.

without extensive dissection. CAS is helpful in identifying the nasofrontal recess, orbital apex, carotid canal, ethmoid roof, optic canal, and the margins of the disease process.

16.4.1 Endoscopic Resection of Common Benign Lesions of the Sinonasal Region and Anterior Skull Base

16.4.1.1 Inverted Papilloma (Schneiderian Papilloma)

Inverted papilloma is one of the most common benign tumors of the paranasal sinuses. This locally aggressive tumor derives its name from the microscopic features that characterize it; its histology reveals the digitiform proliferation of squamous epithelium into the underlying stroma. Patients present with this entity in the fifth to sixth decades of life, with a clearly marked male predominance of 2–4:1 [1–5,28–32]. Classically, the tumor originates from the lateral nasal wall and subsequently involves the contiguous paranasal sinuses. Although no specific symptoms are unique to this entity, unilateral nasal obstruction constitutes the most consistent initially presenting symptom in 71–87% of cases. The potential for malignant transformation is one of the features that characterizes this tumor, with reports ranging from 5 to 13% in some of the studies with larger series of patients [30,31].

Anterior Cranial Base Surgery

The tumor's locally aggressive behavior, high recurrence rate, and potential for malignant transformation are important factors to consider when tailoring a surgical approach to remove these lesions. Most authors agree that incomplete resections constitute the principal cause of recurrence. Some authors have suggested tumor multicentricity as an additional factor to be considered [31,32].

Ideally, surgical treatment should achieve excellent long-term tumor control, have a low complication rate or associated surgical morbidity, and be performed with minimal cost and discomfort to the patients. So far, the consensus has been for surgical resection with wide tumor free margins. Traditionally, this often necessitated a medial maxillectomy or more rarely a craniofacial resection through an external approach [28–32]. However, today more surgeons are favoring a similar degree of resection through a transnasal endoscopic approach (Figure 16.7) [1–5].

For the vast majority of cases, the endoscopic approach is as effective as are external approaches are in the management of inverted papillomas. Even those who advocate the use of transnasal endoscopic excisions offer a very broad range of opinions regarding its limitations. Recommendations range from limiting this approach for the excision of more limited septal or lateral wall lesions to those who advocate for the endoscopic resection of more extensive lesions of the paranasal sinuses. Nevertheless, several generalizations can be made:

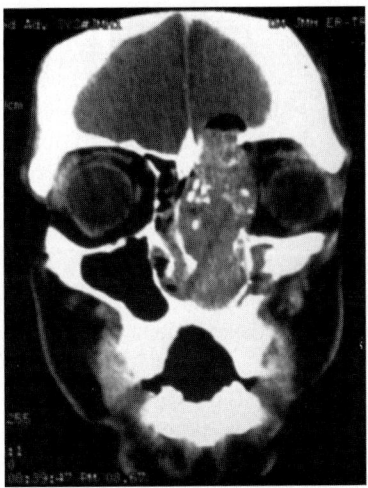

FIGURE 16.7 This coronal CT shows an extensive inverted papilloma with anterior skull base erosion and secondary epidural air. CAS may be used during endoscopic resection of these neoplasms to identify the lateral (orbital) and superior (skull base) boundaries.

A thorough endoscopic evaluation, as well as imaging studies such as CT and/or MRI, are essential for preoperative planning.

Histologically benign, centrally localized tumors seem to constitute the most widely accepted characteristics making endoscopic resections suitable.

The surgical approach is dependent upon the surgeon's experience. Whether or not a surgeon can perform a complete resection undoubtedly depends on his or her experience and skill. In the hands of skilled endoscopists, the use of telescopes to visualize and achieve complete resection of the mass is possible in most cases.

Recurrence seems to occur in an inverse relation to the completeness of tumor removal irrelevant of the elected surgical approach.

Close follow-up will be required for adequate reporting of disease control. This should include long-term serial endoscopic evaluations (>10 years).

In all cases, close postoperative surveillance is essential. Close follow-up and routine utilization of the sinus telescopes allows for early detection of recurrence. In the absence of malignant transformation, recurrent inverted papillomas generally have been seen to exhibit a relatively slow growth rate and small (i.e., millimeters) recurrences can be easily removed in the office setting through endoscopic means. This obviates the need for a subsequent return to the operating room (beyond the initial procedure) in the vast majority of these patients.

16.4.1.2 *Juvenile Nasopharyngeal Angiofibroma*

Juvenile nasopharyngeal angiofibromas (JNAs) are histologically benign, slow-growing, locally invasive, highly vascular tumors that are most frequently found in boys and young men between 14 and 25 years of age [33,34]. The most common presenting symptoms include epistaxis and nasal obstruction. Associated symptoms vary depending on tumoral extension into adjacent structures. Despite their histologically benign nature, rich vascularization gives these tumors the potential for life-threatening complications secondary to bleeding or intracranial extension. The submucosal centrifugal growth makes these lesions obligatorily extradural, even in cases with intracranial extension.

Rarely encountered in adults, it is believed that JNAs exhibit spontaneous regression. In addition, documented cases exist in which subtotal resection or incomplete radiotherapy have come to achieve tumor regression [34]. Whether the tumoral involution observed in these cases was entirely due to spontaneous regression or to devascularization of the residual tumor secondary to surgery or radiation therapy remains unknown.

Indentation of the posterior wall of the maxillary sinus and the superior orbital fissure (the Holmann-Miller sign) is suggestive but not pathognomonic of this entity [35]. Other diagnostic imaging techniques such as CT, MRI, magnetic resonance angiography (MRA), and conventional angiography all have contributed to the improved preoperative assessment of tumor extent, intracranial extension, and feeding vessels. Angiography with preoperative embolization has shown to be a significant adjunct in the management of these lesions reducing intraoperative blood loss and improving intraoperative visualization [7,8,36].

Various modalities of treatment have been proposed for this entity. Radiotherapy has been shown to halt tumor growth [7,37]. However, its effects on the growth of the craniomaxillofacial skeleton, along with its potential carcinogenic effects, should limit its use for surgically unresectable tumors or potentially life-threatening complications.

Surgical excision has been considered curative when complete resection is attained. The surgical goal is to achieve tumor resection with minimal neurological sequelae while minimizing the intraoperative blood loss and postoperative morbidity. In addition, the male craniomaxillofacial skeleton continues to grow until approximately the second decade of life. Hence, soft tissue elevation, maxillofacial osteotomies, and the use of metal plate fixations may potentially lead to subsequent asymmetric growth. These factors have to be considered when selecting a surgical approach for the resection of JNAs. The endoscopic approach offers a potential advantage over most of the external approaches, since the endoscopic approach is minimally disruptive to these developing anatomical structures, but still offers the capacity for adequate long-term disease control.

For cases of JNAs with limited extension to the nasopharynx, nasal cavity, ethmoid and sphenoid sinus, or pterygopalatine fossa, the endoscopic approaches compare favorably with the external approaches [6–8]. Early experience in a relatively small number of patients suggests that adequate tumor control may be attained with minimal disruption to uninvolved soft or bony tissue and little difference in morbidity. It has been noted that tumor recurrence occurs in direct proportion to its clinical stage, with overall recurrence rates being around 10%. The recurrence rate rises in cases with intracranial extension [37,38–40]. In the surgical management of JNAs, CAS may be useful in delineating the boundaries of the pterygomaxillary fossa and identifying the structures adjacent to the tumor margins (such the ICA, cavernous sinus, and clivus).

16.4.1.3 Mucoceles

Mucoceles are gradually expansile, epithelial-lined lesions filled with inspissated secretions. These lesions may erode the bony confines of the nasal cavity with the potential for intracranial or intraorbital penetration. Although many etiologies have also been proposed, mucoceles have been theorized to develop as a direct result of obstruction to the sinus ostium [41,42]. Rapid expansion of the mucocele may occur secondarily to acute infection (mucopyocele) with subsequent rupture that spreads infected material into contiguous orbital or intracranial stuctures.

Several authors have compared endoscopic with external approaches (i.e., Lynch-Howarth and frontal sinus obliteration procedures). Excellent results have been reported utilizing the endoscopic approach with minimal morbidity or complications [9–12]. However, at times this may require an extended frontal or sphenoid sinusotomy to widely marsupialize the cavity [43]. Today, CAS facilitates wide decompression of mucoceles that previously required an external or combined approach because of anatomic limitations and previous surgery. CAS may also be useful during endoscopic marsupialization of mucoceles, in which surgical access would otherwise be difficult because the inflammatory process has altered the standard surgical landmarks. Even mucoceles in the lateral aspect of the frontal sinus can be drained with computer-aided endoscopic techniques. In the event that frontal obliteration is indicated, CAS may also be used to plan the osteotomy cuts [44].

16.4.1.4 Meningoceles and Encephaloceles

Meningoceles or encephaloceles may present in the nose and paranasal sinuses with potentially adverse consequences (Figure 16.8). Cerebrospinal fluid (CSF) rhinorrhea and subsequently meningitis may ensue if these lesions are left untreated. The surgical literature documents many series of patients whose CSF leaks were repaired endoscopically [13–16]. In fact, the endoscopic repair of meningoceles and encephaloceles is attainable in most cases. The successful endoscopic repair of most skull base defects is now possible with one simple outpatient procedure in more than 90% of the patients. The use of CAS also allows identification of the bony and dural defect margins to minimize the chances of inadvertent intracranial resection of brain parenchyma (as in the case of an encephalocele) and subsequent injury to intracranial structures (Figure 16.9).

16.4.1.5 Other Benign Tumors

There have been numerous case reports of histologically benign tumors undergoing successful endoscopic resection. Immature teratomas and fibrous dysplasia

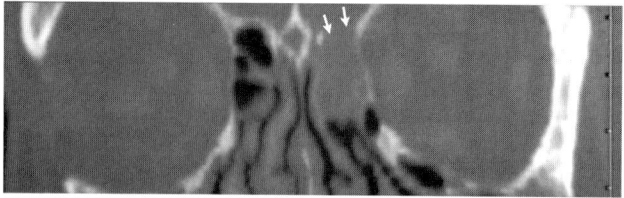

FIGURE 16.8 A meningoencephalocele from the anterior crnail fossa may intrude into the paranasal sinuses. This anterior skull base defect (indicated by the arrow) is well seen on this coronal sinus CT.

Anterior Cranial Base Surgery

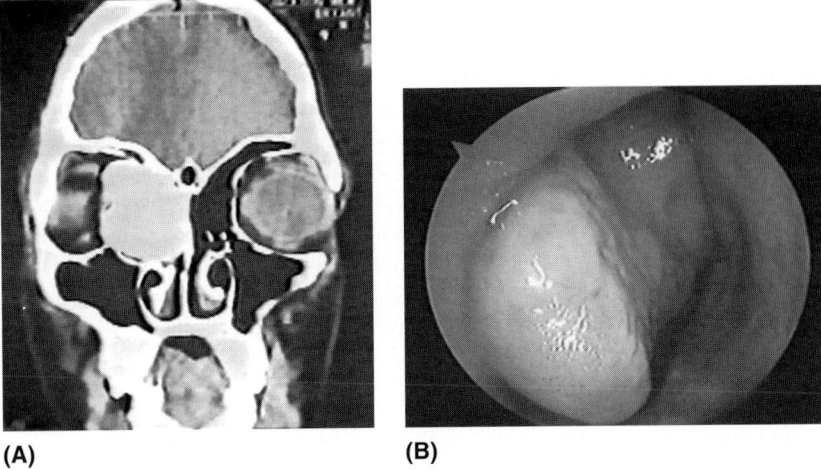

(A) (B)

FIGURE 16.9 (A) CT scans can accurately show the extent of paranasal osteomata. This CT shows a very large ethmoidal osteoma, which was causing significant exophthalmos CAS may be used to identify the boundaries during central debulking of this type of lesion with powered instrumentation. The thinned outer shell can then be safely removed transnasally. (B) Nasal endoscopy in the same patient shows a large submucosal mass that fills most of the superior nasal vault and middle meatus.

have both been treated by endoscopic resection [17,18]. Further generalizations regarding the treatment of these benign lesions cannot be made since no surgeon has had sufficient experience upon which to draw definitive conclusions.

Osteomas of the nasal and paranasal sinus region have also been endoscopically resected. However, most of the published cases report endoscopically assisted external approaches [19,20]. When osteomas are restricted mainly to the medial maxilla or ethmoid sinus, these lesions are thinned with a cutting bur from a central to peripheral direction entirely through an endoscopic approach (Figure 16.9). CAS allows for localization of the orbital and intracranial margins of dissection and thereby facilitates adequate thinning of the osteoma. In this way, the osteoma's outer shell can be easily removed in a piecemeal fashion through the nose.

16.4.2 Endoscopic Resection of Malignant Lesions of the Sinonasal Region and Anterior Skull Base

Until recently, endoscopic resection has been advocated strictly for debulking of malignant neoplasms. Such an approach has been reported for the palliation of sinonasal melanoma; this partial tumor removal can improve the patient's quality of life but not his or her life expectancy [45,46]. More recently, there have been a few reports on endoscopic resection of malignant sinonasal disease [21–24]. All of these have been small case series of patients undergoing endoscopically assisted craniofacial resection. Most of the malignant lesions have been hemangiopericytomas or esthesioneuroblastomas of the anterior skull base.

CAS may be useful in defining the lateral and superior tumor margins of resection at the bony skull base and orbit [47]. Critical neurovascular pedicles may be identified and preserved. As mentioned previously, CAS may not be as useful once the cranial cavity is entered or after the skull base and intracranial structures have been significantly distorted by the surgery, since current CAS systems do not reflect the manipulations induced by the actual surgical procedure.

16.5 CONCLUSION

Over the past several years, minimally invasive endoscopic techniques for the surgical management of sinonasal tumors and anterior skull base lesions have garnered increasing interest. Early reports have suggested that endoscopic techniques are at least comparable to standard approaches and may even offer specific advantages that the standard approaches cannot duplicate. All of these procedures require detailed understanding of critical anatomical relationships, which may be altered by the underlying disease process. CAS offers relatively straightforward ways for better comprehension of these surgical landmarks. CT and MR review at the CAS workstation, coupled with surgical planning and simulation, may actually reduce potential morbidity and enhance surgical results. Furthermore, intraoperative surgical navigation, which provides specific localization information, may provide invaluable guidance for the surgical procedure, especially if the procedure is performed under endoscopic visualization. Strategies that incorporate endoscopic approaches and CAS may emerge as the preferred method for the management of sinonasal tumors and other lesions of the anterior cranial base.

REFERENCES

1. MA Sukenik, RR Casiano. Endoscopic medial maxillectomy for inverted papillomas of the paranasal sinuses: value of the intraoperative endoscopic examination. Laryngoscope 110:39–42, 2000.
2. E Raveh, R Feinmesser, T Shpitzer, E Yaniv, K Segal. Inverted papilloma of the nose and paranasal sinuses: a study of 56 cases and review of the literature. In Isr J Med Sci 32(12):1163–1167, 1996.
3. G Waitz, ME Wigand. Results of endoscopic sinus surgery for the treatment of inverted papillomas. Laryngoscope 102(8):917–922, 1992.

4. WS McCary, CW Gross, JF Reibel, RW Cantrell. Preliminary report: endoscopic versus external surgery in the management of inverting papilloma. Laryngoscope 104(4):415–419, 1994.
5. RH Kamel. Transnasal endoscopic medial maxillectomy in inverted papilloma. Laryngoscope 105(8 Pt 1):847–853, 1995.
6. HZ Tseng, WY Chao. Transnasal endoscopic approach for juvenile nasophoryngeal angiofibroma. Am J Otolarygol 18:151–154, 1997.
7. JJ Fagan, CH Snyderman, RL Carrau, IP Janecka. Nasopharyngeal angiofibromas: selecting a surgical approach. Head Neck 19(5):391–399, 1997.
8. K Ungkanont, RM Byers, RS Weber, DL Callender, PF Wolf, H Goepfert. Juvenile nasopharyngeal angiofibroma: an update of therapeutic management. Head Neck 18: 60–66, 1996.
9. DW Kennedy, JS Josephson, SJ Zinreich, DE Mattox, MM Goldsmith. Endoscopic sinus surgery for mucoceles: a viable alternative. Laryngoscope 99(9):885–895, 1989.
10. NJ Beasley, NS Jones. Paranasal sinus mucoceles, modern management. Am J Rhinol 9:251–256, 1995.
11. MS Benninger, S Marks. The endoscopic management of sphenoid and ethmoid mucoceles with orbital and intranasal extension. Rhinology 33(3):157–161, 1995.
12. VJ Lund. Endoscopic management of paranasal sinus mucocoeles. J Laryngol Otol 112(1):36–40, 1998.
13. RR Casiano, D Jassir. Endoscopic cebrospinal fluid rhinorrhea repair: Is a lumbar drain necessary? Otolaryngol Head Neck Surg 121(6):745–750, 1999.
14. DC Lanza, DA O'Brien, DW Kennedy. Endoscopic repair of cerebrospinal fluid fistulae and encephaloceles. Laryngoscope 106:1119–1125, 1996.
15. EE Dodson, CW Gross, JL Swerdloff, LM Gustafson. Transnasal endoscopic repair of cerebrospinal fluid rhinorrhea and skull base defects: a review of twenty-nine cases. Otolaryngol Head Neck Surg 111(5):600–605, 1994.
16. JA Burns, EE Dodson, CW Gross. Transnasal endoscopic repair of cranionasal fistulae: a refined technique with long-term follow-up. Laryngoscope 106(9 Pt 1):1080–1083, 1996.
17. RL Voegels, W Luxemberger, H Stammberger. Transnasal endoscopic removal of an extensive immature teratoma in a three-month-old child. Ann Otol Rhinol Laryngol 107:654–657, 1998.
18. K Ikeda, H Suzuki, T Oshima, A Shimomura, S Nakabayashi, T Takasaka. Endonasal endoscopic management in fibrous dysplasia of the paranasal sinuses. Am J Otolaryngol 18(6):415–418, 1997.
19. K Al-Sebeih, M Desrosiers. Bifrontal endoscopic resection of frontal sinus osteoma. Laryngoscope 108:295–298, 1998.
20. AM Seiden, YI El Hefny. Endoscopic trephination for the removal of frontal sinus osteoma. Otolaryngol Head Neck Surg 112:607–611, 1995.
21. A Blokmanis. Endoscopic diagnosis, treatment, and follow-up of tumours of the nose and sinuses. J Otolaryngol 23(5):366–369, 1994.
22. N Bhattacharyya, NL Shapiro, R Metson. Endoscopic resection of a recurrent sinonasal hemangiopericytoma. Am J Otolaryngol 18(5):341–344, 1997.
23. ER Thaler, M Kotapka, DC Lanza, DW Kennedy. Endoscopically assisted anter-

ior cranial skull base resection of sinonasal tumors. Am J Rhinol 13(4):303–310, 1999.
24. APW Yuen, KN Hung. Endoscopic cranionasal resection of anterior skull base tumor. Am J Otolaryngol 18(6):431–433, 1997.
25. RR Casiano, W Numa. Efficacy of CT-guidance in residency programs. Laryngoscope (in press).
26. R Metson, M Cosenza, RE Gliklich, WW Montgomery. The role of image-guidance systems for head and neck surgery. Arch Otolaryngol Head Neck Surg 125(10): 1100–1104, 1999.
27. Squamous cell "papillomas" of the oral cavity, sinonasal tract, and larynx. In: JG Batsakis, ed. Tumors of the Head and Neck, 2nd ed., Baltimore: Williams and Wilkins, 1979, pp. 130–143.
28. W Lawson, BT Ho, CM Shaari, HF Biller. Inverted papilloma: a report of 112 cases. Laryngoscope 105(3 pt 1):282–288, 1995.
29. DP Vrabec. The inverted Schneiderian papilloma: a 25-year study. Laryngoscope 104(5 Pt 1):582–605, 1994.
30. MC Weissler, WW Montgomery, PA Turner, SK Montgomery, MP Joseph. Inverted papilloma. Ann Otol Rhinol Laryngol 95(3 pt 1):215–221, 1986.
31. VJ Hyams. Papillomas of the nasal cavity and paranasal sinuses. A clinicopathological study of 315 cases. Ann Otol Rhinol Laryngol 80(2):192–206, 1971.
32. S Bielamowicz, TC Calcaterra, Watson D. Inverting papilloma of the head and neck: the UCLA update. Otolaryngol Head Neck Surg 109(1):71–76, 1993.
33. W Draf. Juvenile angiofibroma. In: LN Sekhar, IP Janecka, eds. Surgery of Cranial Base Tumors. New York: Raven Press, 1993, pp. 485–496.
34. DT Cody (II), LW DeSanto. Neoplasms of the nasal cavity. In: CW Cummings, JM Frederickson, LA Harker, CJ Krause, MA Richardson, DE Schuller, eds. Otolaryngology Head & Neck Surgery, 3rd ed. St. Louis, MO: Mosby-Year Book Inc., 1998, pp. 883–901.
35. CB Hollmann, Miller: Juvenile nasopharyngeal angiofibroma. Am J Roentgenol 94: 292, 1965.
36. TM Siniluoto, JP Luotonen, TA Tikkakoski, AS Leinonen, KE Jokinen. Value of pre-operative embolization in surgery for nasopharyngeal angiofibroma. J Laryngol Otol 107(6):514–521, 1993.
37. BJ Wiatrak, CF Koopmann, AT Turrisi. Radiation therapy as an alternative to surgery in the management of intracranial juvenile nasopharyngeal angiofibroma. Int J Pediatr Otorhinolaryngol 28(1):51–61, 1993.
38. M Jacobsson, B Petruson, P Svendsen, B Berthelsen. Juvenile nasopharyngeal angiofibroma. A report of eighteen cases. Acta Otolaryngol (Stockh) 105(1–2):132–139, 1988.
39. TS Economou, E Abemayor, PH Ward. Juvenile nasopharyngeal angiofibroma: an update of the UCLA experience, 1960–1985. Laryngoscope 98(2):170–175, 1988.
40. LG Close, SD Schaefer, BE Mickey, SC Manning. Surgical management of nasopharyngeal angiofibroma involving the cavernous sinus. Arch Otolaryngol Head Neck Surg 115(9):1091–1095, 1989.
41. C Evans. Aetiology and treatment of fronto-ethmoidal mucocele. J Laryngol Otol 95(4):361–375, 1981.

42. VJ Lund, B Henderson, Y Song. Involvement of cytokines and vascular adhesion receptors in the pathology of fronto-ethmoidal mucocoeles. Acta Otolaryngol (Stockh) 113(4):540–546, 1993.
43. RR Casiano, JA Livingston. Endoscopic Lothrop Procedure: the University of Miami experience. Am J Rhinol 12(5):335–339, 1998.
44. RL Carrau, CH Snyderman, HB Curtin, JL Weissman. Computer-assisted frontal sinusotomy. Otolaryngol Head Neck Surg 111(6):727–732, 1994.
45. JJ Homer, NS Jones, PJ Bradley. The role of endoscopy in the management of nasal neoplasia. Am J Rhinol 11(1):41–47, 1997.
46. VJ Lund. Malignant melanoma of the nasal cavity and paranasal sinuses. Ear Nose Throat J 72(4):285–289, 1993.
47. RL Carrau, HD Curtin, CH Snyderman, J Bumpous, M Stechison. Practical applications of image-guided navigation during anterior craniofacial resection. Skull Base Surg 5:51–55, 1995.

17

Computer-Aided Otologic and Neurotologic Surgery

Eric W. Sargent, M.D., F.A.C.S.
Michigan Ear Institute, Farmington Hills, Michigan

17.1 INTRODUCTION

Otology and neurotology, like sinus surgery, challenge surgeons in ways that make image guidance potentially useful. Both disciplines deal with vital structures whose anatomy may be obscured or altered by disease. The minute structures of the ear, such as the labyrinthine facial nerve and cochlea, test the resolution of currently available computer-aided surgery (CAS) technology.

Like other disciplines, the majority of otologic and neurotologic procedures can be more easily performed *without* CAS using well-established and relatively invariable landmarks. Operations such as stapedotomy, tympanoplasty, tympanomastoidectomy, and labyrinthectomy, for example, benefit little from intraoperative surgical navigation. Other surgical challenges potentially benefit from CAS in extreme circumstances. During cochlear implantation of an ossified or malformed cochlea, for example, CAS surgical navigation can aid in placing the electrode close to the neural elements. In surgery for external auditory canal atresia, CAS may allow delineation of the facial nerve and ossicular mass while drilling proceeds, potentially reducing the risk to these structures.

In the author's experience, procedures in which CAS technology offers the most potential use can be divided into two categories. Cases in which anatomy is distorted by pathology, as in large acoustic tumors, benefit from image guidance. Although not discussed in this chapter, we have used image guidance when removing massive cerebello-pontine angle tumors since CAS can help delineate the tumor/brainstem interface. Cases in which unreliable landmarks obscure vital structures also gain from CAS. Intraoperative surgical navigation is especially useful in these instances. This category includes middle cranial fossa procedures, petrous apex drainage procedures, and retrosigmoid dissection of the internal auditory meatus for acoustic neuroma. CAS would be of little benefit in neurotologic procedures like retrosigmoid vestibular nerve section or vascular decompression where landmarks are clear and the structures of interest are easily visible.

In this chapter, the author's experience with CAS in otology and neurotology will be reviewed so that the reader may understand the applications and potential pitfalls of this technology in otology, neurotology, and lateral skull-base surgery. Two procedures that exemplify the type of otologic operations for which CAS is best suited will be presented. In this regard, CAS, including preoperative surgical planning and intraoperative surgical navigation, has the greatest utility during middle cranial fossa surgery [1] and petrous apex surgery.

17.2 MIDDLE CRANIAL FOSSA SURGERY

Since its reintroduction in 1961 by William House [2], the middle cranial fossa (MCF) approach to the internal auditory canal (IAC) has been used for a variety of indications. For vestibular schwannomas located laterally in the IAC, the MCF approach allows preservation of hearing. For patients with intractable vertigo due to unilateral labyrinthopathy and serviceable hearing, the MCF approach to the vestibular nerve is an alternative to retrolabyrinthine or retrosigmoid vestibular nerve section. It can be used in revision nerve section procedures as well. No matter the indication, however, the MCF approach is a technical challenge.

In the lateral end of the IAC the margin for error is slight. Posterior to the lateral IAC is the ampullate end of the superior semicircular canal (SSC), and anterior to the lateral IAC is the basal turn of the cochlea. Millimeters separate the structures. The facial nerve becomes more superficial in the lateral IAC as it rises to the geniculate ganglion located in the floor of the MCF and is thus more exposed to potential injury. Landmarks are not as apparent in the MCF as in other approaches through the temporal bone, making dissection more difficult.

Without the benefit of CAS, the surgeon may choose a number of strategies to orient the dissection. The greater superficial petrosal nerve may be located in the facial hiatus and traced backward to the geniculate ganglion [3,4]. The IAC may then be located medial to the geniculate ganglion. Alternatively, the superior semicircular canal may be used as the primary landmark and traced forward until the ampullate end is found. This then indicates the position of the superior vestibular and facial nerves [5]. This approach relies on the position of the arcuate eminence on the floor of the MCF to orient dissection. Although in 98% of cases the lateral aspect of the arcuate eminence predicts the underlying lateral limb of the superior semicircular canal, the relationship can vary and the arcuate eminence may be absent in 15% of patients [6]. Yet another approach is to begin drilling in a "safe area" 28 mm from the inner surface of the squamous temporal bone and locating the IAC medially [7].

17.2.1 Technique

Patients with vestibular schwannomas that do not extend more than 5 mm beyond the lip of the porus acusticus, evidence of a superior vestibular nerve tumor, and good preoperative hearing are offered MCF removal of their tumors. Other patients in whom the technique is appropriate include patients with intractable vertigo and unilateral vestibulopathy who desire vestibular nerve section. The author does not use the MCF approach as his primary approach for vestibular nerve section; the retrosigmoid approach is the preferred technique in this instance, unless the patient has failed a prior attempt at nerve section.

On the day prior to surgery, five to seven adhesive markers (fiducial markers) containing a contrast agent are applied to the skin surface in locations that encompass the area of the temporal bone, and a high-resolution noncontrast CT is performed. The dataset is sent to the surgical workstation and patients are instructed to leave the fiducials undisturbed overnight.

On the day of surgery, the patient is positioned in a slightly lateral recumbent position on a bean-bag. Early in our experience, a Mayfield head holder to which we attached the reference arc stabilized the head (Figure 17.1). However, because MCF surgery is performed without the use of muscle relaxant (to allow continuous electromyographic monitoring of the facial nerve), patient movement occasionally caused enough slippage of the head to render the localizer inaccurate. For that reason, the author now uses a small reference arc anchored directly to the calvarium with screws. This method provides reliable registration that cannot be disturbed by patient movement. After anchoring the reference arc, the external fiducial markers are registered and a supplemental registration based on surface contours is performed. The attachment of the reference arc and registration of the fiducial points are performed while other preparations are made for surgery (i.e., starting an arterial line, placing the urinary catheter, placing EMG electrodes) and does not add significantly to the surgical time.

After performing a MCF craniotomy, the brain is retracted with a House-Urban MCF retractor. The floor of the MCF is mapped with the position of the superior semicircular canal, the basal turn of the cochlear, the geniculate ganglion, and IAC marked. Three orthogonal views (sagittal, axial, and coronal)

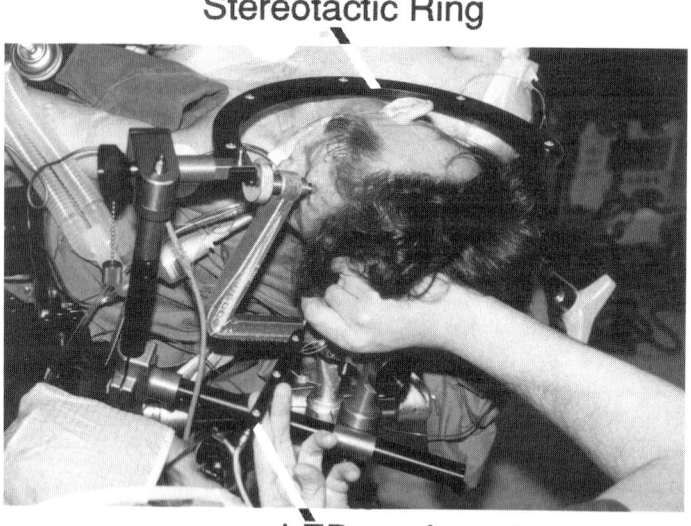

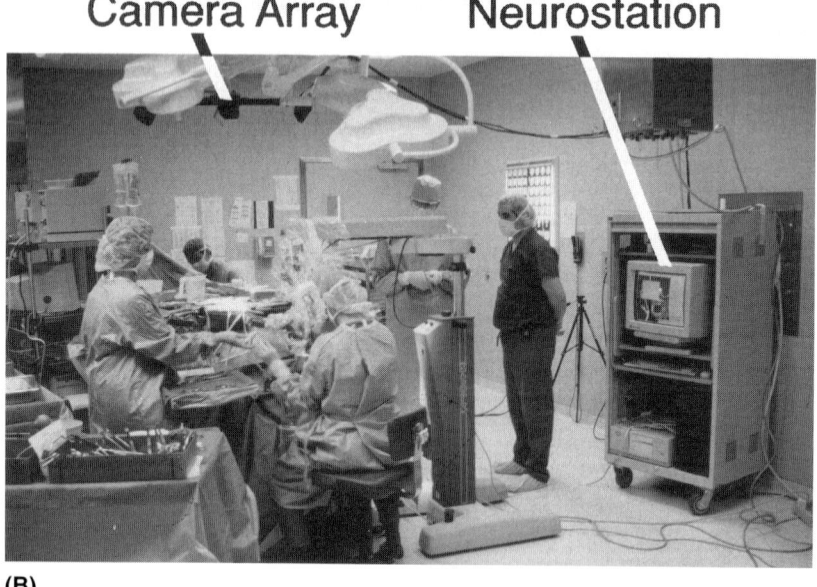

FIGURE 17.1 (A) Patient positioned for middle cranial fossa surgery with image guidance. (B) Operating room arrangement for middle cranial fossa surgery. (From Ref. 1.)

allow three-dimensional orientation of the instrument tip. The IAC is then "bluelined" with the dura left undisturbed until it has been uncovered for 180°. The dura is then opened with an ophthalmic knife and the tumor removed or vestibular nerve cut using standard techniques.

CAS, in the experience of the author, reduces the time required to orient the dissection in the temporal bone during MCF surgery. With attachment of the reference arc directly to the calvarium, the accuracy of the system is increased and remains stable throughout the procedure, even during the rare times when the patient moves.

17.3 PETROUS APEX DRAINAGE PROCEDURES

Petrous apex lesions are relatively rare, usually benign, and typically cystic. The most common lesions are cholesterol granulomas. These locally destructive, expansile lesions can invade the cochlea and labyrinth, causing hearing loss and vertigo. They can also involve Meckel's cave, causing fifth nerve symptoms. Cholesterol granulomas typically arise in well-pneumatized temporal bones as a result of air cell obstruction and foreign body reaction.

Infections of the petrous apex (petrous apicitis) may require drainage. Symptoms of petrous apicitis include boring retro-orbital pain and abducens palsy due to inflammation of Dorello's canal (Gradenigo's syndrome). The condition often arises after mastoidectomy is performed on a draining ear.

A number of approaches can access the petrous apex: transcochlear, infracochlear, infralabyrinthine, transethmoidal/transsphenoidal, or the anterior approaches of Ramadier, Eagleton, and Lempert [8]. The MCF approach can also access the petrous apex, but because it is difficult to establish a drainage tract, it has been largely abandoned for purposes of drainage [9].

For most lesions of the petrous apex, the author favors the infracochlear approach because it readily accesses the air cells anterior to the cochlea. The infracochlear air cells (a region known as the *infracochlear triangle*) are bounded anteriorly by the carotid artery, posteriorly by the jugular bulb, and superiorly by the basal turn of the cochlea. For patients with nonserviceable hearing, the approach can be extended to include the cochlea (the transcochlear approach). If dissection in the infracochlear approach remains inferior to the round window, the cochlea will not be violated and hearing can be preserved. The infracochlear approach can establish a wide tract into the cyst with dependent drainage.

As in MCF surgery, conventional techniques can be used to reliably approach the area of interest. The advantage of CAS is in the fairly common scenario of either an absent or poorly developed infracochlear air-cell tract or a deeply situated or small cyst. In these situations, the author has found that image guidance allows the trajectory of dissection to be monitored and vital structures, such as the horizontal segment of the carotid artery, to be avoided.

17.3.1 Technique

The following case of a petrous apex granuloma illustrates the benefits of CAS. A 35-year-old woman developed numbness, tingling, and intermittent sharp pains on the right side of her face one year before presenting to our institution. Sudden loss of vision in her right eye that spontaneously recovered brought her to the attention of physicians 8 months before seeing the author. Her past medical history included a right myringoplasty 14 years prior to her presentation. About a year before presenting, she had a severe right ear infection. The hearing in her right ear was subjectively impaired.

Evaluated by another surgeon, she was found on MRI (Figure 17.2) to have a right petrous apex cyst with a signal characteristic of a cholesterol granuloma (hyperintensity on T_1 and T_2 and nonenhancement with gadolinium infusion). The cyst impinged the horizontal carotid artery and cavernous sinus. Middle cranial fossa drainage was planned after a temporal bone CT showed no infracochlear air-cell tract. Concerned about the temporal lobe retraction required, she sought evaluation at our institution.

She reported continued fluctuating vision in her right eye and right facial hypesthesia. An audiogram demonstrated normal hearing in the left ear and a moderate neurosensory hearing loss in the right ear with 80% word recognition. Infracochlear drainage was discussed, and the day prior to surgery she underwent a high-resolution CT of the temporal bones with adhesive fiducials applied. On the day of surgery, a reference arc was anchored with three 4 mm long self-tapping screws through a small scalp incision (Figure 17.3). The arc has four detachable reflecting balls that allowing tracking head position during surgery. Registration of the arc and fiducial points was then performed (Figure 17.4). A trajectory for orienting dissection was planned on the workstation (Figure 17.5).

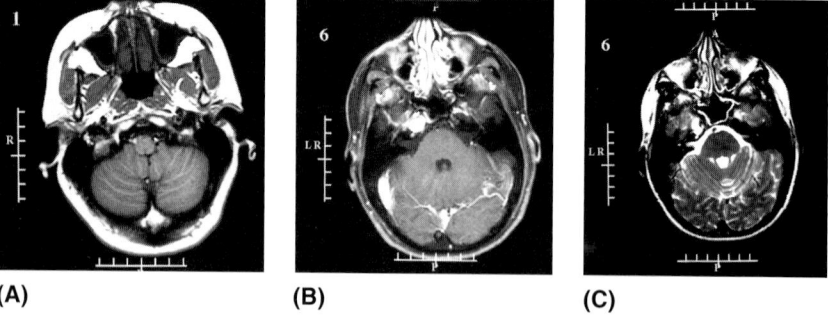

FIGURE 17.2 MRI of petrous apex cyst. (A) T_1-weighted without contrast; (B) T_1-weighted with gadolinium; (C) T_2-weighted.

Computer-Aided Otologic and Neurotologic Surgery

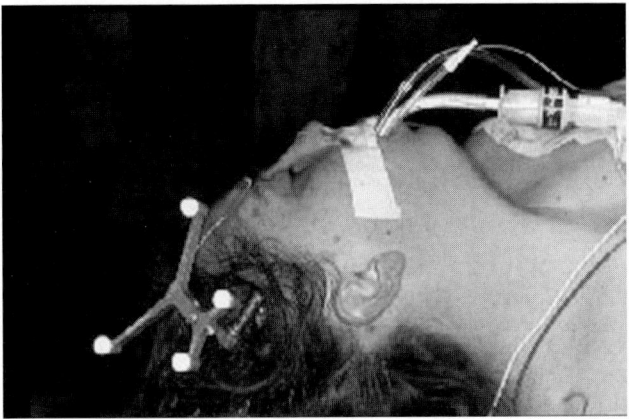

FIGURE 17.3 Reference arc attached to calvarium with 4 mm screws through a small scalp incision.

The surgical field was sterilely prepped and draped. Sterile reflecting balls are placed on the posts of the reference arc (Figure 17.6). Continuous facial nerve EMG was initiated.

Exposure of the hypotympanum was performed using the technique described by Fong et al. (9). A postauricular incision was made and the skin of the posterior external auditory canal was elevated. Approximately 5–6 mm from the

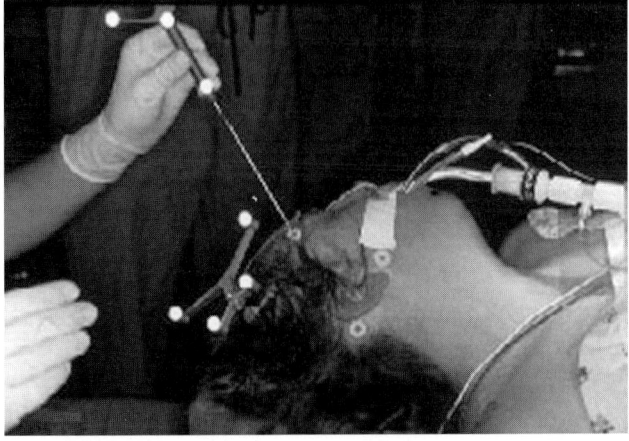

FIGURE 17.4 Registration of reference arc and fiducials.

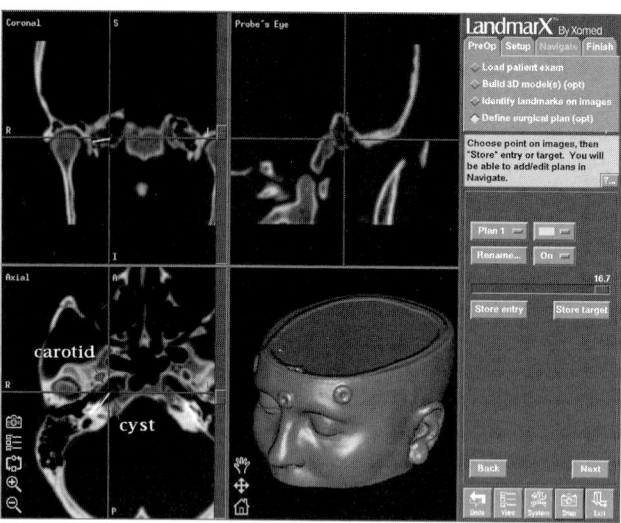

FIGURE 17.5   Planning of trajectory on navigational workstation.

tympanic annulus, the external auditory canal skin was completely transected and a self-retaining retractor placed. Incisions were then made in the remaining canal skin high on the anterior canal wall and at the level of the incudo-stapedial joint. The skin and eardrum were then elevated so that the hypotympanum can be accessed and the eardrum and skin remains attached to the umbo of the malleus. To establish the limits of posterior bone removal and prevent facial nerve injury,

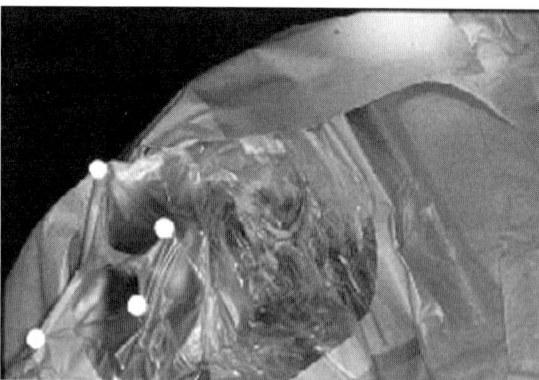

FIGURE 17.6   Surgical field with reference arc.

Computer-Aided Otologic and Neurotologic Surgery

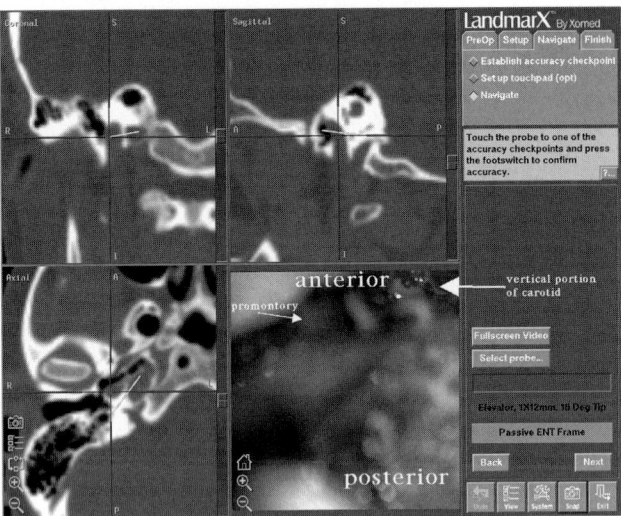

FIGURE 17.7 Skeletonizing the carotid in the infracochlear triangle.

the bone over the chorda tympani was removed with an otologic drill and continuous irrigation. The chorda tympani was followed inferiorly. The inferior external auditory canal bone was removed until the level of the jugular bulb was identified.

Before beginning dissection of the infracochlear triangle, accuracy of the registration of the navigational system was confirmed using landmarks in the middle ear such as the lip of the round window, the stapes, and the bone of the promontory. Drilling then exposed the internal carotid artery and jugular bulb. In this patient's case, the cyst was both deeply situated and the infracochlear air cells were poorly developed, making CAS particularly helpful. (Figures 17.7, 17.8, and 17.9 show the progress of dissection.)

Following surgery, the patient was discharged after an overnight stay. Her visual and facial symptoms resolved completely. An audiogram 2 months after surgery showed no change from her preoperative hearing.

17.4 INSTRUMENTATION

Initially, neurosurgical instruments adapted for the navigational system were used (Figure 17.10) but proved unwieldy in the confines of the ear under the otologic microscope. To overcome these drawbacks, otologic instruments were modified by the author with attachments for the LED array (Figure 17.11). These shorter instruments allow simultaneous dissection and localization under

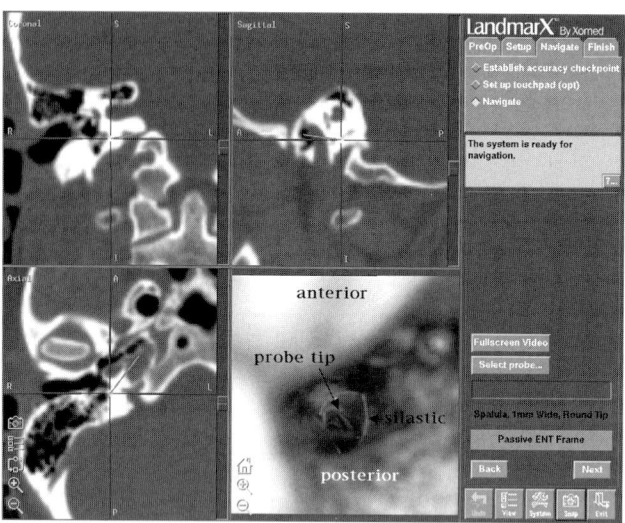

FIGURE 17.8 Introducing silastic into drainage tract after opening cyst.

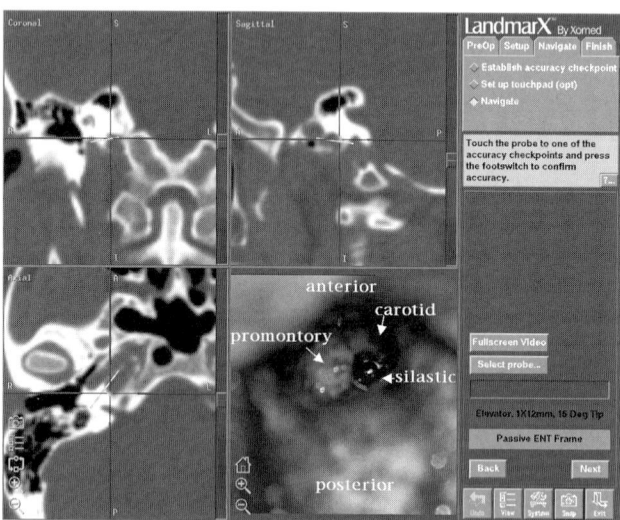

FIGURE 17.9 Completed cyst drainage.

Computer-Aided Otologic and Neurotologic Surgery 307

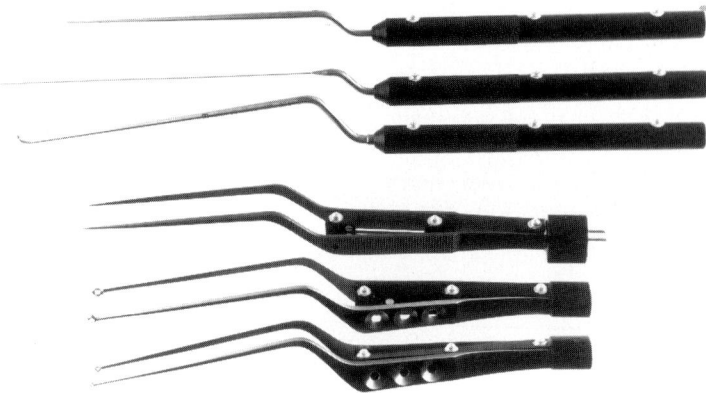

FIGURE 17.10 Modified neurosurgical instruments used in middle cranial fossa surgery.

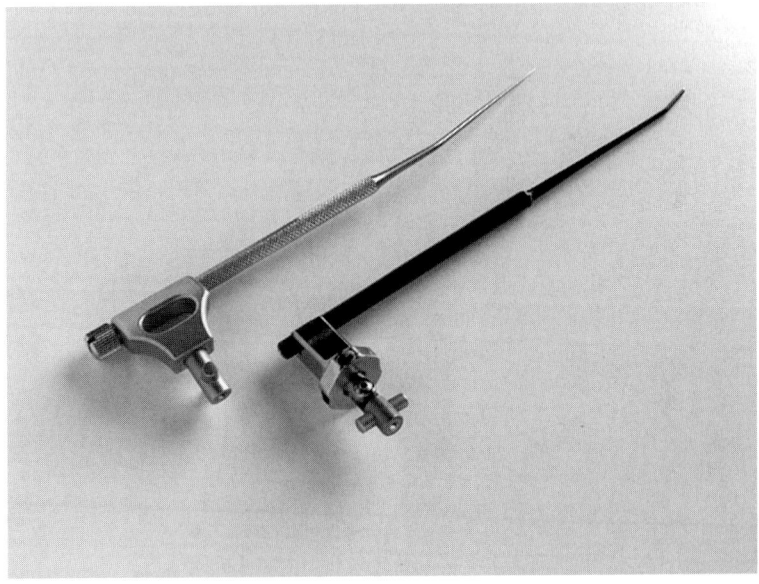

FIGURE 17.11 Modified otologic instrument for surgical navigation. (Courtesy of Medtronic Xomed, Jacksonville, FL)

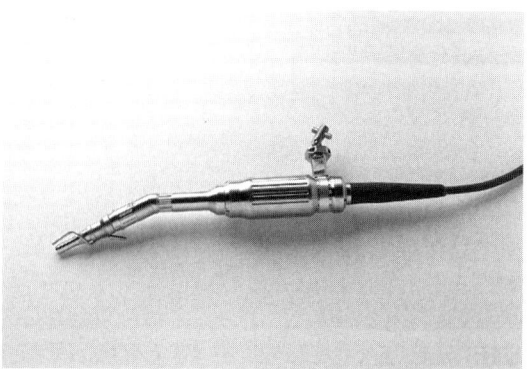

FIGURE 17.12 Drill fitted with mount for LEDs. (Courtesy of Medtronic Xomed, Jacksonville, FL.)

the otologic microscope. The angled straight pick is most useful because the angled handle places the LED array out of the line of sight. Otologic drills have also been fitted with LEDs to allow use with the navigational system (Figure 17.12).

As mentioned previously, early use of the Mayfield head-holder has given way to the direct attachment of the reference arc to the calvarium. The petrous apex drainage case described employed a pedestal stabilized with three screws through a small scalp incision. A recently designed pedestal requiring only one percutaneous screw promises to reduce the time involved with this step as well as eliminating the need for a separate incision with its attendant risk of bleeding and infection (Figure 17.13).

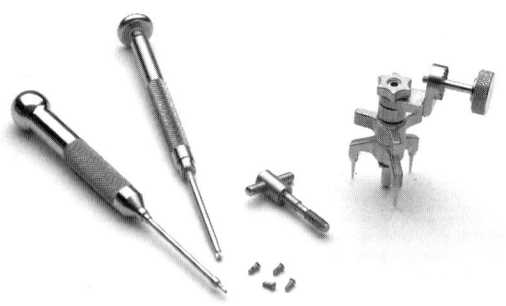

FIGURE 17.13 Single screw pedestal for attachment of reference arc. (Courtesy of Medtronix Xomed, Jacksonville, FL.)

17.5 CONCLUSIONS

Our experience with CAS in the temporal bone and its surroundings has been encouraging. Modification of otologic instruments and simplified attachment of the reference arc to the head with a single screw makes the technology more adapted to the demands of otologic and neurotologic microsurgery. With attachment of the reference arc directly to the skull, calibration and registration remains stable throughout long cases.

The chief advantage of CAS in temporal bone surgery is the rapid and accurate orientation of dissection. Ultimately, time in the operating room is reduced and complications can be avoided. CAS is *not*, however, a substitute for experience, knowledge of anatomy, or surgical judgment.

REFERENCES

1. Sargent EW, Bucholz RD. Middle cranial fossa surgery with image-guided instrumentation. Otolaryngol Head Neck Surg 1997; 117:131–134.
2. House WF. Surgical exposure of the internal auditory canal and its contents through the middle cranial fossa. Laryngoscope 1961; 71:1363–85.
3. House WF. Transtemporal bone microsurgical removal of acoustic neuroma. Arch Otolaryngol 1964; 80:597–756.
4. Glasscock M. Middle fossa approach to the temporal bone. Arch Otolaryngol 1969; 90:41–57.
5. Fisch U. Transtemporal surgery of the internal auditory canal. Adv. Otorhinolaryngol 1970; 17:202–239.
6. Kartush JM, Kemink JL, Graham MD. The arcuate eminence: topographic orientation in middle cranial fossa surgery. Ann Otol Rhinol Laryngol 1985; 94:25–28.
7. Pialoux P, Freyss G. Narch P, deSaint-Macary M, Davaine F. Contributions a l'anatomie stereotaxique du conduit auditif interne et de la premiere portion du facial. Ann Otolaryngol Chir Cerviofac 1972; 89:141–142.
8. Brackmann DE, Giddings NA. Drainage procedures for petrous apex lesions. In: Brackmann DE, C Shelton, Arriaga MA, eds. Otologic Surgery. Philadelphia: W.B. Saunders Company, 1994:566–578.
9. Fong BP, Brackmann DE, Telischi FF. The long-term follow-up of drainage procedures for petrous apex cholesterol granulomas. Arch Otolaryngol Head Neck Surg 1995; 121:426–430.

18

Computer-Aided Tumor Modeling and Visualization

Gregory J. Wiet, M.D.
The Ohio State University College of Medicine and Public Health and Columbus Children's Hospital, Columbus, Ohio

Don Stredney
Ohio Supercomputer Center, Columbus, Ohio

Petra Schmalbrock, Ph.D.
The Ohio State University College of Medicine and Public Health, Columbus, Ohio

18.1 INTRODUCTION

Our goal in this chapter is to provide an update on some of the new and exciting technologies for head and neck tumor visualization. Before this discussion one may ask, "Why is tumor visualization important?" From a surgical perspective, we believe that visualization provides two key elements to understanding the tumor and hence its management: tumor margin and tumor burden. These two elements dictate whether surgical management is possible and, if possible, the approach that should be undertaken. Margin is the local anatomy that is directly affected by the tumor and that may lie within the surgical trajectory. Burden describes the amount of tissue and structures that are directly affected by the abnormal tissue and that may end up being sacrificed to effect a cure. With the advent of more minimally invasive techniques, complete and accurate visualization becomes paramount. Our goal is to develop an interactive visualization environment that provides a better understanding of tumor margin and burden. Over the past 10 years, our focus has been on developing interactive tools for intuitive access to tumor information for head and neck surgeons in the Department of Otolaryngology at The Ohio State University [1–7]. Through innovative software and current and future hardware platforms, we are achieving a more complete and realistic visualization of head and neck tumors. In essence, the result will be an environment much like a cadaver lab, but with the ability to see deep structures without removing covering structures and to manipulate structures without destroying critical relationships. The work will occur in real time and with patient-specific data. We have now extended this technology from the desktop to the Internet for remote collaboration. A complete QuickTime movie of the system can be found at www.osc.edu/Biomed under Past Projects, Interactive Medical Data on Demand, A High-Performance Image-Based Warehouse Across Heterogeneous Environments.

We present our methods for data acquisition and processing, as well as interactive techniques to facilitate tumor visualization for diagnosis, preoperative assessment, and treatment planning, including extirpation. We further discuss implications for synchronous and asynchronous remote collaborations and extensibility to presurgical planning. We conclude with discussions regarding the value of interactive visualizations to exploring and managing treatment options.

18.2 DATA ACQUISITION

As with any computer application, the accuracy of the visualization depends directly upon the quality of data in the system. Current data acquisition techniques do not provide enough resolution that is comparable to what we see in the real world. Despite this limitation, our ability to acquire large amounts of high-resolution patient image data is rapidly increasing. Data sets comprising images $512 \times 512 \times N$ in resolution are common [8]. Recent technology has introduced the next generation of imaging technology capable of delivering resolutions of $1024 \times 1024 \times N$ with unprecedented clarity. Improvements in imaging have increased the use of temporal data sets that demonstrate cognitive function, cardiac function, joint movements, and aspects of development. Although very promising, all these data present an additional problem: storage. Research data and patient records will soon exceed gigabytes in storage needs. At The Ohio State University Medical Center, an estimated 7 terabytes of image data are obtained annually. Currently, shelf life of online image data is limited to 17 days.

Larger and larger data sets not only present storage problems, but they are essentially useless unless they can be rendered and visualized in a timely fashion. Real-time visualizations allow the user to derive structure from motion and gain

Computer-Aided Tumor Modeling and Visualization 313

insight into the configuration of the tumor. Interactive visualizations provide a suite of tools to allow for more intuitive exploration of the information. Furthermore, we see interactive tumor visualizations as ways to manage the visualization of multimodal studies (computed tomography, magnetic resonance, nuclear medicine), facilitate minimally invasive management of tumors, and serve as a communication tool between health care providers. If these ever-increasing data sets are to be visualized in real time, heavy demands will be placed upon both the software and hardware used to process these data. Current technologies can provide interactive visualizations but not without such processes as decimation (removal of data to create a manageable size) or supersampling (introduction of false data to "fill in" defects in the original data). Care must be taken not to remove key data or introduce false data that might alter a diagnosis or treatment plan.

We must address several additional issues in regard to the concepts of tumor margin and burden. Some tumors present defined "capsules" that assist in margin definition, whereas others present poor margin definition. In infiltrative type tumors, margins must be arbitrarily determined using transfer functions that ultimately include healthy tissue that will be sacrificed during extirpation (Figure 18.1). More precise establishment of tumor margin is facilitated by using paramagnetic contrast agents (see below). Comparative studies (with and without contrast) can clarify ambiguous areas. These methods exploit certain characteristics of the tumor such as vascularity, fat content, water content, and density. New methodology will aid in defining tumor margin [9]. Radiolabeled tumor antibodies to epithelial surface antigens and radiolabeled receptor ligands are two examples. The ability to image biochemical processes, such as positron-emission tomography (PET) scanning, has now been used to characterize tumor lesions, differentiate recurrent disease from treatment effects, stage tumors, evaluate the extent of disease, and monitor therapy [10,11]. We use both computed tomography (CT) and magnetic resonance (MR) in our data acquisition, with an increas-

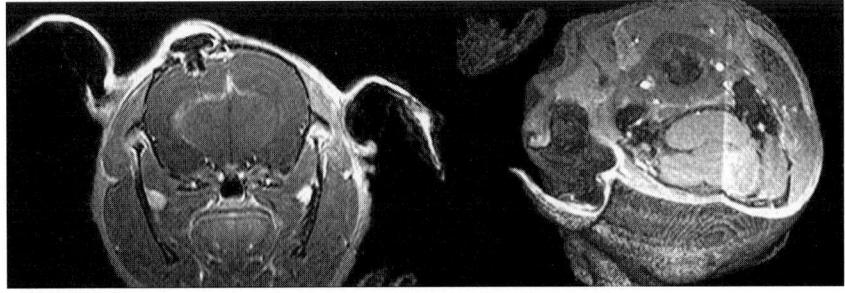

FIGURE 18.1 Image of infiltrative rat lymphoma model.

ing dependence on high-resolution MR because of its higher spatial resolution of soft tissue. Because one of the coauthors (PS) is continually developing new scanning protocols to increase spatial resolution, we will discuss these techniques and show several images of these new modes of data acquisition.

The inner ear and cerebralpontine angle are useful regions to image and demonstrate the capability of these techniques. Our institution acquires high-resolution MR axial images with a 1.5 T MR system (General Electric, Milwaukee, WI) using the standard quadrature head coil. A segmented, interleaved, motion-compensated acquisition in steady state (SIMCAST) sequence provides very high resolution of the region of interest. The SIMCAST sequence is a prototype three-dimensional (3D) gradient echo pulse sequence (8). To avoid potential problems with gross patient motion, we acquire four data sets with different RF phases in an interleaved fashion. For our clinical studies, SIMCAST images are acquired with TR/TE/flip angle of 17 ms/3.5 ms/40 degrees, 22 $\times$ 16 cm FOV, 512 $\times$ 256 matrix size, and 32 slices of 1.2 mm thickness or, more recently, with 0.8 mm slice thickness (interpolated to 0.4 mm). In all cases the SIMCAST images are acquired before contrast injection. Contrast-enhanced T_1-weighted images are acquired after the injection of 10cc Gd-DTPA contrast agent with a 3D spoiled gradient echo sequence [12], using TR/TE/flip angle of 30 ms/4.2 ms/30 degrees, 1 excitation, 20 $\times$ 20 cm FOV, 512 $\times$ 288 matrix size, and 64 slices of 1.5 mm thickness. Both sequences have similar scan times of 7 minutes.

All lesions are clearly depicted with both sequences [13], and tumor volumes can be accurately measured for remarkably small tumors with volumes as low as 0.05 cc (Figure 18.2). Cochlea, vestibule, and semicircular canals are well depicted with SIMCAST, whereas these structures are seen poorly on the T_1-weighted images. The complete course of the 7th and 8th nerves in the CPA and IAC is seen with SIMCAST in normal ears (Figures 18.2 and 18.3).

In patients with small tumors, portions of the vestibulocochlear or facial nerve branches can be seen on axial and reformatted SIMCAST images (Figures 18.2 and 18.4). In some cases, it is possible to observe the nerves displaced by the tumor (Figure 18.4), whereas nerve depiction is usually poor on T_1-weighted images. Lesions were always clearly differentiated from the surrounding high signal CSF, but for some large lesions extending toward the brain stem the tumor/brain boundary is not distinguishable merely by the tissue signal contrast. However, in most cases the tumor margin may be determined from the shapes of the anatomical structures or intervening vessels. Tumor/brain distinction is better on contrasted, enhanced T_1-weighted images; however, because of the low CSF signal on T_1-weighted images, fluid/bone boundaries are poorly defined, and thus the extent of tumor from the fluid spaces into the bony regions may not be as clearly distinguishable.

In our studies, IAC tumor signal was heterogeneous with both the T_1-weighted and SIMCAST sequences in a significant numer of cases. This fact

Computer-Aided Tumor Modeling and Visualization 315

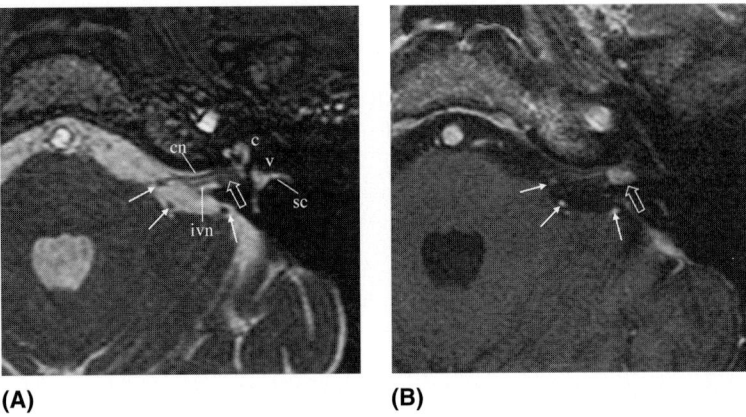

(A) **(B)**

FIGURE 18.2 Incidental finding of a small 0.05 cc IAC mass in an 87-year-old male with vertigo and sudden hearing loss. The mass is clearly identified with SIMCAST (A, open arrow) and with the contrast enhanced study (B, open arrow). Inner ear anatomical structures including the cochlea (c), vestibule (v), and semicircular canal (sc) are clearly seen on the SIMCAST image. These structures are not or only partially seen on the T_1 images. Small vascular structures (arrows) appear dark on SIMCAST and bright on T_1 images. The SIMCAST images also depict the cochlear (cn) and inferior vestibular nerves (ivn), which are isointense with the tumor. Again only a portion of the cochlear nerve is seen on the T_1 images.

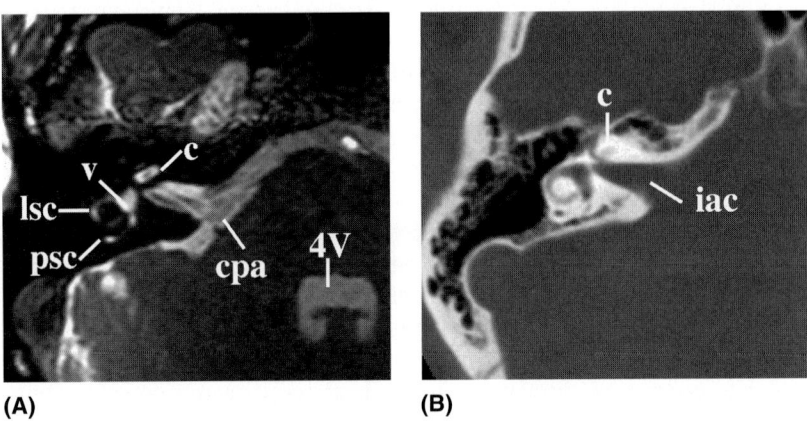

(A) **(B)**

FIGURE 18.3 High-resolution MRI (A) and CT (B) images of a normal subject. Both MRI and CT show the vestibule (v), cochlear (c), and lateral and posterior semicircular canals (lsc, psc), i.e., CT shows the bony outlines and the MRI shows the fluid filled spaces. The CT image also differentiates bone (bright) and air space (dark) in the middle ear and mastoid. However, no further differentiation of fluid and neural structures is achieved with CT. Only MRI can delineate nerves in the internal auditory canal (iac), vascular structures in the cerebellopontine angle (cpa) and the fluid-filled fourth ventricle.

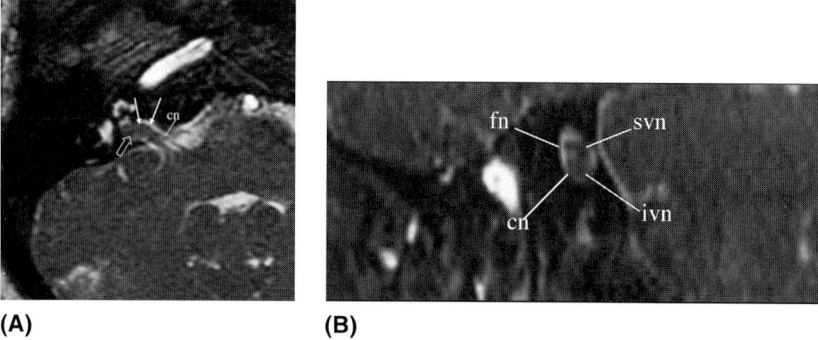

FIGURE 18.4 Original axial (A) and sagittal reformatted (B) SIMCAST images of a 10-year-old patient with a small tumor (0.07 cc, open arrow) emanating from the superior vestibular nerve (as per surgery report). On the axial image, the cochlear nerve can be followed from the brain stem into the internal auditory canal (arrows), where it is pushed anteriorly by the tumor. The inferior branch of the vestibular nerve is seen continuous with the tumor. On the sagittal reformatted image, the facial (fn), cochlear (cn), and superior and inferior nerves (svn, ivn) are clearly distinguishable. The superior vestibular nerve is enlarged and surrounded by low signal tumor. In this patient, hearing preservation was achieved in surgery.

indicates that some of the tumors were probably necrotic, hemorrhagic, or partially cystic. On SIMCAST images cystic tumor regions had higher signal intensity than the brain, helping to distinguish the brain/tumor margin; however, these tumor regions were more difficult to separate from the CSF. Tumors that were partially cystic or necrotic did not enhance homogeneously. This factor led to difficulties in identifying margins between tumor and CSF on the contrast-enhanced images with confidence (Figure 18.5), and such tumor portions were better defined by the SIMCAST studies.

Until such time as the SIMCAST technique can be reliably applied to other areas, we acquire an isotropic volume, employing a short 3DSPGR sequence; that is, we use a T_1-weighted three-dimensional spoiled gradient echo using a TR/TE/FlipAngle of 33 ms/5 ms/45 degrees. The field of view (FOV) of 25 cm provides a voxel resolution of 256 × 128 × 128 and a slice thickness of 2 mm. Fourier interpolation of the data generates isotropic data sets for image processing. This protocol requires 9 minutes of scan time and also allows acquisitions with and without Gd-DTPA, the paramagnetic contrast agent commonly used in MR imaging for imaging tumors.

After the surgeons have initially read MR images to determine tumor location, CT studies are performed when appropriate. CT scans are performed on late-generation scanners, encompassing the specific tumor area to limit radiation

Computer-Aided Tumor Modeling and Visualization

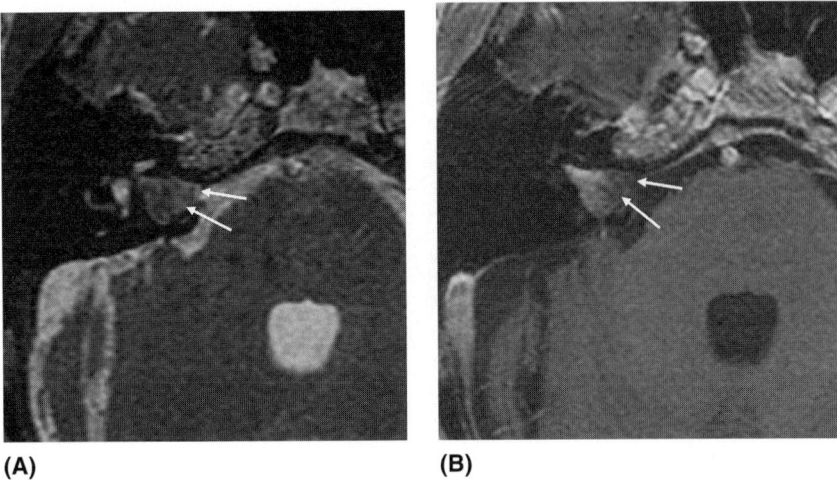

FIGURE 18.5 SIMACAST (A) and contrast enhanced T_1-weighted (B) images of a heterogeneous 0.35 cc internal auditory canal mass in a 75-year-old female. This tumor is well delineated on the SIMCAST image (arrows). However, it does not enhance homogeneously, and, therefore, the tumor margin is not clearly seen on the T_1 image and the tumor size is underestimated.

exposure to the patient with a 2-second scan time at 200 mA and 120 kilovolt peak. The matrix size is 512 × 512, and, whenever possible, gantry tilt is restricted to zero for axial scans. Continuous 1.5 mm sections are obtained using a 1.5 mm slice thickness and 1.5 mm table increments [14].

18.3 DATA PROCESSING

18.3.1 Segmentation

Once transferred to OSC, image data are segmented using various transfer functions, including threshold and slice densities. We have employed neural network–based software (LEGION) [15] to automatically segment structures within the skullbase (Figure 18.6). This software allows one to segment structures within the volume rather than image by image and provides excellent first-pass results. Limited "clean-up" by the user is required in areas where the normal anatomy has been surgically or pathologically altered. The local software, Editmask, provides a robust GUI interface for loading multiple color sections into memory. The user is free to delineate regions of interest (ROIs) in image space, using either a polygon or paint mode. Color image masks are produced with ROIs differentiated with various colors (Figure 18.7). These masks "tag" volume ele-

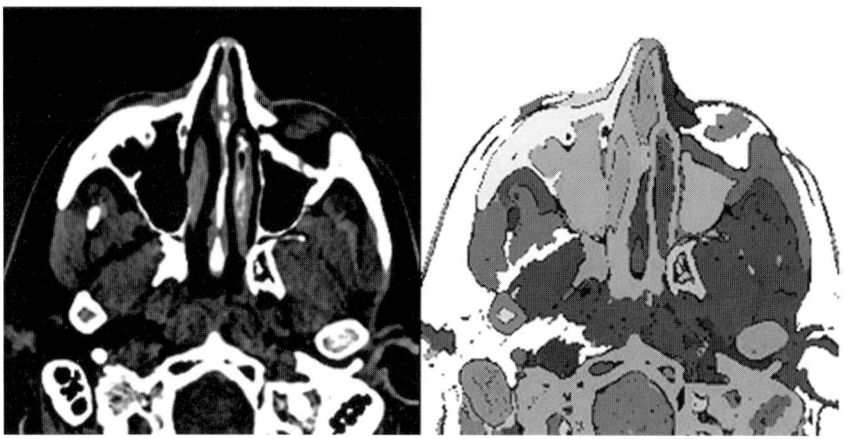

FIGURE 18.6 Left, original axial CT. Right, structural segmentation after first pass with LEGION.

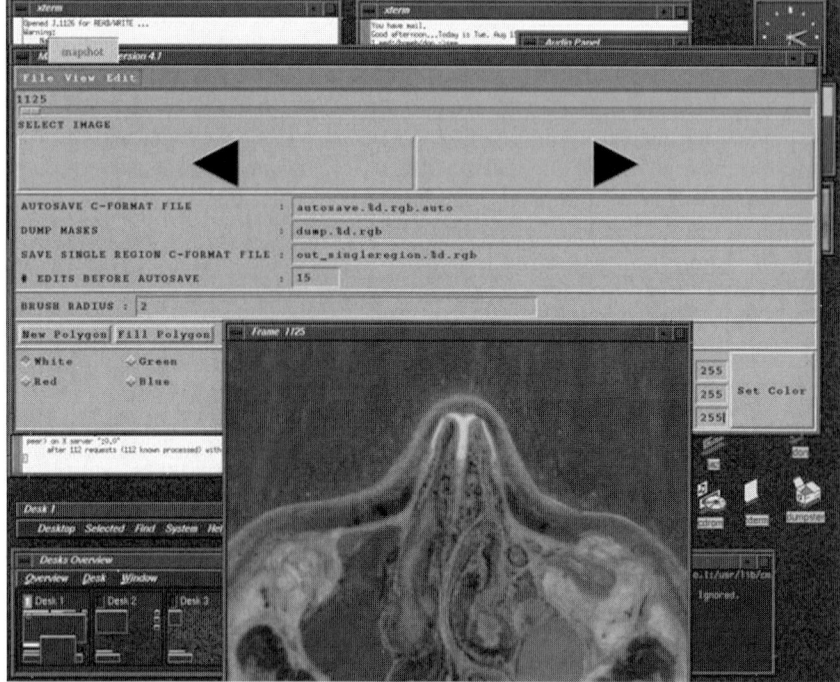

FIGURE 18.7 Graphical user interface for Editmask segmentation application.

Computer-Aided Tumor Modeling and Visualization

ments with structural or functional information, i.e., information that may be useful but is independent of structure.

18.3.2 Multimodal Data Merging

The use of multimodal images allows checks and validations that are critical in determining the extent of the tumor. We have developed techniques to merge these data acquired from different modalities by allowing direct visual manipulation of one volumetric data set with another. One data set is static and serves as a background, allowing the user to position, scale, and rotate another data set. We have employed this technique to merge the data sets acquired at various resolutions (Figure 18.8). This technique obviates the need for fiduciaries.

The following images were acquired from a patient with a sphenoid tumor (Figure 18.9). Binary masks were made for the skull, tumor, vessels, brain, and surrounding structures (Figure 18.10). An image of these components combined can be seen in Figure 18.11.

18.3.3 Rendering: Surface Versus Volume

Two basic approaches to rendering structures are *isosurfaces*, or a polygonal representation that approximates the surface, or *volumetric*, which also approximates the structure, but by discrete volume elements called voxels. Volume repre-

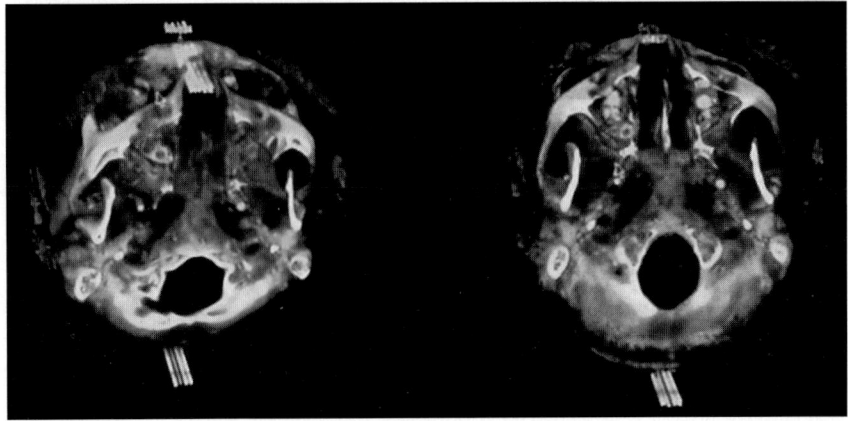

FIGURE 18.8 Image of image file merging environment. The CT volume image file is static, and the MRI image file is being merged to create one multimodal volume image file.

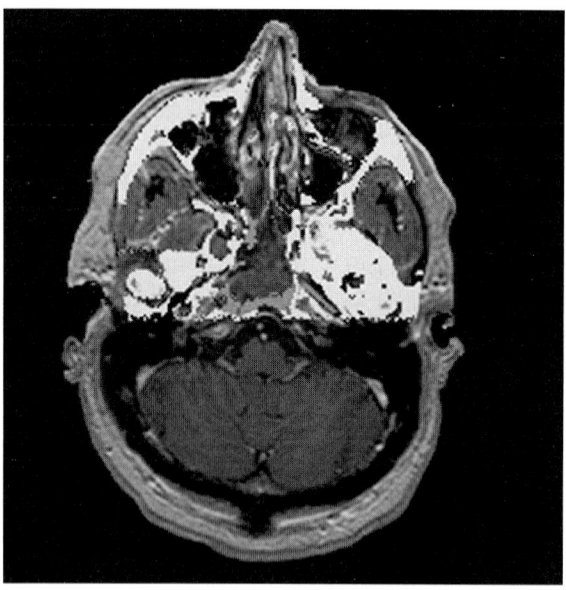

FIGURE 18.9 Merged CT and MRI image data of patient with sphenoid tumor.

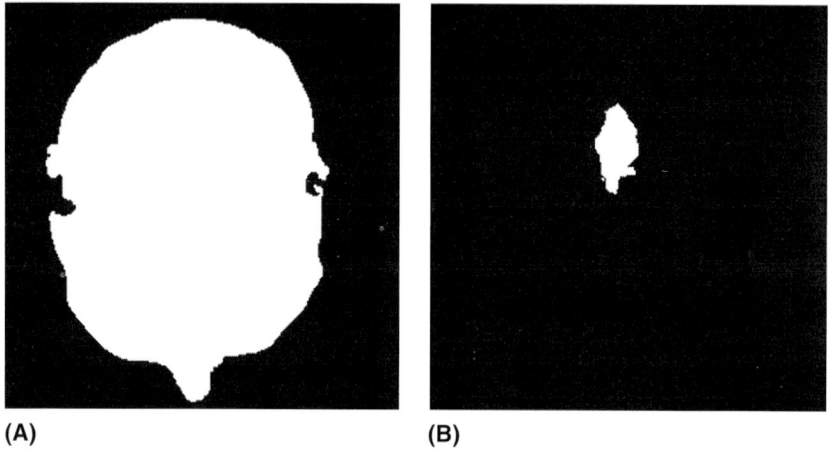

FIGURE 18.10 Binary masks created from segmentation of original data slice of (A) the patient's skin and (B) tumor.

Computer-Aided Tumor Modeling and Visualization

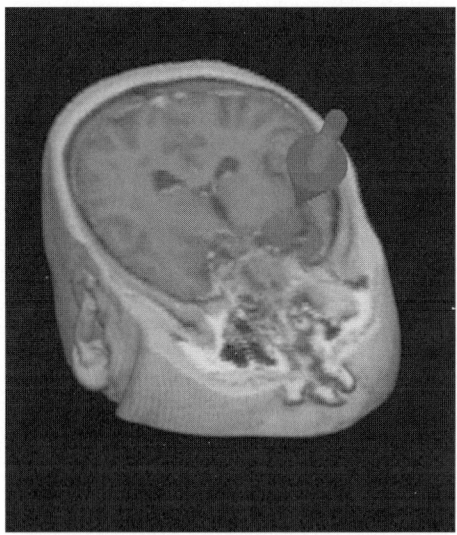

FIGURE 18.11 Volumetric rendering of the composite (merged) data with highlighted tumor and tinting capability performed in the volume.

sentations are derived directly from the imaging data, whereas isosurfaces are derived by a series of image-processing steps. We have chosen to maintain the original integrity of the volume data and use volume representations. There are several reasons for this decision. Originally, volume rendering was computationally expensive, and, for expediency, surfaces were generated to create representations. Many computers had accelerated hardware to facilitate rendering of surfaces. However, recently, 2D and 3D texture memory techniques have evolved, and specialized hardware is becoming more readily available, thus making volume rendering more cost-effective [3,4,6,16–18]. Second, surface rendering allows only a passive exploration of the surface information. While sectioning techniques have been introduced, the overhead for texturing the original information on the newly created cut is computationally expensive and does not lend itself to interactive rates. Volume representation maintains the original intensity information, and techniques for sectioning and removal are straightforward. Finally, it would be easy to generate an overwhelming number of polygons to depict an accurate surface of a complex region such as the skullbase [19], but by using volume representations, we can obviate this expensive step of processing the original data to extract surfaces. Volume rendering expedites the use of more patient-specific data sets and has been used in such high-demand environments as surgical simulations being developed for resident training [20].

18.4 INTERACTIVITY/INTERFACE

Preprocessing and data collection provide a means to an end: the ability of the users to interact with the data. We have extended this beyond the desktop to the Internet to allow multiple, asynchronous users to interact with rendered image data. In this section we will discuss our approach to the user interface as well as our current work in exporting the visualization capability to the Internet. As discussed previously, our goal is to provide real-time interaction with the image data in an intuitive environment.

Hendin and others have presented methods to provide volume rendering over the Internet [21]; however, various restrictions, including interactive latency, limits to viewing orientation, and quality of data representation, exist. Peifer and others have presented a patient-centric, networked relational database for patient-controlled data collection [22], but this work focuses on physiological monitoring, and data sizes and rates are relatively low. Silverstein et al. presented a Web-based system for segmentation of computed tomography images and display via VRML [23]. The authors emphasize the need to access massive high-speed computation to provide resultant images on a desktop computer.

Previous authors have constructed a props-based interface for interactive visualizations in neurosurgery [24]. This work presented a 3D isosurface of the brain with resulting sections from the original images placed in a separate window. We previously explored this approach but found our users preferred the integrated view of the section with the main window [1]. In addition, our users were concerned with issues of scale, i.e., the prop as related to the data, and with physical limitations of the props. Subsequently, we provided an integrated view that allowed the users to focus their attention on the data, while the interfaces allowed them complete utility for orientation and selection, without the use of props.

We have developed a prototype system through unique collaborations among networking and computing specialists, advanced applications developers, and end users (clinicians, researchers, and educators), providing a realistic and initial implementation with scalability to a wide range of applications (healthcare, scientific research, and distance education).

The system provides 3D reconstructions of the volumetric data with the best interactivity possible, given the computing and networking environment. The key issues for delivering representations from high-resolution volumetric data sets are integration/functionality, representational quality, and performance.

Previously we reported on exploiting 3D texture hardware to provide interactive performance over the Internet [6]. Volume rendering using 3D texture mapping hardware treats the volume as a 3D texture [17,18]. A set of image-aligned parallel polygons intersects the volume, and the graphics hardware processes (textures, rasterizes, and composites) the polygons onto the final image.

Computer-Aided Tumor Modeling and Visualization

New techniques render irregular volume grids by computing image-aligned slices, which are polygon meshes constructed by intersecting the irregular grid cells [3,4]. The graphics hardware composites the meshes into the final image. We have continued to develop applications that exploit 3D texture hardware (see below) and present direct applications for use in resident training [20].

The current system configuration contains two parts: the rendering server and the device client. The rendering server is an interactive volume renderer that runs on high-end Silicon Graphics (Mountain View, CA) computers such as the Onyx2™ or Octane™. The rendering software uses OpenGL™ and texture memory to achieve interactive volume-rendering rates. Our software was built upon the 3D texture-based volume rendering software called VRP (Volume Rendering Primer), available from Silicon Graphics, Inc. This code also renders surface geometry, called embedded geometry, defined in an Inventor™ scenegraph file format, simultaneously with volume data.

The device clients connected to an external device control the server. These device clients are used as an intuitive interface to the rendering server. The device client communicates with the rendering server via TCP/IP networking protocol. This system allows a user to control a rendering server from anywhere on the Internet. An example of the device client is the Spaceball™, a manual device that allows the user to orient the data with six degrees of freedom (DOF). The second interface is the Microscribe™, a five DOF device (Figure 18.12). If these elegant

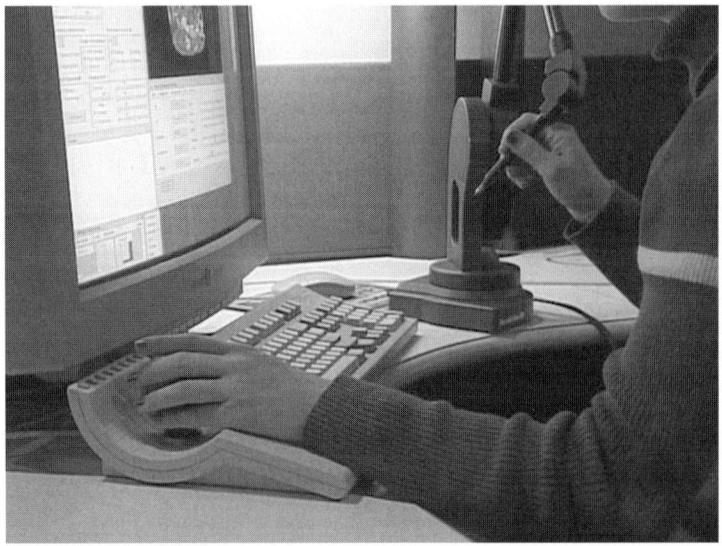

FIGURE 18.12 User during interactive session.

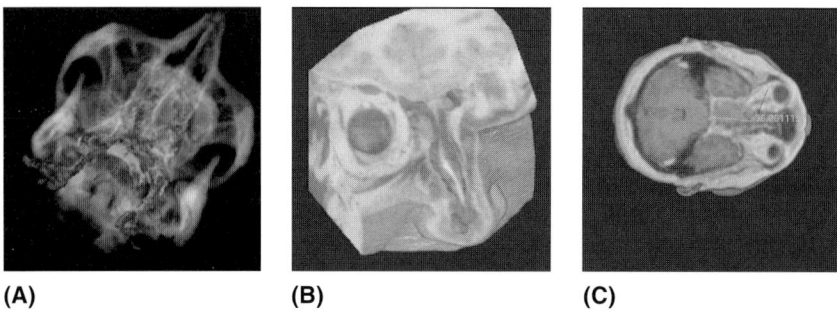

(A) (B) (C)

FIGURE 18.13 (A) Orientation of volume; (B) arbitrary slicing of the volume in real time; (C) Arbitrary removing of data or ''cutting'' from the volume in real time. All are performed in real time.

interfaces are not available, graphical user interface (GUI)–based device simulators are available to provide basic functionality to the user. The system currently supports the following operations:

Orientation. The user can arbitrarily rotate and position a 3D reconstruction of the data (Figure 18.13A).

Arbitrary Slicing. The user can arbitrarily position a plane to reveal underlying structures (Figure 18.13B).

Removal. The user can arbitrarily remove single volume elements for viewing underlying structures (Figure 18.13C). (This function can be changed to provide the addition of volume elements for other applications.)

Tinting. The user can mark specific regions, thus drawing as if on a three-dimensional whiteboard (Figure 18.11).

Morphometrics. The system provides measurement of the underlying structures in 3D.

In addition to allowing one user to control the orientation of the data set and the clipping plane of a rendering server, the system allows others to take control of a server. Users can thus interact in the volumetric environment, similar to a 3D environment. We intend to expand the tinting function to provide hyperlinks to multimedia, including text-, audio-, image-, and movie-formatted data, thus allowing access to more extensive patient information. In addition, with these multimedia objects, the system can allow asynchronous collaborations.

18.5 FUTURE DIRECTIONS

The prototype system demonstrates a shared virtual environment that allows multiple users to interactively manipulate large volumetric data sets across long dis-

Computer-Aided Tumor Modeling and Visualization 325

tances using intuitive interfaces (12–98, OSC-98, CUMREC98). At Internet II in April 1998, network latencies observed between Washington, DC, and the Interface Lab at OSC in Columbus, Ohio, were approximately 1 second. Albeit noticeable, the latencies were tolerable. We have run additional collaborative studies with the Cleveland Clinic Foundation and, most recently, as a telemedicine demonstration with StrongAngel, among OSC, East Carolina University, and Hawaii.

We are implementing the capacity of users to request the system to identify a structure, such as a tumor, with surrounding structures becoming transparent (Figure 18.14). The users can then orient themselves to the structure and then return to the normal view. This utility will assist residents in understanding the relationship of the tumor to surrounding anatomy and will facilitate identifying the optimal choice of surgical approach, resection, and reconstruction.

We have presented our designs for interactive tumor visualizations. As image acquisitions continue to improve in spatial resolution, these systems integrate multimodal acquisitions into succinct, comprehensible formats for direct use by the health care provider. Improvements in hardware-assisted rendering techniques will make cost-efficient desktop systems feasible. Segmentation will continue to provide technical challenges and remains the key barrier for the common use of these systems with more patient-specific data. However, many of the segmentation issues will be obviated by improved spatial acquisitions, contrast enhance-

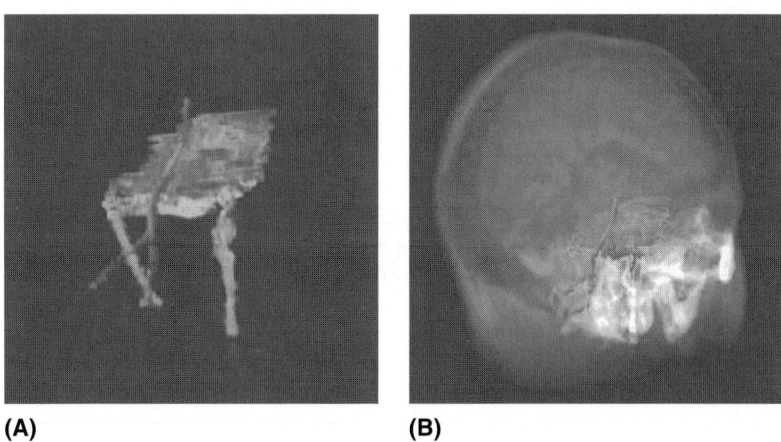

FIGURE 18.14 (A) Volume segmented sphenoid tumor and surrounding vasculature (internal carotids and basilar arteries). (B) Composite image of volume rendered merged data with transparency of skin and brain showing relationship of tumor to skull base and vasculature performed in real time.

ment, multiprotocol acquisitions, and ever-increasing computing and network power.

As hardware and software tools progress, these systems will incorporate more interactions that simulate surgical techniques, thus extending the utility of emerging systems from resident training to presurgical planning on patient-specific data.

ACKNOWLEDGMENTS

This research has been funded under grants from the following sources: The Ohio State University Office of Research, The Department of Otolaryngology, The Ohio State University, Ohio Supercomputer Center, the National Institutes of Health/National Library of Medicine, and the National Institute for Deafness and Communicative Disorders.

The authors gratefully acknowledge the assistance of Dennis Sessanna and Jason Bryan, whose technical expertise has made this work possible, and of Mrs. Pamela Walters and Ms. Barbara Woodall for help with preparation of the manuscript.

REFERENCES

1. Bier-Laning C, Wiet GJ, Stredney D. Evaluation of a high performance computing technique for cranial base Tumor Visualization. In: Fourth International Conference on Head and Neck Cancer, Toronto, 1996.
2. Wiet GJ, et al. Cranial base tumor visualization through high performance computing. In: Weghorst SJ, Sieburg H, Morgan K, eds. Medicine Meets Virtual Reality. Amsterdam: IOS Press, 1996:43–59.
3. Yagel R, et al. Hardware assisted volume rendering of unstructured grids. In: Proceedings of 1996 Symposium on Volume Visualization, San Francisco, 1996.
4. Yagel R, et al. Cranial base tumor visualization through multimodal imaging: integration and interactive display. In: Fourth Scientific Meeting of the International Society for Magnetic Resonance in Medicine, New York, 1996.
5. Wiet GJ, et al. Using advanced simulation technology for cranial base tumor evaluation. In: Kuppersmith R, ed. The Otolaryngologic Clinics of North America. Philadelphia: WB Saunders Company, 1998:369–381.
6. Stredney D, et al. Interactive volume visualization for synchronous and asynchronous remote collaboration. In: Westwood J, et al., eds. Medicine Meets Virtual Reality. Amsterdam: IOS Press, 1999:344–350.
7. Stredney D, et al. Interactive medical data on demand: a high performance image-based approach across heterogeneous environments. In: Westwood J, et al., eds. Medicine Meets Virtual Reality. Amsterdam: IOS Press: 2000:327–333.
8. Kurucay S, et al. A segment interleaved motion compensated acquisition in the steady state (SIMCAST) technique for high resolution imaging of the inner ear. JMRI 1997; (Nov/Dec):1060–1068.

9. Goldsmith SJ. Receptor imaging: competitive or complementary to antibody imaging? In: Seminars in Nuclear Medicine. Philadelphia: WB Saunders Company, 1997:85–93.
10. Hoh CK, et al. PET in oncology: will it replace the other modalities? In: Seminars in Nuclear Medicine. Philadelphia: WB Saunders Company, 1997:94–106.
11. Erasmus JJ, Patz EF. Positron Emission Tomography Imaging in the Thorax. Clin Chest Med 1999; 20:715–724.
12. Vlaadinderbroek MT, DeBoer JA. Magnetic Resonance Imaging. Berlin/Heidelberg: Springer, 1996:167–214.
13. Schmalbrock P, et al. Measurement of internal auditory canal tumor volumes with contrast enhanced T_1-weighted and steady state T_2-weighted gradient echo imaging. AJNR 1999; 20:1207–1213.
14. Davis R, et al. Three-dimensional high-resolution volume rendering of computer tomography data: applications to otolaryngology–head and neck surgery. Laryngoscope 1991; 101:573–582.
15. Shareef N, Wang D, Yagel R. Segmentation of medical data using locally excitatory globally inhibitory oscillator networks. In: The World Congress on Neural Networks, San Diego, CA, 1996.
16. Westover L. Splatting: A Parallel, Feed-Forward Volume Rendering Algorithm. Ph.D. thesis. Chapel Hill, NC: University of North Carolina, 1991.
17. Cabral B, Cam N, Foran J. Accelerated volume rendering and tomographic reconstruction using texture mapping hardware. In: Symposium on Volume Visualization, Washington, D.C., 1994.
18. Van Gelder A, Kim K. Direct volume rendering via 3D texture mapping hardware. In: Proceedings of the 1996 Volume Rendering Symposium, 1996.
19. Stredney D, et al. A Comparative analysis of integrating visual representations with haptic displays. In: Westwood J, et al., eds. Medicine Meets Virtual Reality. Amsterdam: IOS Press, 1998:20–26.
20. Wiet GJ, et al. Virtual temporal bone dissection simulation. In: Westwood, et al., eds. Medicine Meets Virtual Reality. Amsterdam: IOS Press, 2000:378–384.
21. Hendin O, John NW, Shocet O. Medical volume rendering over the WWW using VRML and Java. In: Westwood J, et al., eds. Medicine Meets Virtual Reality. Amsterdam: IOS Press, 1998:34–40.
22. Peifer J, Sudduth B. A patient-centric approach to telemedicine database development. In: Westwood J, et al., eds. Medicine Meets Virtual Reality. Amsterdam: IOS Press, 1998:67–73.
23. Silverstein J, et al. Web-based segmentation and display of three-dimensional radiologic image data. In: Westwood J, et al., eds. Medicine Meets Virtual Reality. Amsterdam: IOS Press, 1998:53–59.
24. Hinckley K, et al. The Props-based interface for neurosurgical visualization. In: Morgan KS, et al., eds. Medicine Meets Virtual Reality. Amsterdam: IOS Press, 1997: 552–562.

19

Head and Neck Virtual Endoscopy

**William B. Armstrong, M.D., and
Thong H. Nguyen, M.D.**
*University of California, Irvine, Orange, and Veterans Affairs
Medical Center, Long Beach, California*

19.1 INTRODUCTION

Virtual endoscopy (VE) can be broadly defined as the reconstruction and rendering of two-dimensional (2D) data to create a realistic depiction of the inner walls of a hollow organ or tubular structure. The term is not technically accurate, since it is not a true "endoscopic" procedure and it is not a "virtual" experience, which is more accurately defined as immersing the observer within a three-dimensional (3D) real-time interactive environment. In its current form, VE allows the observer to review a predetermined flight path through the imaged organ system [1,2]. However, the term "virtual endoscopy" has become so commonly used, it has become a *de facto* terminology to describe radiographic techniques that provide an undistorted intraluminal view that emulates the view seen by an endoscopist.

Development of VE is the result of the convergence of advances in surgical endoscopy, radiology, and computer science and technology. Each of these professions has contributed to the nascent field of VE. The early nineteenth century witnessed the development of laryngoscopy, starting with Bozzini's attempts to use extracorporeal light to view luminal cavities of the body in 1809 [3]. Subsequently, the mirror laryngoscope, head mirror, and external sources of illumination were developed. From these primitive devices, developed in the early to mid-nineteenth century, major advances in lighting, optics, flexible fiberoptics, and documentation techniques have made endoscopic procedures indispensable to the modern practice of otolaryngology. Endoscopic applications have expanded from their origins in the upper respiratory and digestive tract to the nasal cavity and sinuses and more recently to imaging the middle ear [4–7].

In parallel to advances in direct and indirect visual endoscopy, radiology has also undergone a no less impressive revolution. From the time of the first radiographs, attempts have been made to develop cross-sectional imaging techniques. Plain x-ray tomography was one of the early techniques that provided some anatomical and pathological details, but images were generally blurry and its low resolution limited its usefulness. The development of computed tomography (CT) by Hounsfield and Cormack (co-recipients of the 1979 Nobel Prize in Medicine) revolutionized the ability to visualize fine anatomical details previously inaccessible without surgical intervention. Although the mathematical foundations for image reconstruction that underlie planar reconstruction were published by Radon in 1917 [8], it was not until the 1970s that the medical application of his work was realized by development of the CT scanner. Since that time, the quality of CT scans has steadily improved as scanning speed and resolution have increased. The cost per scan has decreased. As a result, CT has become a standard and indispensable imaging tool.

Magnetic resonance imaging (MRI) has undergone a similar revolution using magnetic and radiofrequency energy to discriminate tissues based on differences in hydrogen content and recovery from induced magnetic field perturbations. Both CT and MRI studies produce a large number of cross-sectional images. A significant drawback of these studies is the requirement of the person reading the studies to mentally form a 3D reconstruction of the individual cross-sectional slices. This skill is not equally possessed by all persons and is especially difficult with complex anatomical structures or pathology.

Techniques for 3D reconstruction were adapted for medical use from technology developed for nonmedical applications, including flight simulation, terrain guidance, computer science, and defense applications, in an attempt to improve visualization of complex anatomical structures and pathological abnormalities (9,10). These 3D-reconstruction algorithms have been used in the head and neck region to provide renderings of complex craniofacial defects [11–15], visualization of the larynx [16–18], data for the manufacture of prosthetic implants for craniofacial defects, and guidance for surgical planning [19,20].

David Vining and others have taken endoscopic imaging and radiology down a new path by manipulating the noninvasive radiographic information provided from axial CT data to simulate the endoluminal view provided by fiberoptic endoscopy, thereby producing novel radiographic "endoscopic" images [21,22]. VE is a noninvasive radiographic technique that allows visualization of intraluminal surfaces by 3D perspective renderings of air/tissue or fluid/tissue interfaces

Head and Neck Virtual Endoscopy

using axial CT, MRI, and, recently, ultrasound data [23–25]. VE is widely applicable throughout the body, and a number of organ systems have been studied, including the esophagus [26,27], stomach [28,29], small bowel [30–32], colon [22,33–35], genitourinary tract [36–38], tracheobronchial tree [21,39], vascular structures [40–43], nervous system [44–48], the temporal bone [49–52], paranasal sinuses [23,53–58], and upper respiratory tract [59–63]. A summary of the anatomical regions under investigation is displayed in Table 19.1.

19.2 VIRTUAL ENDOSCOPY TECHNIQUES

It is important to understand the essential distinction between 3D image reconstructions produced with software that does not incorporate the concept of perspective into the image reconstructions, and perspective-rendering methods used to produce VE studies. Perspective is an artistic term that describes techniques used to represent the spatial relationships of objects, as they would appear to the eye when viewed on a 2D surface. A simple illustration of perspective representation is shown in the two cubes in Figure 19.1. The cube on the left (Figure 19.1A) is drawn without incorporation of perspective to produce a representation of an object that appears three-dimensional, but relative sizes are not taken into account. The size of the posterior face of the cube is the same as the front face surface. The cube on the right (Figure 19.1B) depicts a decrease in the size of the apparent posterior surface of the cube, which seems to be viewed from a further distance than the front surface. This second illustration is more representative of what the human visual system would normally perceive. The 3D reconstruction techniques that do not incorporate perspective use an orthogonal or parallel ray-casting technique to display the 3D image onto a 2D plane; this approach assumes that the object is viewed from a remote distance in space [64,65]. When viewed from long distances, the light rays reflected from an object are nearly parallel, and use of parallel ray-casting techniques to display the image does not produce significant distortion (Figure 19.2A). Using parallel ray projections to produce 3D reconstructions is mathematically and computationally much simpler, but the view generated is not conducive to close-up viewing. Attempts to obtain a magnified view results in a larger view of a smaller portion of the structure. This situation is analogous to using the zoom feature on a copy machine. The image is larger and appears closer, but the field of view is extremely narrow because of limitations imposed by the reconstruction algorithm.

Perspective rendering techniques attempt to simulate the properties of the human eye by taking into account divergence of light rays between the eye and different portions of a given object, differences in the size of objects viewed from different distances, the field of view of the human eye or camera lens, and the effects of lighting, shading, and reflections. Figure 19.2 graphically illustrates differences between parallel ray reconstruction (Figure 19.2A) and perspective

TABLE 19.1 Virtual Endoscopy: Anatomical Regions of Clinical Investigation

Otolaryngology
  Trachea
  Larynx
  Pharynx
  Otological structures
    middle ear
    cochlea
    vestibular system
  Nasal cavity and paranasal sinuses
Pulmonology
  Bronchoscopy
Vascular Surgery
  Carotid artery
  Aorta
  Renal artery
Gastroenterology
  Esophagus
  Stomach
  Small bowel
  Biliary tract
  Colon
Urology
  Renal calyces
  Ureter
  Bladder
  Evaluation of bladder reconstructions
Neurosurgery
  Spinal canal
  Intracranial vasculature
  Cerebral ventricular system
  Aneurysm mapping
Gynecology
  Uterus
  Fallopian tubes
Orthopedic surgery
  Major joint spaces

Head and Neck Virtual Endoscopy

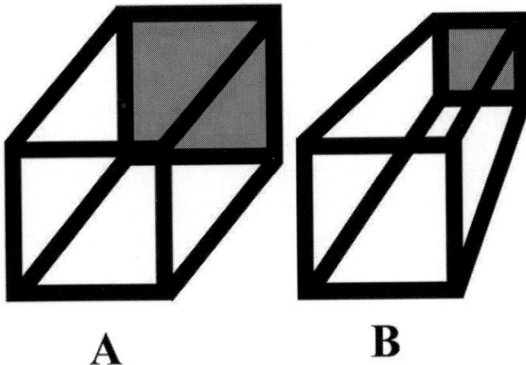

FIGURE 19.1 Depiction of cube without and with incorporation of perspective. (A) Cube is constructed to depict the appearance without incorporation of perspective. The front and back (shaded) surfaces are of equal size. (B) Cube incorporates the concept of perspective. The more distant posterior surface is depicted as smaller to account for the increased distance from the viewpoint.

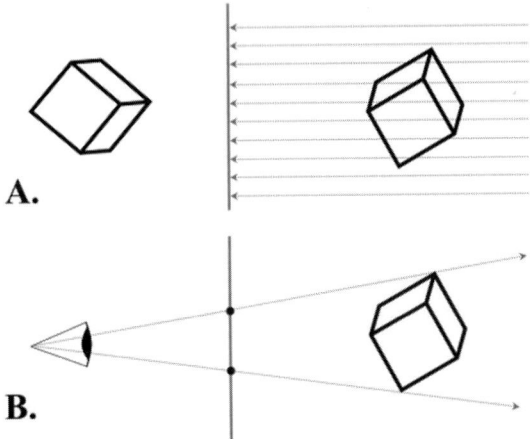

FIGURE 19.2 Parallel ray vs. perspective rendering of 3D structures. (A) Parallel rays projected onto a planar surface to simulate nonperspective rendering. There is a linear transposition of data from the 3D cube onto the 2D plane. (B) Divergence of light rays from the eye or camera lens on the left to the surface of the cube. The relative position of sampled points on the object will vary depending on their relative position in space and distance from the viewpoint.

rendering (Figure 19.2B). In parallel ray reconstruction, the parallel light rays pass through the object and map onto the planar surface with one-to-one correspondence, irrespective of distance from the viewpoint. In contrast, in perspective reconstruction, the relative position of the points mapped along the diverging rays projected from the viewpoint mapped onto a 2D plane varies by distance from the viewpoint, resulting in changes in the apparent size based on distance from the viewpoint. By mimicking the optical properties of the human visual system in a fashion similar to the ways in which an artist creates a painting with cues to relative size and distance, the perspective rendering software can create a realistic appearing simulation of an endoscopic visualization from cross-sectional data.

Four major steps are required to create a VE study. Cross-sectional data are first acquired by either spiral CT or MRI and transferred to a 3D workstation. These data are then processed to construct a 3D model of the imaged structure for the third step. Next, individual perspective rendered images are created. In this step, a series of rendered images along a selected pathway are generated and linked together in the final step to produce a simulated flight path. A number of technical variables at each of the above steps need to be understood, as they will affect the ultimate quality of the studies.

19.2.1 Data Acquisition

The majority of VE studies currently utilize CT data, and the majority of this discussion will concentrate on processing CT data. Advances in CT technology, especially the development of spiral (helical) CT scanners, has enabled rapid acquisition of high-resolution CT scans. Because spiral CT data are rapidly acquired in a continuous fashion, there is no interval gap or misalignment of successive slices from patient motion. Interval gap and image misalignment can be problematic in conventional CT scanners. Parameters affecting the quality of spiral CT studies include collimation width of the x-ray beam, table translation speed, image reconstruction interval, and the length of the anatomic region covered by the examination, which will be discussed briefly below.

The collimation width is a principal determinant of the resolution in the longitudinal axis. In general narrow collimation widths of 1–2 mm are used in examinations of the head and neck. Translation speed indicates how rapidly the body is moved through the scanner, while the gantry containing the x-ray tubes and detectors rotate at a fixed rate. Translation is generally expressed in terms of pitch factor, defined as:

$$\text{Pitch factor} = [\text{table speed (mm/sec)} \div \text{collimation (mm)}] \times \text{gantry rotation period (sec)}$$

Head and Neck Virtual Endoscopy

The distance to be covered by the study must also be taken into account with spiral CT studies. X-ray tube heating limits the available time to obtain a scan without interruption to allow x-ray tube cooling. When collimation width and pitch are small, a shorter distance is covered in a given scanning period. Ideally, a very narrow collimation width and small pitch would be selected to provide the highest possible resolution, but this limits the distance that can be scanned without interruption to allow x-ray tube cooling.

Since scanning is performed in a continuous fashion, the data are manipulated using interpolation algorithms to reconstruct a series of axial slices. The number and spacing between slices is specified by the reconstruction interval. Selection of an optimal reconstruction interval is important because it is also an important determinant of the longitudinal resolution of the final VE images [67]. Appropriate selection and balancing of collimation width, pitch, and reconstruction interval are all necessary to obtain a high-quality VE imaging study. Optimization of these variables has largely been a heuristic exercise, although several researchers have attempted to use phantoms to determine optimal scanning values [17,32,63]. In our practice, for VE evaluations of head and neck neoplasms or airway compromise, spiral axial CT imaging is typically performed from the skull base to the thoracic inlet using iodinated intravenous contrast with the patient breathing in a relaxed manner (breath holding physiologically distorts the glottic and supraglottic anatomy). We have found the following parameters to provide high-quality data for endoscopic renderings:

Collimation thickness = 2 mm
Pitch factor = 1.5–2.0
Reconstruction interval = 1–2 mm

19.2.2 Data Processing for 3D Reconstruction

The axial image data are transferred to a dedicated computer workstation and processed using image rendering software. Prior to constructing VE images, a 3D model of the data is constructed to first generate a 3D data set that can be analyzed by the rendering software. The processing methods to generate the 3D model differ based on the software used, and several manufacturers have developed and made commercially available their own proprietary software (*Voxel View*®/*Vitrea*®, Vital Images Inc., Fairfield, IA; *Voyager*™, Marconi Medical Systems, Cleveland, OH; *3D Navigator*, GE Medical Systems, Milwaukee, WI). Two general methods are used to prepare image data for perspective rendering: shaded surface display (SSD) and the more advanced volume reconstruction techniques used in volume rendering software.

SSD techniques rely on identification and selection of surface feature data to construct a 3D model of the lumen surface. This is accomplished by a process of segmentation that requires selecting voxels of desired intensities for inclusion into the data set. A 3D surface model containing the voxels located on the surface of the imaged object is reconstructed, and extraneous data are eliminated. SSD has the advantage of requiring less computational power to process the image data, but the rendered images have increased artifacts such as floating pixels and surface discontinuities. Because data are eliminated, information about submucosal tissues is not available.

In contrast to SSD, volume rendering software systems assign a color and opacity to each voxel in the entire data set based on the intensity of the image data. For CT scans, intensity is the attenuation expressed in Hounsfield units, while for MRI scans, intensity is the signal intensity. If desired, manual or automated segmentation of the data can also be performed prior to image rendering to highlight desired structures for incorporation into the VE image (see Ref. 49). Volume rendering has the advantage of retaining all available data, which can be selected and ultimately utilized by altering opacity, color, and lighting effects in the rendering program. Although volume rendering requires considerably more computational power, no information is lost during the reconstructions, and this method of image processing is becoming more popular as computer hardware costs decrease.

19.2.3 Perspective Rendering

The next step in generation of a VE study is to visualize the digital 3D reconstruction in a manner similar to that of the human eye through the use of perspective rendering software. Although all objects imaged will be finally displayed on a 2D surface (either hard copy, films, or monitor screen), the perspective effect created by the graphics software gives the object the impression of three-dimensional depth of field.

The perspective rendering software programs provide a number of tools to emulate visualization of the imaged object. These tools mimic human visual perception of real objects. Software tools allow selection of viewpoint and view direction, view angle (which alters perceived magnification), and lighting effects (intensity and direction of light). Color and opacity can also be altered as described earlier. Skillful manipulation of these imaging tools allows the operator to produce single frame radiographic images that visualize the anatomical structures from almost any direction, distance, magnification or lighting angle. Figure 19.3 shows the first frame of a VE study, looking superiorly into the trachea. The subglottic larynx is visible in the distance.

19.2.4 Animation of VE Images

After generation of the first viewpoint is performed, the flight path for the study is selected either manually or semiautomatically using programmed algorithms

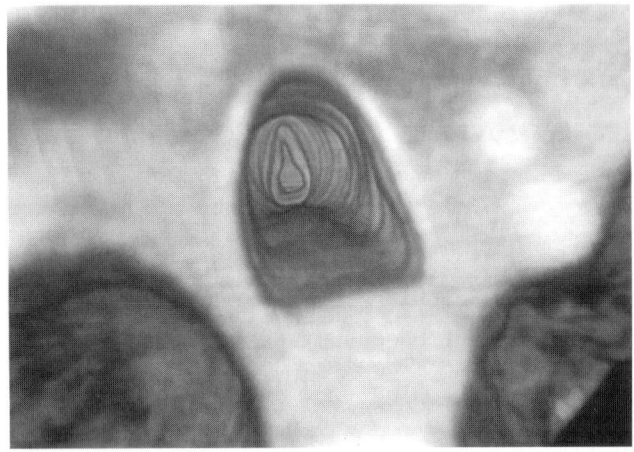

FIGURE 19.3 Virtual endoscopic still frame depicting the trachea and subglottic larynx with cut-away of the thoracic cavity. This image was constructed using perspective volume rendering technique, incorporating all image data as demonstrated in the cut-away view through the thorax. Although submucosal details are not visible through the lumen in this projection, alteration of opacity could be performed to visualize the relational anatomy of the great vessels, thyroid gland, and other structures adjacent to the tracheal lumen.

[68–70]. At selected points along the flight path, the operator acquires images using the selected viewing parameters. The flight path consists of a sequential collection of perspective rendered images incrementally acquired at specified points along the flight path. Flight paths can be viewed as an animated movie that simulates flying through the patient; this approach emulates the experience of an endoscopic examination. The operator can control playback rate and view the study in forward or reverse direction along the predetermined path. Each key frame of the movie is a representation of a viewpoint, view direction, and view angle, and the quality of the study is dependent on the appropriate selection of each of these image components along the entire flight path.

The flight paths generated by VE provide a simulated endoscopic examination. The current technology is not real-time and is not interactive. In order to provide a true virtual reality experience, it is necessary to produce real-time image rendering and display at 30 frames per second (standard frame rate for viewing video) and update the images interactively in response to operator changes in position and view direction within 100 msec (preferably within 10 msec) to provide the sense of immediate response to operator instructions. Current computational power on commercially available workstations does not come close to realizing these requirements, but given the rapid pace of increased computational power, this will be possible in the foreseeable future.

19.3 CLINICAL APPLICATIONS OF VIRTUAL ENDOSCOPY

Since the first clinical reports of VE in the colon and bronchi [21,22,39], VE techniques have been developed for a wide variety of organ systems, including the upper and lower digestive tracts, the biliary tree, the urogenital system, the central nervous system, vascular structures, and major joint spaces (Table 19.1). Although VE has been applied to a number of areas of the body, the techniques are still relatively primitive, and clinical indications for use are still being assessed, while VE techniques and methodology are undergoing rapid evolution. By no means has the full potential of VE been explored. Evaluation of VE in every major organ system and the continued rapid pace of innovation and evolution of the technology indicate that VE will rapidly evolve and will advance beyond the realm of research and become a standard tool in clinical practice. Just how, when, and where VE will play its role remains to be defined.

In the head and neck region pilot studies have been completed at a number of sites. These early studies, which will be described below, have demonstrated the ability of VE to visualize anatomical structures and pathological lesions in a manner similar to that of optical endoscopic examinations. These early studies have provided valuable information necessary to further refine and define the applicability of VE in clinical diagnosis, surgical planning and treatment, and integration with other technologies and teaching applications.

19.3.1 Temporal Bone and Middle Ear

The middle ear and mastoid cavity do not lend themselves to direct (noninvasive) examination beyond limited visualization of the middle ear contents through an intact and (sometimes) semitransparent tympanic membrane. The use of rigid telescope endoscopy to evaluate the middle ear has become popular in recent years [4]. However, the technique requires perforation or reflection of the tympanic membrane. Virtual otoscopy can noninvasively provide information about the middle ear and has the advantage of visualization of structures from any desired perspective. The middle ear is normally aerated, making it a potentially good site to study using VE, but the small size of the middle ear space and structures within are technical impediments to adequate virtual representation.

Frankenthaler et al. [49] recently demonstrated successful mapping of the temporal bone using VE. Their group was able to successfully visualize middle ear and mastoid structures using perspective volume rendering techniques. Their methodology required both manual and automatic segmentation of images to iso-

Head and Neck Virtual Endoscopy

late and outline the important anatomical structures of interest (ossicles, facial nerve, internal carotid artery, etc.), but it added significantly to the time required to produce images. Although the manual segmentation process was very labor intensive, it provided valuable data. In the temporal bone, simple visualization of the surface morphology of the mastoid cavity and middle ear spaces is relatively easy because of large differences in attenuation between air and soft tissues. However, much more clinically relevant information can be provided by clearly representing the subsurface anatomy of the critical temporal bone structures, including the facial nerve, cochlea, membranous labyrinth, carotid artery, and jugular bulb as described earlier. The ability to visualize the deep, bone-encased structures and to display anatomical relationships with the same view obtained at surgery could provide the surgeon with preoperative diagnostic information and contribute to an enhanced understanding of the anatomical and pathological details that will be encountered at surgery.

VE of the middle and inner ear has been studied very little so far, and its eventual utility remains to be seen. A number of potential otological applications may become available with advances in image acquisition and processing techniques. Detailed evaluation of the cochlea and semicircular canals for persons with vertigo, imaging of the cochlea in cochlear implant candidates, evaluation of congenital atresias or ossicular dislocations, and evaluation and postoperative follow-up of cholesteatomas are all potential future applications. A recent study that provides a dramatic illustration of the potential of VE in otology is provided by Diamantopoulos et al. [71]. MR VE examination of a normal subject was able to display the cochlea, oval window, vestibule, common crus, and the semicircular canals using perspective volume rendering techniques. The ability to accurately image and visualize the anatomy of the cochleovestibular structures with high resolution provides a clear illustration of the untapped potential of VE for diagnosis, teaching, and research applications.

19.3.2 Nasal Cavity and Paranasal Sinuses

The nasal cavity is more accessible to direct visualization than the middle ear, and optical endoscopy of the sinuses is a standard diagnostic modality for the otolaryngologist. However, current endoscopic techniques only allow visualization of the orifices of the maxillary, sphenoid and frontal sinuses, and unless unusually patent or surgically enlarged, direct visualization into the sinuses is not possible. Axial and/or coronal CT studies are used to evaluate sinus pathology and visualize the bony and soft tissue anatomy adjacent to the paranasal sinuses. The images serve both as a preoperative diagnostic tool and an anatomical roadmap during surgery to prevent inadvertent injury to critical structures adjacent to the sinuses during endoscopic surgical procedures. Accurate correlation of the anatomy seen through the telescope at surgery with CT data requires the surgeon to mentally reconstruct the cross-sectional data to precisely determine proximity to vital structures; this considerable skill may only be acquired with experience.

As with other anatomical sites where there is a need to provide accurate 3D reconstructions of complex anatomical structures; VE of the nasal cavity and paranasal sinuses could be a very useful clinical tool. Potential applications of VE in the nasal cavity and sinuses include providing supplemental data to augment standard CT and MR studies, assist presurgical planning, use as an adjunctive tool for intraoperative navigation, and for postoperative monitoring. Gilani et al. (54) have demonstrated high-resolution depictions of the nasal cavity and paranasal sinuses, the ability to view anatomy with unique perspectives, and ability to "look into" the paranasal sinuses with VE [54]. In addition to simply creating an endoscopic visualization of the sinus anatomy, Hopper et al. [56] were able to perform "virtual tissue removal" by first constructing VE reconstructions of the nasal cavity and subsequently electronically removing the middle turbinate and uncinate process. They demonstrated that electronic tissue removal mimicked the findings demonstrated at actual surgery and allowed complete visualization of the infundibulum and the planned surgical site. The importance of their findings should not be discounted. Their work demonstrated the use of VE not only as a novel method to realistically visualize anatomical structures, but also as a tool for planning and rehearsal of surgical procedures. Further refinement could allow surgeons to preoperatively perform complete rehearsals of planned operations at a computer workstation. This ability has potential teaching applications for students as well as for skilled surgeons prior to performing advanced procedures.

19.3.3 Larynx and Pharynx

Several studies have demonstrated the feasibility of VE to evaluate pharyngeal and laryngeal anatomy and pathology. Yumoto et al. provided clear demonstration of the potential of VE to visualize normal anatomy and pathological changes in a series of two normal cases and 10 diseased subjects [72]. They demonstrated that their reconstructed images provided supplemental diagnostic information in cases of vocal cord paralysis but did not provide additional information to axial CT images in the cases of laryngeal cancer. Recently, Fried et al. reported on three cases of VE using CT and MRI data to produce virtual reconstructions [60]. In one of these cases, they demonstrated the ability to fuse the CT and MRI image data into one combined image and utilize this merged data to produce VE images. Using the same techniques reported for temporal bone imaging [49], segmentation of important structures was performed to provide a reconstruction of not only surface anatomy, but also structures surrounding the larynx. These images were stacked to form a 3D structure and subsequently imported into a VE software program to construct endoscopic renderings. Although the process

Head and Neck Virtual Endoscopy

was very labor intensive, it demonstrated the potential not only to visualize the surface anatomy of the lumen, but also to also view the submucosal structures, evaluate tumor extent, and visually display tumor interaction with surrounding structures.

19.3.3.1 Anatomical Delineation

We recently reported our experience using VE for evaluation of head and neck neoplasms in a series of 21 patients with head and neck tumors who underwent VE as part of their diagnostic evaluation [59]. VE flight paths were constructed from spiral CT images obtained during tumor staging workup, and images were compared to findings on axial CT images, flexible, and rigid endoscopic findings. VE images were constructed to provide luminal contour detail only. Overall, normal anatomy was clearly seen at all locations in the majority of cases. There was, however, variability in the quality of images at different sites. VE was able to display tracheal and subglottic anatomy not well visualized by standard mirror or flexible fiberoptic examination. The semirigid structure of the trachea allowed for excellent visualization of the tracheal rings, the cricoid cartilage contour, and the mucosal contour of the undersurface of the true vocal cords. Figure 19.4 displays superior (Figure 19.4A) and subglottic (Figure 19.4B) views of the true vocal folds; the subglottic view clearly provides a unique visualization of the undersurface of the true vocal cords. Nasopharyngeal anatomy was also clearly delineated with VE. Fine anatomical details such as the fossa of Rosenmüller, torus tubarius, the posterior choanae, the posterior aspects of the inferior turbinates, and the nasopharyngeal walls were clearly delineated in the majority of the patients (Figure 19.5). Both the trachea and nasopharynx have in common a relatively rigid framework that is generally patent and does not tend to collapse in the normal state. Laryngeal anatomy was also generally well visualized by VE. The true vocal folds, false folds, arytenoids, aryepiglottic folds, and epiglottis were all well seen in the majority of cases. The laryngeal ventricles were not well seen in most cases in our study, most likely because of the selected flight path, field of view, and angulation of the virtual camera. It is likely that variation of the flight path would allow better delineation of this area. For example, Yumoto et al. produced sagittal cutaway views of the medial laryngeal surfaces, which displayed the ventricles clearly [72]. Image quality at the tongue base, vallecula, and pyriform sinuses was more variable. Several anatomical factors contributed to this variability. Posterior displacement of the tongue base, apposition of the tip of the epiglottis on the posterior pharyngeal wall, and collapse of the soft palate and/or lateral pharyngeal walls all contributed to obliteration of the lumen, rendering contour delineation imprecise and unreliable in many patients. Apposition of mucosal surfaces in many studies limited resolution of the normal anatomy. This resulted from inability to discern surface contour when two surfaces are touching each other. Figure 19.6 shows the apparent melding of apposed

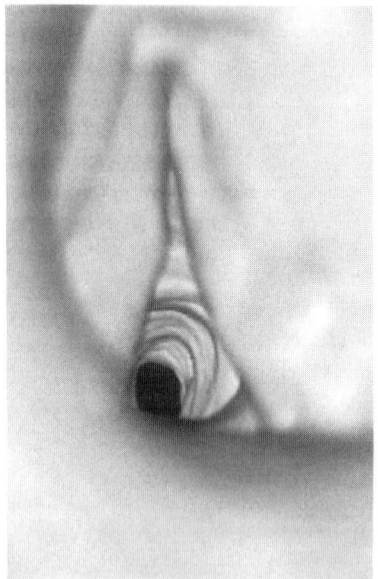

(A)

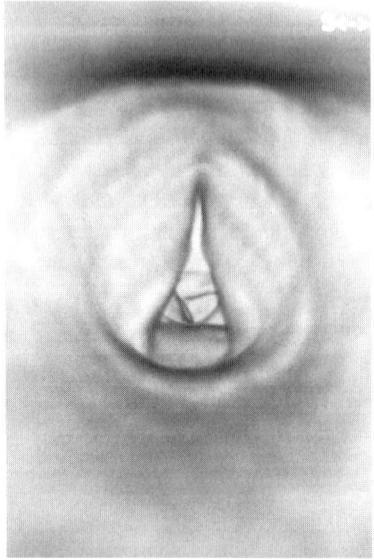

(B)

FIGURE 19.4 Laryngeal anatomy: (A) superior view; (B) subglottic view of normal larynx.

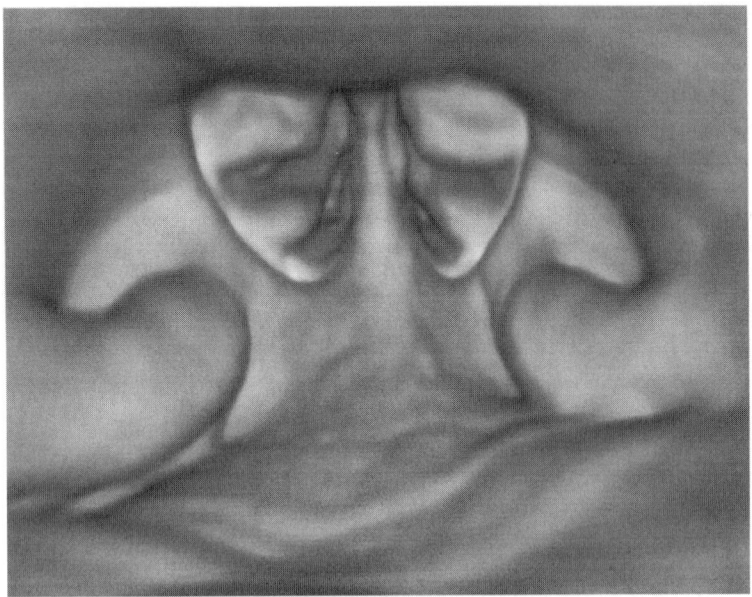

FIGURE 19.5 In this view of nasopharynx from below, note detailed depiction of fossa of Rosenmüller, torus tubarius, vomer, and posterior choanae. Due to the rigid structure of the nasopharynx, high-quality images of the surface features can be reliably obtained.

tissues at the epiglottis (Figure 19.6A) and uvula (Figure 19.6B). With the exception of superior ability to visualize the subglottis from an inferior perspective, limitations of VE were similar to those obtained by standard visual examination techniques in the conscious patient. In the hypopharynx, distension of the pharyngeal walls is necessary to visualize the surface anatomy, either by performing a valsalva maneuver in the awake patient, which is a standard part of our flexible endoscopic examination routine, or manual distension of the tissues during operative endoscopic procedures under general anesthesia. Performance of a valsalva maneuver during image acquisition for VE may improve image quality, but it will likely require an additional sequence of scans, since breath holding will forcefully close the glottis, degrading the image quality of the true and false vocal folds.

19.3.3.2 Tumor Assessment

The ability to delineate tumor extent using VE also varied by anatomical location, and the same anatomical constraints that limited visualization of normal anatomy using VE also affected visualization of tumors. Subglottic tumor extension was

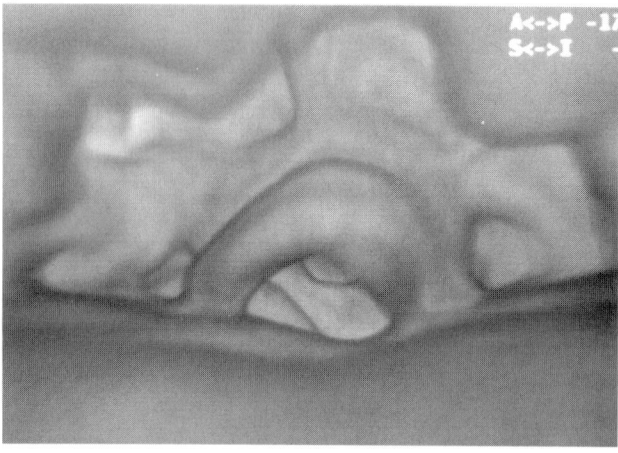

(A)

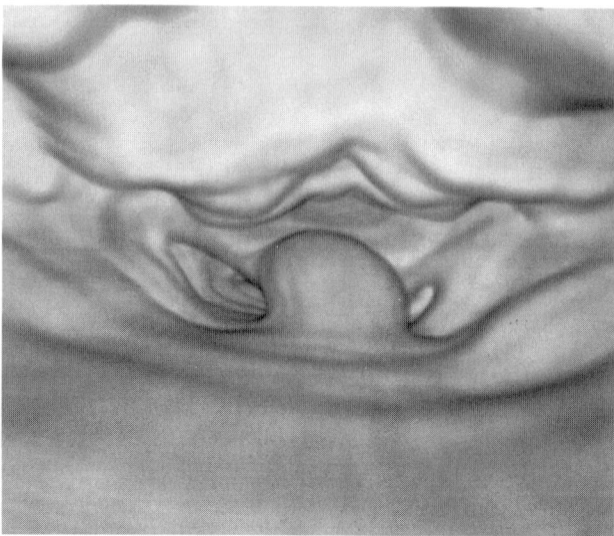

(B)

FIGURE 19.6 Apposition of mucosal tissues in airway. Apposition of the epiglottis (A) and uvula (B) demonstrate how abutment of tissues results in a loss of distinction between the two independent surfaces at the interface and artifactual distortion of the anatomical appearance.

clearly identified as blunting or mass effect at the anterior commissure, and laryngeal tumors were generally well visualized, with the exception of small mucosal T-1 glottic tumors that could not be distinguished from normal mucosa and were missed by both axial CT and CT VE. Visualization of supraglottic tumors was also generally accurate. Figure 19.7 shows a VE image of a T-2 epiglottic SCCA viewed from above. Visualization of the laryngeal surface of the epiglottis, which can also be difficult with rigid direct laryngoscopy, was also suboptimal with VE in our study. The laryngeal surface of the epiglottis lies in a plane nearly parallel to the visual axis of standard endoscopic examinations, making visualization of the surface difficult. However, visualization may be improved with different viewing angles designed to specifically image the laryngeal surface of the epiglottis. Tumors of the hypopharynx and oropharynx were less well visualized, and pyriform sinus tumors were especially problematic, just as they are with other noninvasive diagnostic techniques that do not distend the pyriform sinus. Although in some patients the images were able to show the hypopharyngeal anatomy, tumor visualization and assessment proved difficult. Tumors of the posterior pharyngeal wall could be visualized, but if there was apposition of redundant mucosal folds, visualization was limited. In the hypopharynx, gravity, apposition of mucosal surfaces, and pooled secretions decrease resolution and account for the loss of contour definition. Mucosal contour changes were visualized by VE, but subtle mucosal irregularities could not be appreciated, limiting the sensitivity

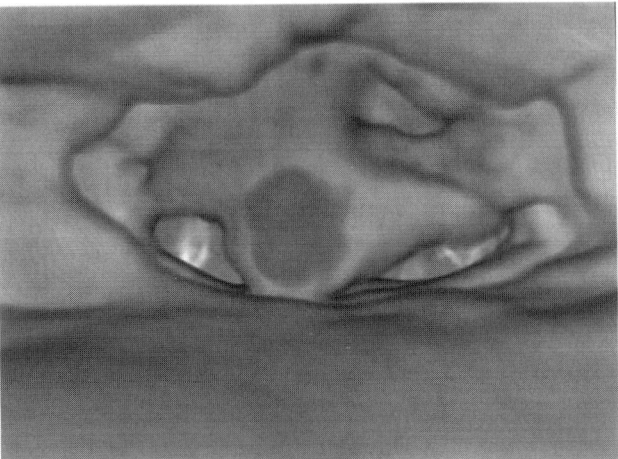

FIGURE 19.7 T-2 squamous cell carcinoma of the superior portion of the laryngeal surface of the epiglottis. Tumor is shown extending along the superior margin and along the laryngeal surface of the epiglottis.

TABLE 19.2 Factors Impairing VE Image Quality

Flat mucosal or submucosal lesions
Apposition of two mucosal surfaces (pyriform sinus, tongue base, epiglottis, soft palate)
Bulky tumors apposing multiple mucosal surfaces
Pooling of secretions
Motion (swallowing, phonation, breathing, arterial pulsation)

of the technique, especially for smaller tumors. Factors leading to impaired visualization of normal anatomy and tumors are summarized in Table 19.2.

19.3.3.3 Evaluation of Airway Obstruction

Burke et al. published their experience using CT VE to evaluate 21 patients with airway obstruction resulting from a variety of causes including laryngotracheomalacia, tracheal masses, glottic webs, innominate artery compression, and vocal fold immobility [73]. They found that VE was as accurate as optical endoscopy for evaluation of fixed stenoses. Correct diagnosis was made in 95% of fixed obstructions, and VE accurately depicted the extent of the lesion seen by optical endoscopy in all but one case. VE was better able to assess the length of tracheal tumors than optical endoscopy. However, the technique was not accurate for evaluation of dynamic obstructions from tracheomalacia, vocal fold immobility, and innominate artery compression of the trachea. This initial study revealed areas for further study and improvement. Their group proposed evaluation of gated examinations timed for respiration and/or heartbeat and infusion of contrast to aid evaluation of dynamic obstructions.

VE of the upper airways shows significant promise for evaluation of the trachea and subglottic larynx and is useful for evaluation of fixed airway obstructions. In addition, the technique may provide information that can aid in staging of persons unfit for operative endoscopy under general anesthesia. Current techniques allow resolution that can image contour deformities, but no color information or indication of vascularity is provided, and the resolution is not precise enough to demonstrate subtle mucosal irregularities that are characteristic of smaller tumors. Nevertheless, this technology is in its infancy, and improvements in resolution and image processing may greatly improve the resolution capabilities of VE.

19.4 ADVANTAGES AND LIMITATIONS OF VIRTUAL ENDOSCOPY

VE has a number of inherent advantages (Table 19.3). First and foremost, VE is a noninvasive technique and has been successfully applied to depict anatomy

TABLE 19.3 Advantages and Limitations of VE

Advantages
   Noninvasive imaging technique
   Ability to use CT, MRI, or ultrasound data
   3D representation of complex anatomy with perspective
   Ability to view lesions from any angle without lens angle distortion
   Visualization past tight stenoses
   Visualization of luminal irregularities
   Objective noninvasive documentation of response to therapy
Limitations
   Limited resolution of mucosal defects
   No color information
   No texture information
   No tissue obtained for diagnosis
   Anatomical visualization variable by location
   Limited ability to evaluate tumor invasion
   Time requirement to construct flight path
   Radiation exposure (CT)
   Cost

and pathological changes at a number of sites in both the head and neck region and the entire body. VE imaging provides a realistic depiction of complex radiographic anatomy in a manner that is more familiar to clinicians [16,20,74], and virtual reconstructions when seen side by side with corresponding axial images facilitates the clinician's 3D interpretation and understanding of both normal anatomy and pathological changes. VE is a very flexible technique that is not subject to the same limitations as visual endoscopic techniques. There is no lens-angle distortion, and the virtual camera can be maneuvered in any desired direction, magnification, and field of view. This allows visualization of anatomy from unique perspectives and the ability to bypass anatomical obstructions that cannot be traversed using standard optical endoscopy techniques.

    Clinically, a number of areas in the head and neck region show great potential for utilization of VE. Assessment of airway obstruction is one area where VE has been demonstrated to be a helpful adjunctive study. VE is an excellent tool for evaluation of luminal incursions, making it useful for evaluation and follow-up for lesions of the subglottic larynx and trachea. It is especially helpful in situations where there is significant narrowing that precludes safe passage of an endoscope through the obstruction and for evaluation of patients medically unfit for general anesthesia. The airways have been studied much more extensively than other areas of the head and neck, but early studies in the sinuses and the temporal bone are encouraging and have stimulated further research to better define how and when VE can be applied at these sites.

VE is a flexible and powerful technology that is widely applicable to a number of medical and nonmedical applications. Perspective image rendering requires high-resolution cross-sectional image data that is an accurate anatomical representative of the imaged structure. The ability to perform VE is independent of imaging modality, but the resolution, precision, and inherent contrast differences between tissues are important inherent properties of the imaging modality that determine the quality of the VE study. There is no limitation on the scale of applicability of these techniques. Perspective rendering techniques have applications in flight simulation, terrain mapping, and manufacturing on a large scale and microscopic applications on a very small scale. For example, 3D reconstruction techniques have been applied to image subcellular anatomy using data obtained from confocal microscopic examinations [65,75]. Along with the flexibility to adapt VE to different imaging modalities, VE image data is inherently portable and can be transferred to other computers for further study and manipulation. The portability of the data can facilitate additional applications of VE. The image data are also objective, and comparison of subsequent VE studies is easy to perform. Optical endoscopic examinations do not share this advantage unless the study is recorded onto videotape or digital media. The presence of a permanent record of the examination makes VE potentially very useful for posttherapy follow-up of clinical response or detection of recurrence or relapse following treatment. It may also be able to obviate the need for repeated surgical endoscopy in certain cases. Medical student and physician education and preoperative surgical planning are two logical applications suggested in other studies [54,74,76].

Although VE has several important advantages over operative endoscopy and can accurately delineate many lesions, there are a number of disadvantages and limitations to this imaging modality (Table 19.3). Perhaps most important is that, although VE provides excellent contour definition, fine mucosal irregularities, vascularity, and color are not depicted [63]. These characteristics are often critical for detection and delineation of the extent of tumors, thus subtle mucosal or submucosal lesions cannot be detected by VE. Contrast resolution is inherently limited by the type of data obtained. For CT, only data reflecting x-ray absorption are recognized—not the vibrant colorful appearance of the tissues seen visually. Although collimations as thin as 1 mm with pitch ratio of 1 can be attained with current spiral CT scanners, the resolution is still not refined enough to delineate subtle mucosal details visible to the human eye. A second major drawback of VE is lack of tissue for diagnosis, which is a critical requirement in the evaluation of potential malignant neoplasms. Successful imaging is dependent upon at least some lumen patency, and when there is collapse of soft tissues or abutment of tumor against the opposite mucosal wall, image quality decreases markedly, just as occurs with flexible endoscopic examinations.

The cost of constructing and interpreting VE images is a barrier to acceptance of this diagnostic modality. We found generation of VE sequences for our initial examinations took more than one hour with supervision by a neuroradiologist, but with experience this time rapidly decreased to approximately 20 minutes by a skilled CT technologist. This finding is similar to that reported by Rodenwadt et al. [63]. VE also requires specialized hardware and software, which represent a significant capital expenditure. Efforts are underway by a number of groups to develop automated and semiautomated methods to speed up the creation of VE studies [60,70,77]. Automation of image segmentation and flight path generation are areas of focus to improve the speed to complete the examinations, and in the near future many of the functions currently performed by the physician or technologist at the imaging workstation may be automated.

19.5 FUTURE CHALLENGES

A number of challenges need to be met before widespread incorporation of VE into clinical practice can occur. There has been extensive evaluation of VE throughout the body, and a number of preliminary studies in the head and neck region have been completed. The indications for VE and an understanding of the strengths and limitations of VE are rapidly being acquired, but additional study is necessary to further define the utility of current applications for VE as well as to discover new applications for this imaging tool. Areas where VE is likely to play a greater role in the future are clinical education and integration with other technologies. VE use will expand as technology improves, costs decrease, and the new applications of VE are discovered.

19.5.1 Improvement of VE Study Quality and Speed

Several technical hurdles limit the utility of VE, and attention is focused on these problems. The quality of the raw image data will reflect the quality of the final VE study. CT, MRI, and ultrasound rely on different physical properties to display tissue contrast and have different contrast and spatial resolutions. A current limitation of VE studies is they do not have the resolution necessary to show the fine mucosal details that provide texture clues visible to the naked eye. Increased spatial resolution may improve this somewhat, but a significant enhancement of resolution will be necessary. MRI has the advantage of acquiring images without ionizing radiation, but the usefulness of MRI for generation of VE is limited by the increased time to acquire images and lower tissue resolution. MRI has better soft tissue contrast resolution than CT, which allows more precise segmentation of anatomical structures and potentially improved discrimination of soft tissues and tumor margins. Use of CT and MRI data together may provide better contrast and resolution of deep tissues than either study alone. Initial experience fusing CT and MRI data is promising, but significant refinement is required to allow seamless merging of image data [60]. For MRI to assume a more prominent role in VE, advances in MRI technology to allow more rapid imaging and processing will be necessary. There is considerable interest in fast scanning techniques such as fast spiral MRI, echo planar imaging, and fast low-angle shot MRI, which decrease scanning time to 50 msec or less [78,79]. Although fast scanning MRI techniques are currently receiving great attention in myocardial imaging and other applications where rapid acquisition is critical [78,79], the contrast and spatial resolution as well as signal to noise ratios currently available do not provide adequate image quality to produce usable VE studies at this time.

Data segmentation is a critical step before image rendering occurs, and also one of the most difficult. Segmentation is simply classification of the image data to allow discrimination of different features. CT attenuation and MRI signal intensity values are generally used in the segmentation process. Unfortunately, these values alone often do not allow precise discrimination of vital anatomical structures or tumor margins, and manual or semiautomated segmentation of anatomical structures is performed to specifically select desired anatomical features. It is a tedious task to manually outline individual anatomical structures, and current semiautomated segmentation programs rely on the skill of the operator to properly select the anatomic regions of interest. Automation and improved accuracy of the data segmentation process will greatly simplify generation of VE studies and decrease cost [23].

Along with automation of segmentation processes, automation of flight path determination and VE frame acquisition along the flight path will greatly speed the process and decrease study costs. Manual flight path generation and image acquisition has a learning curve that must be mastered before studies can be efficiently produced, but the process involves repetitive manual selection of position, view direction, view angle, and lighting. Algorithms to partially automate the process have been developed, but further improvements are necessary before they can be completely automated to dependably generate useful flight paths [68–70]. By removing the repetitive steps in the imaging process and increasing automation, protocols could eventually be developed to allow the technicians currently performing CT and MRI scans to efficiently perform VE studies. This is a necessary prerequisite for VE to be cost-effective.

The next logical advancement of VE after development of automated data segmentation and flight path generation is the development of true virtual reality simulations that will radiographically support real-time navigation throughout the body (analogous to the concept of miniaturization and travel throughout the body depicted in the 1966 movie *The Fantastic Voyage*). It is not difficult to conceive that an operator will be able to access a computer workstation, set the camera angle, and manipulate a joystick to navigate throughout the imaged data set in real time. As described earlier, this will require advances in software as well as

Head and Neck Virtual Endoscopy

increased computational power of several orders of magnitude to perform segmentation and render images in real-time. Given the persistent exponential increases in computing power since the invention of the transistor, the time until this dream can be realized is not as far off as many would think.

19.5.2 Potential Future Applications

It is extremely difficult and foolhardy to predict the future, and attempts to forecast how VE will advance and how it will be applied in coming years will probably be no more successful than predicting the direction of the economy or forecasting the weather. The further out one looks, the less predictable the result. Nevertheless, VE is a flexible tool that provides a unique way to visualize anatomy and pathological changes, and this flexibility indicates that it can be adapted to a wide variety of applications. There are several exciting areas where further study and development of VE will likely lead to valuable clinical applications for otolaryngologists in the future.

19.5.2.1 Development of Teaching Applications

The visualizations produced by VE can be used in a variety of educational applications, ranging from teaching normal anatomy to medical students to evaluating complex anatomical variations and pathology by seasoned clinicians. VE images can be viewed in conjunction with standard axial, coronal, and sagittal images to provide radiologists and clinicians additional views that enhance the understanding of normal and abnormal anatomy. VE data can be incorporated into computerized atlases cataloguing normal and pathological cases. Integration with virtual reality software applications could allow immersion into the anatomical structures to facilitate learning of complex 3D anatomical relationships. These cases could also be integrated with the virtual human project data sets provided by the National Library of Medicine. This is a set of complete digital models of the human body constructed from high-resolution cross-sectional images of human male and female cadavers. CT, MRI, and anatomical cross-sectional data are available for the entire body with 3D resolution of approximately 1 mm. These data can be downloaded off the Internet and processed using image rendering software [65,80].

19.5.2.2 Surgical Simulators

Surgical training is another application where VE can play a role [76]. Hopper et al. demonstrated electronic tissue removal from paranasal sinus VE studies to simulate surgical intervention and visualize deeper structures with the VE study [56]. With further advances, it will become possible to perform rehearsals of complete operations at a workstation using patient-specific data prior to taking the patient to the operating room. The use of surgical training simulators (see Chapter 7) for teaching and skill assessment is also undergoing rapid development [55,81–83]. Surgical simulators provide an interactive 3D virtual reality environment that also allows real-time interaction and tactile feedback (haptics) to endoscope or instrument manipulation within the virtual environment. This allows the virtual surgeon not only to visualize, retract, cut, and cauterize tissues, but also to receive tactile feedback that is a critical part of the surgical experience. One simulator system developed for endoscopic sinus surgery utilizes data from the visible human data set to construct a virtual environment [83]. It may be feasible to adapt surgical simulators to incorporate VE data and construct a library of simulations based on patient-specific VE studies. Having a number of patient-specific databases could allow creation of a portfolio of different scenarios a surgeon is likely to encounter, in a fashion analogous to different weather conditions or equipment malfunctions provided to aircraft pilots in flight simulators. This has the potential to enhance the realism of surgical simulators to improve teaching and is an area that is largely unexamined at this time.

19.5.2.3 Additional Potential Applications

CT and MRI data are used in stereotactic systems in the operating room for anatomical localization. Current systems display 3D location on a monitor showing composite axial, coronal, and sagittal images. It is possible that integrating VE data and currently available stereotactic software used intraoperatively to provide precise 3D anatomical localization in real time might enhance the utility of these localization systems. Positional information obtained using stereotactic image localization techniques could be utilized to merge optical images seen through the endoscope with radiographic VE images to form a composite image. In fact, the SAVANT surgical navigation platform (CBYON, Palo Alto, CA), a system that is currently available, can register endoscopic images generated by perspective volume rendering of preoperative data with the view through a standard nasal telescope. In this system, the SAVANT tracks telescope position and registers the virtual endoscopic view to the real work endoscopic view. This may allow the surgeon to potentially see through the tissues in the operative field. Jolesz et al. demonstrated a simple application of the concept of image-guided endoscopy in a patient with a retropharyngeal tumor requiring endoscopy-guided intubation [77]. A small electromagnetic sensor was attached to the tip of a fiberoptic endoscope. The endoscope was introduced with an endotracheal tube, and the position of the tube tip was registered to data from a VE study. The progress of the intubation was monitored using data obtained from the VE study to guide the endotracheal tube placement.

Computerized radiation therapy treatment planning systems may also be able to incorporate VE data to enhance the speed and accuracy of radiation treat-

Head and Neck Virtual Endoscopy

ment planning. Potential applications include selection of treatment fields, planning beam paths, and monitoring of treatment response.

Robotic or remote (telepresence) surgery is an exploding technology that is starting to be applied clinically [84–88]. It is conceivable that VE information can be successfully incorporated with computerized surgical systems to allow telepresence surgery. There are many unexplored areas where VE could be utilized to enhance the effectiveness of existing technologies.

Poor contrast resolution between tissues is a limiting factor with imaging modalities in current use. The limited ability to define tumor from normal or inflamed tissues and difficulties encountered trying to separate anatomical structures from the surrounding tissue are technical hurdles that limit the quality of VE studies. One new technology that may eventually be able to improve tissue resolution is MR spectroscopy (MRS). MRS has the potential to noninvasively discriminate between normal and malignant tissues based on functional properties of the tissues. Studies in the prostate [89–92], breast [93], and cervical lymph nodes [94] demonstrate successful spatial discrimination of tumor from normal tissues. If very specific high-resolution discrimination of tumor margins becomes possible with MRS, there is potential for incorporation into VE to map tumors and evaluate potential recurrences.

19.6 SUMMARY

VE provides a new way of visualizing anatomy and pathological changes and represents the convergence of advances in optical endoscopy, radiology, and computer science and technology to provide a realistic visualization of radiographic anatomy with the viewpoint of a person inside the imaged structure. The methodologies behind VE combine techniques from the fields of computer graphics and image processing to provide realistic perspective views of cross-sectional image data applicable to a wide variety of both medical and nonmedical applications. VE is perhaps best thought of as an adaptable and flexible imaging tool that provides a new way to view anatomy and pathological changes.

Three-dimensional perspective rendering of luminal anatomy has been tested in a number of body sites, and the technique is rapidly evolving. New applications are being evaluated, and the advantages and disadvantages of this new technology are being assessed. VE has potential clinical applicability in a number of areas in the head and neck region. Further advances in technique and marriage of VE with other technologies, including surgical localization systems, surgical simulators, computerized radiation therapy equipment, telepresence surgery applications, and MR spectroscopy, to name a few, may eventually make VE an indispensable tool for future generation of clinicians. It is difficult to predict how VE will evolve and how it will ultimately be utilized, but it is very likely that this new technology will play an increasing role in clinical medicine in the future.

REFERENCES

1. Rogers LF. A day in the court of lexicon: virtual endoscopy [editorial; comment] [see comments]. Am J Roentgenol. 171:1185, 1998.
2. Johnson, C. D., Hara, A. K., and Reed, J. E. Virtual endoscopy: what's in a name? [see comments]. Am J Roentgenol 171:1201–1202, 1998.
3. Zeitels SM. Premalignant epithelium and microinvasive cancer of the vocal fold: the evolution of phonomicrosurgical management. Laryngoscope 105:1–51, 1995.
4. Bottrill ID, Poe DS. Endoscope-assisted ear surgery. Am J Otol 16:158–163, 1995.
5. Youssef TF, Poe DS. Endoscope-assisted second-stage tympanomastoidectomy, Laryngoscope 107:1341–1344, 1997.
6. Silverstein H, Rosenberg S, Arruda J. Laser-assisted otoendoscopy. Ear Nose Throat J 76:674–676, 678, 1997.
7. Good GM, Isaacson G. Otoendoscopy for improved pediatric cholesteatoma removal. Ann Otol Rhinol Laryngol. 108:893–896, 1999.
8. Deans SR. The Radon Transform and Some of Its Applications. New York: Wiley, 1983.
9. Gobbetti E, Scateni R. Virtual reality: past, present and future. Studies Health Technol Inform 58:3–20, 1998.
10. Kaltenborn KF, Rienhoff O. Virtual reality in medicine. Methods Inform Med 32:407–417, 1993.
11. Altobelli DE, Kikinis R, Mulliken JB, Cline H, Lorensen W, Jolesz F. Computer-assisted three-dimensional planning in craniofacial surgery. Plastic Reconstruct Surg 92:576–585; discussion 586–587, 1993.
12. Marentette LJ, Maisel RH. Three-dimensional CT reconstruction in midfacial surgery. Otolaryngol Head Neck Surg 98:48–52, 1988.
13. Vannier MW, Conroy GC, Marsh JL, Knapp RH. Three-dimensional cranial surface reconstructions using high-resolution computed tomography. Am J Phys Anthropol 67:299–311, 1985.
14. McEwan CN, Fukuta K. Recent advances in medical imaging: surgery planning and simulation. World J Surg 13:343–348, 1989.
15. Zonneveld FW, Lobregt S, van der Meulen JC, Vaandrager JM. Three-dimensional imaging in craniofacial surgery. World J Surg 13:328–342, 1989.
16. Zinreich SJ, Mattox DE, Kennedy DW, Johns ME, Price JC, Holliday MJ, Quinn CB, Kashima HK. 3-D CT for cranial facial and laryngeal surgery. Laryngoscope 98:1212–1219, 1988.
17. Zeiberg AS, Silverman PM, Sessions RB, Troost TR, Davros WJ, Zeman RK. Helical (spiral) CT of the upper airway with three-dimensional imaging: technique and clinical assessment. Am J Roentgenol 166:293–299, 1996.
18. Silverman PM, Zeiberg AS, Sessions RB, Troost TR, Davros WJ, Zeman RK. Heli-

cal CT of the upper airway: normal and abnormal findings on three-dimensional reconstructed images. Am J Roentgenol 165:541–546, 1995.
19. Eppley BL, Sadove AM. Computer-generated patient models for reconstruction of cranial and facial deformities. J Craniofacial Surg 9:548–556, 1998.
20. Eisele DW, Richtsmeier WJ, Graybeal JC, Koch WM, Zinreich SJ. Three-dimensional models for head and neck tumor treatment planning. Laryngoscope 104:433–439, 1994.
21. Vining DJ, Liu K, Choplin RH, Haponik EF. Virtual bronchoscopy. Relationships of virtual reality endobronchial simulations to actual bronchoscopic findings. Chest 109:549–553, 1996.
22. Vining DJ, Shifrin RY, Grishaw EK. Virtual colonoscopy (abstr). Radiology 193:446, 1994.
23. Rubin GD, Beaulieu CF, Argiro V, Ringl H, Norbash AM, Feller JF, Dake MD, Jeffrey RB, Napel S. Perspective volume rendering of CT and MR images: applications for endoscopic imaging. Radiology 199: 321–330, 1996.
24. Yuh EL, Jeffrey RB, Jr., Birdwell RL, Chen BH, Napel S. Virtual endoscopy using perspective volume-rendered three-dimensional sonographic data: technique and clinical applications. Am J Roentgenol 172:1193–1197, 1999.
25. Heunerbein M, Ghadimi BM, Gretschel S, Schlag PM. Three-dimensional endoluminal ultrasound: a new method for the evaluation of gastrointestinal tumors [see comments]. Abdom Imag 24:445–448, 1999.
26. Lambert R. Diagnosis of esophagogastric tumors: a trend toward virtual biopsy. Endoscopy 31:38–46, 1999.
27. Blezek DJ, Robb RA. Evaluating virtual endoscopy for clinical use. Digital Imag 10:51–55, 1997.
28. Ogata I, Komohara Y, Yamashita Y, Mitsuzaki K, Takahashi M, Ogawa M. CT evaluation of gastric lesions with three-dimensional display and interactive virtual endoscopy: comparison with conventional barium study and endoscopy [see comments]. Am J Roentgenol 172:1263–1270, 1999.
29. Springer P, Dessl A, Giacomuzzi SM, Buchberger W, Steoger A, Oberwalder M, Jaschke W. Virtual computed tomography gastroscopy: a new technique. Endoscopy 29:632–634, 1997.
30. Lewis BS. Enteroscopy. Gastrointest Endosc Clin North Am 10:101–116, 2000.
31. Wood BJ, O'Malley ME, Hahn PF, Mueller PR. Virtual endoscopy of the gastrointestinal system outside the colon. Am J Roentgenol 171:1367–1372, 1998.
32. Rogalla P, Werner-Rustner M, Huitema A, van Est A, Meiri N, Hamm B. Virtual endoscopy of the small bowel: phantom study and preliminary clinical results, Eur Radiol 8:563–567, 1998.
33. Royster AP, Fenlon HM, Clarke PD, Nunes DP, Ferrucci JT. CT colonoscopy of colorectal neoplasms: two-dimensional and three-dimensional virtual-reality techniques with colonoscopic correlation. Am J Roentgenol 169:1237–1242, 1997.
34. Morrin MM, Farrell RJ, Raptopoulos V, McGee JB, Bleday R, Kruskal JB. Role of virtual computed tomographic colonography in patients with colorectal cancers and obstructing colorectal lesions. Dis Colon Rectum 43:303–311, 2000.

35. Kay CL, Kulling D, Hawes RH, Young JW, Cotton PB. Virtual endoscopy—comparison with colonoscopy in the detection of space-occupying lesions of the colon [see comments]. Endoscopy 32:226–232, 2000.
36. Nolte-Ernsting CC, Krombach G, Staatz G, Kilbinger M, Adam GB, Geunther RW. [Virtual endoscopy of the upper urinary tract based on contrast-enhanced MR urography data sets]. Fortschr Geb Röntgenstr Neuen Bildgebenden Verfahren 170:550–556, 1999.
37. Stenzl A, Frank R, Eder R, Recheis W, Knapp R, zur Nedden D, Bartsch G. 3-Dimensional computerized tomography and virtual reality endoscopy of the reconstructed lower urinary tract. J Urol 159:741–746, 1998.
38. Frank R, Stenzl A, Frede T, Eder R, Recheis W, Knapp R, Bartsch G, zur Nedden D. Three-dimensional computed tomography of the reconstructed lower urinary tract: technique and findings. Eur Radiol 8:657–663, 1998.
39. Ferretti GR, Vining DJ, Knoplioch J, Coulomb M. Tracheobronchial tree: three-dimensional spiral CT with bronchoscopic perspective. J Comput Assist Tomogr 20:777–781, 1996.
40. Liu JB, Goldberg BB. 2-D and 3-D endoluminal ultrasound: vascular and nonvascular applications. Ultrasound Med Biol 25:159–173, 1999.
41. Neri E, Caramella D, Falaschi F, Sbragia P, Vignali C, Laiolo E, Viviani A, Bartolozzi C. Virtual CT intravascular endoscopy of the aorta: pierced surface and floating shape thresholding artifacts. Radiology 212:276–279, 1999.
42. Neri E, Caramella D, Bisogni C, Laiolo E, Trincavelli F, Viviani A, Vignali C, Cioni R, Bartolozzi C. Detection of accessory renal arteries with virtual vascular endoscopy of the aorta. Cardiovasc Intervent Radiol 22:1–6, 1999.
43. Davis CP, Ladd ME, Romanowski BJ, Wildermuth S, Knoplioch JF, Debatin JF. Human aorta: preliminary results with virtual endoscopy based on three-dimensional MR imaging data sets. Radiology 199:37–40, 1996.
44. Fellner F, Fellner C, Beohm-Jurkovic H, Blank M, Bautz W. MR diagnosis of vein of Galen aneurysmal malformations using virtual cisternoscopy. Comput Med Imag Graph 23:293–297, 1999.
45. Boor S, Resch KM, Perneczky A, Stoeter P. Virtual endoscopy (VE) of the basal cisterns: its value in planning the neurosurgical approach. Minimally Invasive Neurosurg 41:177–182, 1998.
46. Fellner F, Blank M, Fellner C, Beohm-Jurkovic H, Bautz W, Kalender WA. Virtual cisternoscopy of intracranial vessels: a novel visualization technique using virtual reality. Magn Resonance Imag 16:1013–1022, 1998.
47. Auer LM, Auer DP. Virtual endoscopy for planning and simulation of minimally invasive neurosurgery. Neurosurgery 43:529–537; discussion 537–548, 1998.
48. Marro B, Galanaud D, Valery CA, Zouaoui A, Biondi A, Casasco A, Sahel M, Marsault C. Intracranial aneurysm: inner view and neck identification with CT angiography virtual endoscopy. J Comput Assist Tomogr 21:587–589, 1997.
49. Frankenthaler RP, Moharir V, Kikinis R, van Kipshagen P, Jolesz F, Umans C, Fried MP. Virtual otoscopy. Otolaryngol Clin North Am 31:383–392, 1998.
50. Karhuketo TS, Dastidar PS, Laasonen EM, Sipilea MM, Puhakka HJ. Visualization of the middle ear with high resolution computed tomography and superfine fiberoptic videomicroendoscopy. Eur Arch Oto-rhino-laryngol 255:277–280, 1998.

51. Seemann MD, Seemann O, Englmeier KH, Allen CM, Haubner M, Reiser MF. Hybrid rendering and virtual endoscopy of the auditory and vestibular system. Eur J Med Res 3:515–522, 1998.
52. Seemann MD, Seemann O, Bonael H, Suckfeull M, Englmeier KH, Naumann A, Allen CM, Reiser MF. Evaluation of the middle and inner ear structures: comparison of hybrid rendering, virtual endoscopy and axial 2D source images. Eur Radiol 9: 1851–1858, 1999.
53. De Nicola M, Salvolini L, Salvolini U. Virtual endoscopy of nasal cavity and paranasal sinuses. Eur J Radiol 24:175–180, 1997.
54. Gilani S, Norbash AM, Ringl H, Rubin GD, Napel S, Terris DJ. Virtual endoscopy of the paranasal sinuses using perspective volume rendered helical sinus computed tomography. Laryngoscope 107:25–29, 1997.
55. Hilbert M, Meuller W. Virtual reality in endonasal surgery. Studies Health Technol Inform 39:237–245, 1997.
56. Hopper KD, Iyriboz AT, Wise SW, Fornadley JA. The feasibility of surgical site tagging with CT virtual reality of the paranasal sinuses. J Comput Assist Tomogr 23:529–533, 1999.
57. Morra A, Calgaro A, Cioffi V, Pravato M, Cova M, Pozzi Mucelli R. [Virtual endoscopy of the nasal cavity and the paranasal sinuses with computerized tomography. Anatomical study]. Radiol Med 96:29–34, 1998.
58. Rogalla P, Nischwitz A, Gottschalk S, Huitema A, Kaschke O, Hamm B. Virtual endoscopy of the nose and paranasal sinuses. Eur Radiol 8:946–950, 1998.
59. Gallivan RP, Nguyen TH, Armstrong WB. Head and neck computed tomography virtual endoscopy: evaluation of a new imaging technique. Laryngoscope 109:1570–1579, 1999.
60. Fried MP, Moharir VM, Shinmoto H, Alyassin AM, Lorensen WE, Hsu L, Kikinis R. Virtual laryngoscopy. Ann Otol Rhinol Laryngol 108:221–226, 1999.
61. Aschoff AJ, Seifarth H, Fleiter T, Sokiranski R, Georich J, Merkle EM, Wunderlich AP, Brambs HJ, Zenkel ME. [High-resolution virtual laryngoscopy based on spiral CT data]. Radiologe 38:810–815, 1998.
62. Giovanni A, Nazarian B, Sudre-Levillain I, Zanaret M, Moulin G, Vivarrat-Perrin L, Bourliaere-Najean B, Triglia JM. [Geometric modeling and virtual endoscopy of the laryngo-tracheal lumen from computerized tomography images: initial applications to laryngo-tracheal pathology in the child]. Rev Laryngol Otolo Rhinol 119: 341–346, 1998.
63. Rodenwaldt J, Kopka L, Roedel R, Margas A, Grabbe E. 3D virtual endoscopy of the upper airway: optimization of the scan parameters in a cadaver phantom and clinical assessment. J Comput Assist Tomogr 21:405–411, 1997.
64. Beaulieu CF, Rubin GD. Perspective rendering of spiral CT data: flying through and around normal and pathologic anatomy. In: Fishman EK, Jeffrey RB, eds. Spiral CT: Principles, Techniques, and Clinical Applications, 2nd ed. Philadelphia: Lippincott-Raven, 1998, pp. 35–52.
65. Lichtenbelt B, Crane R, Naqvi S. Introduction to Volume Rendering. Upper Saddle River, NJ: Prentice Hall, 1998.
66. Napel S. Basic principles of spiral CT. In: Fishman EK, Jeffrey RB, eds. Spiral CT:

Principles, Techniques, and Clinical Applications, 2nd ed. Philadelphia: Lippincott-Raven, 1998, pp. 3–15.
67. Brink JA. Technical aspects of helical (spiral) CT. Radiol Clin North Am 33:825–841, 1995.
68. Paik DS, Beaulieu CF, Jeffrey RB, Rubin GD, Napel S. Automated flight path planning for virtual endoscopy. Med Phys 25:629–637, 1998.
69. Summers RM. Navigational aids for real-time virtual bronchoscopy. Am J Roentgenol 168:1165–1170, 1997.
70. Kumar S, Asari KV, Radhakrishnan D. Real-time automatic extraction of lumen region and boundary from endoscopic images. Med Biol Eng Comput 37:600–604, 1999.
71. Diamantopoulos II, Ludman CN, Martel AL, O'Donoghue GM. Magnetic resonance imaging virtual endoscopy of the labyrinth. Am J Otol 20:748–751, 1999.
72. Yumoto E, Sanuki T, Hyodo M, Yasuhara Y, Ochi T. Three-dimensional endoscopic mode for observation of laryngeal structures by helical computed tomography. Laryngoscope 107:1530–1537, 1997.
73. Burke AJ, Vining DJ, McGuirt WF, Jr., Postma G, Browne JD. Evaluation of airway obstruction using virtual endoscopy. Laryngoscope 110:23–29, 2000.
74. Pototschnig C, Veolklein C, Dessl A, Giacomuzzi S, Jaschke W, Thumfart WF. Virtual endoscopy in otorhinolaryngology by postprocessing of helical computed tomography. Otolaryngol Head Neck Surg 119:536–539, 1998.
75. Robb RA. Virtual (computed) endoscopy: development and evaluation using the visible human datasets.: http://www.mayo.edu/bir/nlmpaper/robb_pap.htm, 1996.
76. Wiegand DA, Page RB, Channin DS. The surgical workstation: surgical planning using generic software. Otolaryngol Head Neck Surg 109:434–440, 1993.
77. Jolesz FA, Lorensen WE, Shinmoto H, Atsumi H, Nakajima S, Kavanaugh P, Saiviroonporn P, Seltzer SE, Silverman SG, Phillips M, Kikinis R. Interactive virtual endoscopy [see comments]. Am J Roentgenol 169:1229–1235, 1997.
78. Wiesmann F, Gatehouse PD, Panting JR, Taylor AM, Firmin DN, Pennell DJ. Comparison of fast spiral, echo planar, and fast low-angle shot MRI for cardiac volumetry at .5T. J Magn Reson Imag 8:1033–1039, 1998.
79. Davis PL. Principles of magnetic resonance imaging. In: Moss AA, Gamsu G, Genant HK, eds. Computed Tomography of the Body with Magnetic Resonance Imaging, 2nd ed., Vol. 3. Philadelphia: Saunders, 1992.
80. The national library of medicine's visible human project.: http://www.nlm.nih.gov/research/visible/visible_human.html, 2000.
81. Edmond CV, Jr, Heskamp D, Sluis D, Stredney D, Sessanna D, Wiet G, Yagel R, Weghorst S, Oppenheimer P, Miller J, Levin M, Rosenberg L. ENT endoscopic surgical training simulator. Stud Health Technol Inform 39 518–528, 1997.
82. Weghorst S, Airola C, Oppenheimer P, Edmond CV, Patience T, Heskamp D, Miller J. Validation of the Madigan ESS simulator. Stud Health Technol Inform 50:399–405, 1998.
83. Rudman DT, Stredney D, Sessanna D, Yagel R, Crawfis R, Heskamp D, Edmond CV, Jr, Wiet GJ. Functional endoscopic sinus surgery training simulator. Laryngoscope 108:1643–1647, 1998.
84. Wagner A, Millesi W, Watzinger F, Truppe M, Rasse M, Enislidis G, Kermer C,

Ewers R. Clinical experience with interactive teleconsultation and teleassistance in craniomaxillofacial surgical procedures. J Oral Maxillofacial Surg 57:1413–1418, 1999.
85. Satava RM. Emerging technologies for surgery in the 21st century. Arch Surg 134: 1197–1202, 1999.
86. Rininsland H. ARTEMIS. A telemanipulator for cardiac surgery. Eur J Cardio-Thorac Surg 16 (suppl 2): S106–S111, 1999.
87. Hill JW, Holst PA, Jensen JF, Goldman J, Gorfu Y, Ploeger DW. Telepresence interface with applications to microsurgery and surgical simulation. Stud Health Technol Inform 50:96–102, 1998.
88. Bowersox JC, Shah A, Jensen J, Hill J, Cordts PR, Green PS. Vascular applications of telepresence surgery: initial feasibility studies in swine. J Vasc Surg 23:281–287, 1996.
89. Kim JK, Kim DY, Lee YH, Sung NK, Chung DS, Kim OD, Kim KB. In vivo differential diagnosis of prostate cancer and benign prostatic hyperplasia: localized proton magnetic resonance spectroscopy using external-body surface coil. Magnet Reson Imag 16:1281–1288, 1998.
90. Garcaia-Segura JM, Saanchez-Chapado M, Ibarburen C, Viaano J, Angulo JC, Gonzaalez J, Rodraiguez-Vallejo JM. In vivo proton magnetic resonance spectroscopy of diseased prostate: spectroscopic features of malignant versus benign pathology. Magn Reson Imag 17:755–765, 1999.
91. Tran TK, Vigneron DB, Sailasuta N, Tropp J, Le Roux P, Kurhanewicz J, Nelson S, Hurd R. Very selective suppression pulses for clinical MRSI studies of brain and prostate cancer. Magne Reson Med 43:23–33, 2000.
92. Males RG, Vigneron DB, Star-Lack J, Falbo SC, Nelson SJ, Hricak H, Kurhanewicz J. Clinical application of BASING and spectral/spatial water and lipid suppression pulses for prostate cancer staging and localization by in vivo 3D 1H magnetic resonance spectroscopic imaging. Magn Reson Med 43:17–22, 2000.
93. Cheng LL, Chang IW, Smith BL, Gonzalez RG. Evaluating human breast ductal carcinomas with high-resolution magic-angle spinning proton magnetic resonance spectroscopy. J Magn Reson 135:194–202, 1998.
94. Star-Lack JM, Adalsteinsson E, Adam MF, Terris DJ, Pinto HA, Brown JM, Spielman DM. In vivo 1H MR spectroscopy of human head and neck lymph node metastasis and comparison with oxygen tension measurements. Am J Neuroradiol 21:183–193, 2000.

20

Computer-Aided Facial Plastic Surgery

Daniel G. Becker, M.D.
University of Pennsylvania, Philadelphia, Pennsylvania

Madeleine A. Spatola, M.A.
Thomas Jefferson University Medical School, Philadelphia, Pennsylvania

Samuel S. Becker, M.F.A.
University of California at San Francisco Medical Center, San Francisco, California

20.1 INTRODUCTION

The most obvious example of the nearly universal incorporation of computer technology into facial plastic surgical practices is office software and computer systems, which provide valuable benefit for the surgical practice seeking to deliver efficient state-of-the-art care. Computer technology is playing an increasing role in communication with patients and colleagues and also in education. In the area of photodocumentation—a critical component in facial plastic surgery—digital technology now provides an alternative to the time-tested 35 mm single lens reflex (SLR) camera. Digital photography and computer photo archiving are allowing easier storage and retrieval of photographic images for improved documentation, self-education, and communication. Computer imaging has become increasingly commonplace as a preoperative educational tool and a surgical planning tool. The World Wide Web has become an increasingly important forum for communication and education.

As computer technology has caught up with the needs and dreams of surgeons, increasingly it is finding significant applications in the operating room. Continuing technological advances—some anticipated, others not—will undoubtedly lead to continued improvements in facial plastic surgical care. As we become increasingly reliant on computer technology, it is critical that we understand its potential and also its potential pitfalls, such as medicolegal issues. Understanding the rapidly occurring developments in computer technology may allow facial plastic surgeons to prepare for the office and operating room of the future. In this chapter, we discuss the current and potential future status of computer technology in facial plastic surgery.

20.2 PLASTIC SURGICAL OFFICE SOFTWARE

Office software has become so integrated into physician practices that it is often overlooked in discussions of computers in otolaryngology and facial plastic surgery. Zupko and Toth provide an overview of important considerations in the selection of a computer system that meets the specific practice needs of the facial plastic surgeon [1]. They point out the importance of having an organized approach, especially when one considers that there are approximately 1000 practice management systems available nationwide. Zupko and Toth describe what they perceive to be the facial plastic surgeon's specific practice needs: namely, a need for niche marketing strategies; a need to track patient relationships from the first telephone call, to the appointment, to surgery, and postoperatively; a need to track skin care product use and sales; a need to track in-office OR inventory; financial control given the cash nature of cosmetic surgery; and computer imaging. They emphasize the need for an integrated system that incorporates all of these factors.

Hodnett described important guidelines for the facial plastic surgery practice seeking new office software [2]. He felt that office software must have the following features: it must be Windows based (Microsoft Corporation, Bellevue, WA), it must be Y2K compliant, and it must be able to integrate easily with present and future programs. In addition, Hodnett proposed that the software should easily customize materials (such as forms) for the patient, that it should decrease the need for the patient to ask questions before and after surgery, and that it should simplify the tasks of the office staff. The author felt that an office software program should be able to track patient information, including demographical information (such as the geographic origin of patients) and practice parameters (such as the percentage of patients who seek consultation and ultimately proceed to surgery). A knowledgeable sales force with immediate technical and customer support was also deemed vital. The software should have comprehensive database capabilities to accommodate the critical need for comprehensive reports in practice management. Lastly, the author emphasized that the software company should provide a copy of the software in the office on floppy disk or CD-ROM, because the practice could be stranded if the computer's hard drive fails.

Quatela et al. [3] reviewed important considerations in plastic surgical office software. They pointed out a number of important practical considerations, including the need for an adequate network server, the ability of the system to quickly compile and analyze reports, electronic scheduling and mailing, and electronic billing link to insurance companies. They noted that the Health Care Financing Administration indicated that by 2002 insurance companies and state providers will only accept electronic claims [3,4].

20.3 DIGITAL PHOTOGRAPHY, COMPUTER IMAGING, AND PHOTOARCHIVING

Photographic images in facial plastic surgery play a critical role in photodocumentation, patient education, preoperative planning, and self-education [5–8]. Consistent, uniform, high-quality photography allows the best opportunity for critical self-assessment and self-education by surgeons. Uniform photographs are essential for legal documentation of surgical events and outcomes. Furthermore, an increasingly sophisticated patient population often asks to see photographic examples of a surgeon's work, providing an added incentive for the surgeon to produce high-quality, uniform, professional images that reflect the surgeon's attention to detail. However, perusal of most medical journals suggests widespread and significant persisting deficiencies in photographic quality.

Equipment, lighting and background, film selection, and a standardized photographic technique are critical aspects of achieving satisfactory images (Figure 20.1, Table 20.1). Multiple reports discuss the essential elements of professional photography for facial plastic surgery [5–8]. Digital cameras are becoming increasingly less expensive and offer increasingly better quality; they also have significant advantages with regard to ease of image storage and retrieval [6]. Miller et al. compared a number of currently available digital cameras [8].

Photographic storage may be more cost-effective and efficient with digital systems. Ease of storage and image retrieval are important considerations. A busy plastic surgical practice may accumulate as many as 2 million images over a 30-year surgical practice [5]. Storage of such a large volume of traditional 35 mm slides requires a significant amount of space, in contrast to a similar number of digital images.

Patients seeking cosmetic surgery now often expect preoperative imaging. Improvements in hardware and software have allowed great increases in speed

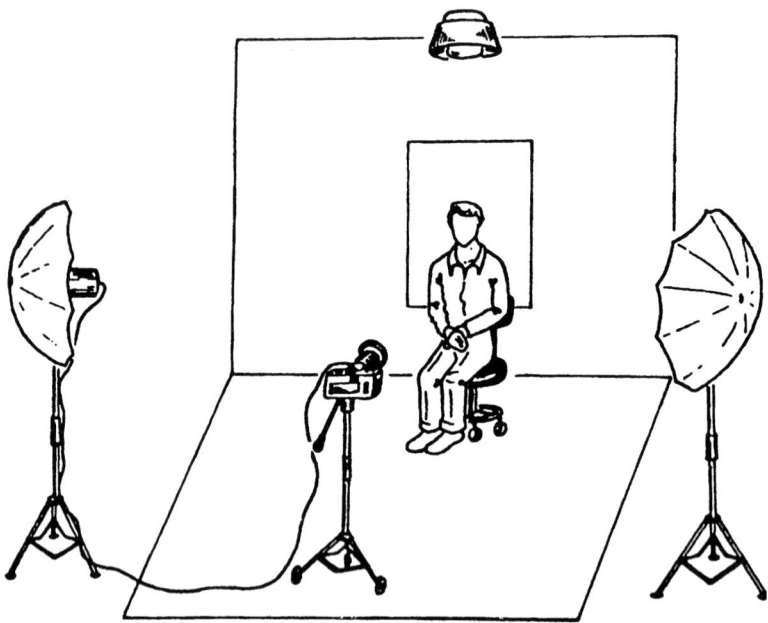

FIGURE 20.1 Diagrammatic photographic setup. The patient is seated in front of the photographic background on a chair with a back support. The chair rotates so that patient positioning may be optimized. The camera may be mounted on a mobile tripod, or it may be hand-held by the photographer. The camera is connected to synchronized lights; a "kicker" light overhead and behind the patient is optional.

and accuracy in patient imaging. This can facilitate doctor-patient communication and has the potential to help provide realistic patient expectations. Indeed, Papel and Jiannetto report that a literature search (through 1998) revealed no lawsuits directly involving computer imaging [9]. They suggest that conservative utilization of computer imaging by the facial plastic surgeon may actually reduce liability and promote communication.

Typically, a patient presenting to the plastic surgeon will undergo preoperative photography. Either at the time of the initial visit (or at a later visit), the plastic surgeon or a staff member will review the proposed changes in the patient's physical appearance on the patient's computerized image. It must be carefully explained to the patient that this exercise is nothing more than another form of communication. In this way, digital photography helps ensure that both the surgeon and the patient share similar surgical goals. Indeed, computer imaging, when accompanied by appropriate explanation, provides the opportunity for improved patient-doctor communication.

TABLE 20.1 Photographic Guidelines for Specific Surgical Procedures

Image	Focal length
Rhinoplasty	
Full face	1:7
Right and left lateral	1:7
Right and left oblique	1:7
Base or submental view	1:3 and 1:5
Blepharoplasty	
Full face	1:7
Eyes to camera	1:4
Eyes closed, at rest	1:4
Eyes looking up	1:4
Rhytidectomy	
Full face	1:10
Right and left lateral	1:10
Right and left oblique	1:10
(shirt or blouse collar pulled back to see collar bone)	
Browlift	
Same as blepharoplasty	
Otoplasty	
Full face	1:10
Right and left lateral	1:10
Back of head	1:10
Submental vertex	1:10
Antihelix of ears	1:3
Hair transplant	
Full face	1:10
Right and left lateral	1:10
Back of head	1:10
Top of head	1:10
Forehead	1:5
Scars	
Close-up views important, but full-face views must also be obtained.	

The surgeon or staff member should explain to the patient that computer-based morphing cannot take into account certain unpredictable factors that are a part of the practice of surgery. The patient is "analog" and not "digital;" so the results of an actual surgery can in no way be predicted or represented in advance by a computer "simulation." The imaging is simply a way for both the patient and doctor to share an image of the surgical goal. Of course, this process can be a reassuring exercise for both the patient and the surgeon. Patients typically understand this simple concept; some surgeons incorporate provisions that address this disclosure into a consent form.

Papel and Jiannetto also noted recent technological advances that have significantly enhanced the value of computer imaging in the facial plastic surgery practice [9]. Miniaturization, portability, increased speed, and decreased cost have made computer imaging more accessible (Figure 20.2). Indeed, while Koch and Chavez estimated that 10% of cosmetic surgeons owned computer imaging systems in 1998 [10], it has been projected that up to 45% of cosmetic surgeons will own them by 2001 [11]. The imaging process may facilitate presurgical planning and clarification of the surgeon's own thought processes. Various "expert system modules," such as the Gunter Rhinoplasty Module (Mirror Imaging Systems), may aid the surgeon in selecting an effective technique for a particular deformity. These algorithms reflect a database that summarizes the approach of a particular expert or the consensus approach of a panel of experts in a variety of clinical situations [9,12]. These systems may be most useful for resident surgeons and novice surgeons.

Chand conducted a survey of 50 facial plastic and reconstructive surgeons in the United States and Canada [13]. In this group, 61% of the 44 respondents reported that they use computer imaging in their practice, but most respondents use the technology for "selected" patients only. Interestingly, there was no correlation between years in practice and the use of a computer-based system.

20.4 COMPUTERS IN SLIDE PRODUCTION AND PRESENTATIONS

Computer software for presentations have transformed traditional slide presentations into an elaborate multimedia events [14]. The production of slides is no

---

20.2 Patient presenting for rhinoplasty (A) who requested pre-operative computer imaging simulation (B). The imaging was done on a laptop personal computer using an inexpensive software program. The photographic slide was scanned into the computer using a ScanJet ADF with Slide Adapter (Hewlett-Packard, Palo Alto, CA). The image was then altered using SuperGoo morphing software (ScanSoft, Peabody, MA). Transfer of the image into the computer via the slide scanner and then into Kai's SuperGoo degrades the image quality somewhat. This degradation in image quality may be disadvantageous, especially when compared against dedicated high resolution digital cameras, which directly acquire the digital image. However, the senior author prefers the slight fuzziness of the computer simulation image. The fuzzy image seems to reinforce the point that the computer morphing is simply a helpful communication tool regarding the goals of surgery, and that it is not designed in any way to suggest a guaranteed or exact result. The postoperative result shown for this patient (C).

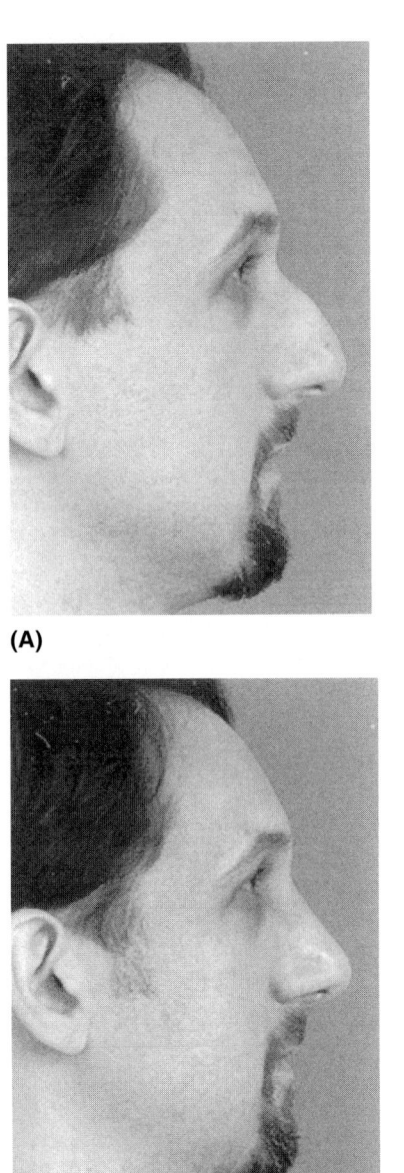
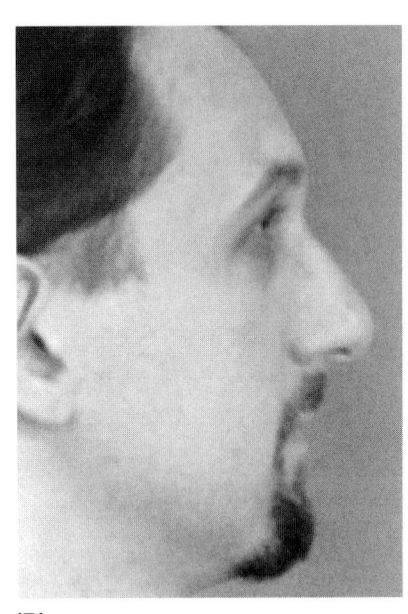

(A)

(B)

(C)

longer a time-consuming and expensive process. Digital cameras and digital scanners allow easy input of pictorial information that can dramatically enhance a presentation. New digital projection equipment will support a direct electronic link to the presenter's PC, increasing the flexibility of presentations, which now can be altered at a moment's notice. Indeed, it is important to note that dynamic visual aids have a dramatic and measurable effect on audience recall [15]. While the business world has fully adopted these advances, the medical community has been slower to make the transition to these presentation methods.

20.5 COMPUTER-BASED LONG-DISTANCE EDUCATION

Meyers summarized the increasing use of the Internet and the World Wide Web for distance education, both of patients and of facial plastic surgeons [16]. He notes a recent report indicating that 22.3 million adults, or nearly 40% of American adults online, used the Internet to seek health-related information [17]. In addition, online journals are proliferating. Several journals offer a website with supplemental materials to the journal. For example, the *Archives of Facial Plastic Surgery*, an American Medical Association journal and the official publication of the American Academy of Facial Plastic & Reconstructive Surgery and the International Federation of Facial Plastic Surgery Societies, has expanded its content at its web site (http://www.ama-assn.org/facial).

Available electronic textbooks offer immediate, up-to-date information enhanced with audio and video. The first comprehensive textbook of facial plastic and reconstructive surgery is online at http://www.emedicine.com.

Meyers described online chat rooms and discussion groups for facial plastic surgery [16]. FACEnet was established at the University of Colorado Health Sciences Center in 1995 for facial plastic surgeons and has over 250 participants. (For more info about FACEnet, please contact Facenet-request@lists.uchsc.edu). FACEnet members submit questions or cases to colleagues for online advice or consultation.

Several university departments of Otolaryngology–Head and Neck Surgery have posted an online syllabus and grand rounds, including topics in facial plastic and reconstructive surgery. Meyers recommended the website of Baylor College of Medicine as an excellent example (http://www.bcm.tmc.edu/oto) [16].

Online continuing medical education, while still in its infancy, is developing rapidly. Nevertheless, some sites already have extensive offerings, such as America's Health Network (http://www.ahn.com), the Virtual Lecture Hall (http://www.vlh.com), and others.

Meyers also highlighted several excellent basic science and clinical information websites. He points to the Visible Human Project, a computer-accessible database of over 13,000 images that comprise the National Library of Medicine

Visible Humans. By visiting the National Library of Medicine site (http://www.nlm.nih.gov/pubs/factsheets/visible human.html), surgeons can study human facial anatomy in a number of formats [16].

Surgical simulators offer enormous potential for teaching complex facial plastic surgery procedures. Meyers reported that the Center for Human Simulation at the University of Colorado has developed simulators for a few selected surgical procedures. These simulators allow surgeons to practice on virtual patients or body parts without the cost and risk of using live patients [16].

20.6 THE INTERNET IN FACIAL PLASTIC SURGERY

The Internet offers easy unrestricted access to an incredible volume of information. For this reason it has become a vital tool in the facial plastic surgical practice [18]. The American Academy of Facial Plastic Surgery (AAFPRS), the American Academy of Otolaryngology–Head and Neck Surgery (AAO-HNS), and the American Rhinologic Society (ARS), as well as other professional organizations, have recognized that the Internet can dramatically help communication among surgeons, members, patients, and the general public. For this reason, many websites, including the AAFPRS site (www.aafprs.org), the AAO-HNS site (www.entnet.org), and the ARS site (www.american-rhinologic.org), offer services to members and nonmembers alike (Figure 20.3). Mendelsohn and Hilger reported that the AAFPRS site received approximately 220,000 hits per month from more than 50,000 visitors in 1999 [19]. At the AAFPRS site, the most commonly visited nonmember areas are the "Procedures," "Facial Plastic Surgery Today," and "Find a Surgeon" sections.

Larrabee and Eggert [20] describe their experience with the World Wide Web. They concluded that the Internet is the medium of the future for physician-patient communication and that sooner or later every facial plastic surgeon will need a web presence to maintain a viable clinical practice. Approximately 40% of the U.S. adult population accesses the Internet, and this number continues to grow. The Internet is a valuable way to provide information to current and potential patients and to provide general information to the public. Importantly, Larrabee and Eggert emphasized that e-mail interactions with patients and potential patients should be limited until privacy and medicolegal issues are resolved.

Wall and Becker [21] reported on the growing presence of facial plastic surgery sites on the Internet. They noted that a search on the Microsoft Network's search engine on August 22, 1999, for "plastic surgery" and "facial plastic surgery" identified 39,469 and 5718 sites, respectively. The search parameter "facelift" yielded 12,031 sites, while the search term "rhinoplasty" produced 2923 sites. These numbers reflect an ever-expanding number of people turning to the Internet as a source for medical information. One report noted that 64.2 million

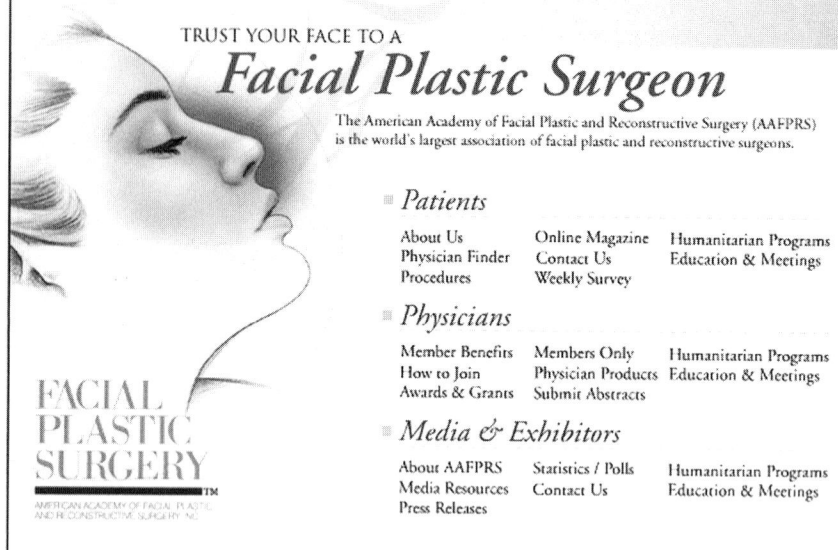

FIGURE 20.3 The American Academy of Facial Plastic and Reconstructive Surgery (AAFPRS) home-page. (www.aafprs.org.)

Americans routinely use the Internet for data retrieval [22]. Additional growth in this usage may be anticipated.

Chand conducted a survey of 50 facial plastic and reconstructive surgeons in the United States and Canada [13]. In this survey, 91% of the 44 respondents reported that they maintain an e-mail address, and 64% have a practice web site. Interestingly, 43% of the sites provided "information only," while the remaining sites permitted users to ask questions that may be answered in a delayed fashion.

Internet-based patient education applications have also been implemented. Murphy has discussed the option of in-office computer for interactive computer programs that serve to make the patient an informed member of the decision-making team [23]. This software can improve the doctor-patient interaction and reduce patient anxiety. This approach may be considered a supplement to or even a replacement for standard videotapes, which some physicians use for patient education. Computer-based instruction offers a significant advantage since the interactive patient education programs are generally thought to yield the highest rate of information retention of any information-delivery system. In order to facilitate their use, these programs may be transitioned to an Internet-based system, which offers the potential for near universal adoption.

Telemedicine, the provision of health care consultation and education using telecommunication networks that communicate information between remote providers and expert mentors offers tremendous opportunities but needs to overcome significant impediments. The widespread availability of the Internet has shifted most telemedicine efforts to this medium, rather than dedicated network facilities. While telemedicine technology may provide easy rapid access to both generalized and specialized medical care (including facial plastic surgical consultation), technical, financial, and legal restrictions must be addressed before telemedicine becomes more widespread in facial plastic surgery [24].

Telemedicine's initial emphasis had been the provision of general medical services in areas where medical services are limited; however, today, there may be an an even greater need for subspecialty services, since today's medical system often restricts access to medical and surgical specialists. Sclafani and Romo [24] identified a number of challenges in telemedicine, including the need to (1) define the settings in which telemedicine will benefit patients, (2) balance the benefits of an ''in-person'' consultation with the theoretical efficiency of a telemedicine encounter, (3) determine the most appropriate type of telemedicine transmission (telephone, high-speed line, or Internet), (4) define the clinical and technical requirements necessary to provide enough information of sufficient detail to make accurate diagnosis and treatment plan, (5) ensure confidentiality of the electronic medical record, and (6) develop a program that accommodates both legal and financial restrictions.

20.7 OUTCOMES RESEARCH

In his discussion of outcomes research in facial plastic surgery, Goldberg emphasized that a powerful database is central to any coordinated assessment in health care [25,26]. Computer technology makes possible the efficient and organized accumulation and processing of data to measure the patient experience; this information can then be applied to the analysis and improvement of patient care. This type of quality assurance is as important in facial plastic surgery as in any other medical discipline.

Health-related quality-of-life (HRQOL) questionnaires that focus on aspects of general health can be used in this sort of analysis. The short-form 36 (SF-36) has become popular because of its ease of administration and proven reliability across many diseases. However, to measure factors that relate more specifically to a particular disease process, survey instruments, known as disease-specific HRQOLs, have been proposed. However, development of these questionnaires is difficult, and the use of an existing and proven instrument such as SF-36 is often preferable.

Klassen et al. used the SF-36 and two other questionnaires preoperatively and postoperatively in patients undergoing aesthetic surgery [27]. Their study suggested that patients undergoing aesthetic surgery began at a lower level of social and psychological functioning and had improvements in health status postoperatively. The study also demonstrated that general health status instruments offered a reliable, valid, and independent method of evaluating aesthetic plastic surgical interventions.

20.8 SURGICAL APPLICATIONS

Citardi and Kokoska have reviewed developments in computer-aided surgery (CAS) techniques in craniomaxillofacial surgery [28]. While originally developed for stereotactic localization during neurosurgical procedures, CAS systems have an increasing role in craniomaxillofacial surgery due to their ability to provide insight into complex three-dimensional anatomic relationships. CAS provides an opportunity for three-dimensional image analysis that traditional plain radiographs and CT scans cannot produce.

The concept of CAS surgical navigation promotes a revolutionary approach to surgery. Preoperative data is currently uncoupled from the patient and the surgery and must be related by the surgeon to the actual anatomy. In the CAS surgical navigation paradigm, preoperative images, planning, simulation, and actual surgery are integrated. The software tools may be used not just in surgical planning but also intraoperatively. Further developments may create an unexpected impact on aesthetic and functional aspects of facial plastic and reconstructive surgery.

The heart of computer-aided surgery systems are the computer workstations that house the patient's imaging data and facilitate data manipulation. The computer system allows stereotactic surgical navigation, so that the position of the patient and surgical instruments may be tracked in three-dimensional space in the operating room. Precise tracking is essential for accurate intraoperative information. Current technology relies on electromagnetic tracking (Visualization Technologies, Woburn, MA) or on optical tracking (CBYON, Palo Alto, CA; Zeiss/Linvatec-Hall, Surgical Largo, FL; Medtronic Surgical Navigation Technology, Louisville, CO). All systems noted above have been adapted to use in otorhinolaryngology–head and neck surgery.

Computer-aided surgery provides a potential advance over intraoperative C-arm fluoroscopy, which some surgeons have advocated for facial fracture reduction. Kokoska presented their cadaver experience on the use of computer-aided surgery for the precise reduction of zygoma fractures. [29]. She reported an improved degree of accuracy of fracture reduction using CAS in this study.

Computer-Aided Facial Plastic Surgery

Cephalometric analysis can be a useful guide during selected surgical procedures. However, it has important limitations because it relies on the two-dimensional analysis of three-dimensional structures. The usefulness of cephalometrics is based on the quantification of specific anatomical relationships by measuring the distance between points or the geometric angles between lines. Computer-aided cephalometrics can now be performed on digitalized plain radiographs with specific software packages (Orthognathic Treatment Planner, Pacific Coast Software, Huntington Beach, CA) [28].

Computer-aided computed tomography (CT) based cephalometrics can provide both two-dimensional and three-dimensional volumetric information. This can provide more three-dimensional information than is now routinely applied during these cases. As computer-aided surgery develops, this provides an opportunity to improve the surgeon's ability to perform the best possible reconstruction [28]. Indeed, in the area of cosmetic surgery, one might speculate that computer software could allow individualized modeling of precise implants, such as chin or malar implants, that could be specifically tailored to the patient to achieve the specific goals.

Computer-generated three-dimensional models and computer simulation of surgery (e.g., anticipated location of osteotomies) may facilitate more effective, less morbid surgery. Computer software for this kind of work has not yet been optimized but should be technically possible [28].

Computer-aided surgical navigation has been extensively developed for neurosurgical procedures, sinus surgery, and spine surgery. CAS navigation systems can follow the position of specific surgical instrumentation in the surgical field. Application of this technology to craniomaxillofacial surgery can be challenging because this sort of surgery was not considered in the development and design of most CAS systems. Intraoperative CAS remains a promising area of development.

Another area of ongoing development is "real-time" CT- and MRI-guided surgical navigation. This approach is obviously expensive and logistically challenging, although technological advances may facilitate its application and reduce the cost.

The application of CAS surgical navigation technology to facial plastic surgery is still in its infancy. Nonetheless, Rosen suggests in his discussion on the application of advanced surgical technologies for plastic and reconstructive surgery that advances in computer animation techniques, virtual reality, and graphic interfaces may soon allow complex preoperative electronic modeling [30]. For example, in planning a reconstruction of a nasal defect with a midline forehead flap, a specialized helmet and electronic gloves may allow the surgeon to plan and simulate the ideal shape for the flap. The surgeon may actually be able to see and feel the reconstructed nose.

The limbs provide a simpler model for computer simulation, and so much of the current work in computer simulation has focused on this area. In one report, a computer-generated model of a hip joint with muscle and tendon actuators was used to predict the outcome of hip arthroplasties (total hip joint replacements) [31].

Achieving a useful computer model will require taking human animation beyond simulating surface skin geometry but will require accurate computer depiction of the complex human system. Larrabee and Galt compared a two-dimensional computer simulation of human skin to pigskin to analyze flap advancements [32]. Others have reported on the use of computer modeling to analyze Z-plasty, orthognathic surgery, and other plastic surgical procedures [31–34]. Even these relatively simple constructs require fairly complex computer programs. Because the complexity of facial anatomy magnifies the challenges of surgical simulation, this work should be considered the early stages in this area.

Just as flight simulators are a proven means of training pilots, surgical simulators provide the opportunity for training experiences with decreased cost and increased safety. In addition, simulators may provide invaluable "planning" opportunities for complex cases. Moreover, as with flight simulators, simulation of infrequent but highly hazardous scenarios provides experience that would otherwise be unavailable. Furthermore, one can expect that as the systems become increasingly sophisticated, they may provide useful information intraoperatively.

20.9 OFFICE AND OPERATING ROOM OF THE FUTURE

Miller and Mendelsohn have speculated about the potential office of the future [35]. Extrapolating today's technology, they "let their imaginations wander . . . into the realm of scientific speculation and science fiction" to envision incredible changes in the way computer technology affects both their personal and professional lives over the next 50 years. The authors see a critical turning point to be the secure storage and transfer of information that is accessible to anyone who is granted the authority. Wireless technology will allow unprecedented networking and communication between patients and physicians.

The authors describe "Mrs. Jones" and her decision to have a facelift in the year 2050. Her voice-activated personal digital assistant (PDA) scans the Internet; the "text-to-speech" option allows her to listen to the information while she is driving. She decides to proceed and asks her PDA to find a local facial plastic surgeon who has been in practice 10 years, performs primarily facelifts, has a "success" rate of greater than 95% and a limited complication rate. (The authors speculate that the governmental authorities will require this sort of information as part of a quality assurance and performance improvement plan.) She peruses a few websites and decides to schedule an appointment with your office. The details are all taken care of electronically, and she receives personalized directions to your office via e-mail. Her chart has been completed electronically from her health database, and any additional necessary questions are also included in her e-mail. On the day of her consultation, you are running 20 minutes late and your office computer automatically informs your remaining patients via e-mail.

During your visit, you answer additional questions and also review the before and after holographic simulations. She decides to proceed. Her preoperative instructions are e-mailed to her, her postoperative medications are electronically sent to her pharmacy, and all financial transactions are completed electronically. Except for the day of surgery and the first postoperative visit, her remaining postoperative visits are handled via Web-based teleconference.

Will the future patient-physician interactions follow that vision? Today, nobody can answer that question; however, it is clear that computer-based technologies are forging dramatic changes in health care delivery. Additional changes can be expected.

REFERENCES

1. Zupko KA, Toth CL. Selecting a computer system that meets your practice needs. Facial Plast Surg Clin North Am 8(1):13–24, 2000.
2. Hodnett R. Tips for software selection. Facial Plast Surg Clin North Am 8(1):25–28, 2000.
3. Quatela VC, Sabini PA, Williams DL. Review of plastic surgical office software. Facial Plast Surg Clin North Am 8(1):5–11, 2000.
4. www.health.state.ny/nysdoh.
5. Becker DG, Tardy ME. Standardized photography in facial plastic surgery: pearls & pitfalls. Facial Plast Surg 15(2):93–100, 1999.
6. Kokoska MS, Thomas JR. 35 mm and digital photography for the facial plastic surgeon. Facial Plast Surg Clin North Am 8(1):35–44, 2000.
7. Wall SJ, Kazahaya K, Becker SS, Becker DG. 35 mm versus digital photography: comparison of photographic quality and clinical evaluation. Facial Plast Surg 15(2):101–110, 1999.
8. Miller PJ, Light J. A comparison of digital cameras. Facial Plast Surg 15(2):111–118, 1999.
9. Papel ID, Jiannetto DF. Advances in computer imaging/applications in facial plastic surgery. Facial Plast Surg 15(2):119–126, 1999.
10. Koch RJ, Chavez A. Medicolegal aspects of imaging and internet communications. Facial Plast Surg 15(2):139–144, 1999.
11. Koch RJ, Chavez A, Dagum P, Newman JP. Advantages and disadvantages of computer imaging in cosmetic surgery. Dermatol Surg 24:195–198, 1998.
12. Pieper SD, Laub Jr DR, Rosen JM. A finite-element facial model for simulating plastic surgery. Plast Reconstr Surg 96(5):1100–1105, 1995.
13. Chand MS. Survey: computer technology in facial plastic surgery practices. Facial Plast Surg Clin North Am 8(1):1–4, 2000.

14. Watson D, Sorenson S. Computers in slide production & presentations. Facial Plast Surg Clin North Am 8(1):1–9, 2000.
15. Lindstrom RL. Business Week Guide to Multimedia Presentations. Berkeley, Osborne McGraw-Hill, 1994.
16. Meyers AD. Recent advances in facial plastic and reconstructive surgery distance education. Facial Plast Surg Clin North Am 8(1):61–64, 2000.
17. Wall Street Journal. www.doctorsmedicinediseasesgalore.com, B1 June 10, 1999.
18. Kriet JD, Wang TD. The Internet and the World Wide Web. Facial Plastic Surgery 15(2):145–148, 1999.
19. Mendelsohn JE, Hilger P. The AAFPRS website. Plastic Surgery 15(2):1999, 149–152.
20. Larrabee WF, Eggert E. One physician's experience on the Web. Facial Plast Surg Clin North Am 8(1):81–84, 2000.
21. Wall SJ, Becker DG. Physician websites in facial plastic surgery. Facial Plast Surg Clin North Am 8(1):85–90, 2000.
22. Turner S, Ellwanger S. Spring 1999 Cyberstats. MediaMark Research, www.mediamark.com.
23. Murphy KR. Computer-based patient education. Facial Plast Surg Clin North Am 8(1):73–80, 2000.
24. Sclafani AP, Romo T. A brave new world: telemedicine and the facial plastic surgeon. Facial Plast Surg 15(2):153–160, 1999.
25. Goldberg AN. Outcomes research in facial plastic surgery. Facial Plast Surg Clin North Am 8(1):91–96, 2000.
26. Ellwood PM. Shattuck Lecture—outcomes management: a technology of patient experience. N Engl J Med 318:1549, 1988.
27. Klassen A, Jenkinson C, Fitzpatrick R, Goodacre T. Measuring quality of life in cosmetic surgery patients with a condition-specific instrument: the Derriford scale. Br J Plast Surg 51:380, 1988.
28. Citardi MJ, Kokoska MS. Computer-aided craniomaxillofacial surgery. Facial Plast Surg Clin North Am 8(1):97–106, 2000.
29. Kokoska MS. The role of computer-aided surgery in reduction of zygoma fractures. Presentation, American Academy of Facial Plastic and Reconstructive Surgery Spring Meeting, May 13, 2000.
30. Rosen JM. Advanced surgical technologies for plastic & reconstructive surgery. Facial Plast Surg Clin North Am 8(1):107–116, 2000.
31. Delp SL, Loan JP, Basdogen C, et al. Surgical simulations: an emerging technology for military medical training. Military Telemedicine On-Line Today, IEEE Press, 1995, pp. 29–34.
32. Larrabee WF, Galt JA. A finite element model of skin deformation. III: The finite element model. Laryngoscope 96:413, 1986.
33. Kawabata H, Kawai H, Masada K, et al. Computer-aided analysis of Z-plasties. Plast Reconstr Surg 83:319, 1989.
34. Laub DR Jr. Use of a finite element facial model for computer simulation of cleft lip repair. Presented at the New England Plastic Surgical Society, Boston, May 1995.
35. Miller PJ, Mendelsohn J. Office of the future. Facial Plast Surg Clin North Am 8(1):29–34, 2000.

21
Software-Enabled Cephalometrics

Martin J. Citardi, M.D.
Cleveland Clinic Foundation, Cleveland, Ohio

Mimi S. Kokoska, M.D.
Indiana University School of Medicine, Indianapolis, Indiana

21.1 INTRODUCTION

Before the advent of computer-assisted surgery (CAS) technology, orthognathic surgeons developed techniques for the quantitative analysis of standardized plain films of the craniomaxillofacial skeleton. Over the years these efforts developed into the discipline of cephalometrics. Although the relevance of cephalometrics may seem diminished by contemporary diagnostic imaging modalities, cephalometrics still provides useful information for surgery of mandible and midface. Furthermore, the rationale for cephalometrics also may guide the development of CAS applications for craniomaxillofacial surgery.

21.2 TRADITIONAL CEPHALOMETRICS

Cephalometrics provides a systematic method for the measurement of specific maxillary, mandibular, occlusal, and soft-tissue relationships [1–3]. This information may serve to guide accurate diagnosis of the anatomical relationships that underlie midface and mandibular anomalies. Cephalometrics also facilitates preoperative planning. After surgery, cephalometrics may be utilized for the objective assessment of surgical outcomes.

The consideration of the specific techniques of cephalometric analysis is beyond the scope of this discussion; however, it is appropriate to review briefly the mechanics of cephalometric analysis. Cephalometrics may be split into a phase of image acquisition and a phase of image review.

During image acquisition, a plain film x-ray is obtained. The plain film radiographs for cephalometrics have been standardized, since all plain film radiography produces some image distortion and magnification. Fixation of the subject-to-film distance and the x-ray source-to-subject distance minimizes both distortion and magnification, but it cannot eliminate this problem. Set distances for these variables does yield a constant error and hence a large degree of reproducibility. This has been deemed an acceptable compromise. In addition, a cephalostat must be used for patient placement for cephalometric x-rays. The cephalostat is simply a standarized head holder that fixes the patient's head at three or more points; this device obviously enhances reproducibility.

During image review, the surgeon actually traces specific landmarks on the film. These landmarks define specific anatomical points. Then the surgeon draws lines between the points; clinical experience has demonstrated that these lines portray useful anatomical information. Next, angular and linear measurements based upon these lines are performed. These measurements may then be compared to normative data. Through this process, patterns of anatomical relationships become apparent; recognition of these patterns directly influences preoperative surgical planning. These patterns also guide the postoperative assessment of maxillofacial surgery.

Although cephalometrics has been widely utilized for many decades, it does have several important limitations. In fact, these potential issues have been recognized for many years in the orthognathic and plastic surgery literature. As already noted, plain x-ray radiography produces some image enlargement; standardized techniques reduce the practical impact of this problem [4]. In addition, the projection of three-dimensional structures onto a two-dimensional planar surface introduces additional image distortion [5]. Finally, a variety of human errors can influence cephalometric measurements. Identification of landmarks on the lateral x-ray can be problematic [6,7]; inaccurate identification inevitably compromises the accuracy of any measurements [8].

21.3 SOFTWARE APPLICATIONS FOR TRADITIONAL CEPHALOMETRICS

As one may anticipate, digital imaging has been applied to cephalometrics. For these software programs, the standard plain x-ray must be digitized so that it can be reviewed on the computer workstation. For instance, the Orthognathic Treatment Planner (OTP, Pacific Coast Software, Huntington Beach, CA) facilitates computer-based cephalometrics. Some of these programs also offer options for surgical planning, including predictions for final surgical results.

Several reports have focused on the accuracy and clinical utility of this type of software. When reviewing the literature, it is important to realize that the critical threshold is clinical significance. Experience has shown that the relative accuracy/inaccuracy of plain films, hand tracing, etc. are acceptable for current surgical applications. In this regard, traditional cephalometrics has an error margin that has been considered acceptable according to practical experience. If cephalometrics software packages produce results within this error margin, then it is considered acceptable.

Plain x-ray digitization can introduce extraneous image magnification and distortion; however, digitization procedures, using a specific protocols designed to reduce such errors, have been demonstrated to be accurate and reproducible for the vast majority of cephalometric parameters [9]. The predictive accuracy of the software has also been examined. The Quick Ceph Image (Orthodontic Processing, Coronado, CA) can calculate values of cephalometric parameters before or after orthognathic surgery. The predictive data produced by Quick Ceph and actual measurements after orthognathic surgery have been shown to be statistically equivalent for most parameters; for parameters in which statistically significant differences between predicted and actual values were noted, the magnitude of the differences was less than that commonly ascribed to traditional cephalometric tracings [9]. From a practical standpoint, Quick Ceph was equivalent to standard cephalometrics for these parameters. Most reports have emphasized that Quick Ceph, as well as Dentofacial Planner (Dentofacial Software, Toronto, Canada), provide good predictive data for a population of patients across a variety of parameters; however, some landmarks seem to possess a wide range of variation, and the software does a poor job of modeling soft-tissue changes after surgery [10].

Several factors contribute to the limitations of software applications for traditional cephalometrics. Interestingly, some of these issues reflect general issues with cephalometrics. Magnification and distortion of the original x-ray, during its initial acquisition as well as during digitization, may produce errors. Human errors in identifying landmarks may also influence cephalometric calculations. Software protocols usually have rounding functions. Although such rounding may seem insignificant for a given value, the rounding of multiple parameters may compromise accuracy. The software programs rely upon specific methods for modeling; if the premises for such methods are incorrect, the resultant models will be incorrect. Users of the software assume that the modeling approaches are reliable; however, this may not be true.

21.4 LESSONS FROM TRADITIONAL CEPHALOMETRICS

Because of advanced imaging technologies (such as CT with model reconstruction), it may seem reasonable to downplay the significance of traditional cephalometrics; however, such a maneuver really dismisses the significance of cephalometrics. Despite its limitations, numerous surgeons have recognized the value of cephalometrics: cephalometrics provides a relatively objective means for quantitative analysis of the craniomaxillofacial skeleton. This information may guide the diagnosis of congenital and acquired anomalies and assist surgical planning for the correction of these anomalies. Lastly cephalometrics can be used for the documentation of postoperative results. Even if traditional cephalometrics is eventually supplanted by other technologies, its objectives should influence its successor technologies.

The formal approaches for cephalometrics compensate for its intrinsic limitations. In many ways these standardized protocols resemble corresponding protocols for computed tomography (CT) scans for CAS systems. Furthermore, the cephalostat provides orientation for the craniomaxillofacial skeleton during plain x-ray acquisition. Although the cephalostat is not a frame used for CAS surgical navigation, the concepts for both are similar, since both the CAS frame and the cephalostat provide orientation.

21.5 TOWARD A NEW UNDERSTANDING OF CEPHALOMETRICS

Traditional cephalometrics seeks to develop quantitative information about complex maxillomandibular anatomical relationships. The approach relies upon standardized plain films that are then analyzed in specific fashion. In this way, cephalometrics provides information about the occlusal relationships and the adjacent maxillomandibular facial skeleton. Surgeons can rely upon this knowledge for preoperative diagnosis and planning as well as postoperative monitoring of surgical outcomes.

As described above, traditional cephalometrics has intrinsic challenges that relate to image distortion and magnification during image acquisition as well as human errors. Importantly, cephalometrics relies upon two-dimensional representations of three-dimensional structures. The super-positioning of multiple structures on a single two-dimensional image may obscure image information. At the very least the image is difficult to comprehend, and at worst the image is incomplete.

Because CAS shares many of its objectives and basic premises with traditional cephalometrics, the application of CAS to cephalometrics is logical;

Software-Enabled Cephalometrics

in fact, CAS-derived cephalometrics may offer critical advantages by merging CAS technologies and cephalometrics principles. Although the linkage of CAS and cephalometrics has not been formally recognized, CAS applications in craniomaxillofacial surgery have been reported numerous times over the previous 15 years. In these efforts, computer modeling has been used to create three-dimensional models of various craniomaxillofacial deformities and then these models were used for surgical planning. These approaches all rely upon high-resolution CT scans that provide excellent three-dimensional anatomical data, but the entire process has been qualitative, rather than quantitative.

CAS-based cephalometrics should seek to apply traditional cephalometrics' emphasis upon a systematic, quantitative analysis of image data. Although it is not yet a recognized discipline, the goal of CAS-based cephalometrics is a computer-based system for the quantitative assessment of CT image data.

What are the advantages of this approach? Stated simply, CT scans offer more precise anatomical data than corresponding plain films. For this reason, CT has emerged as the preferred imaging modality for preoperative planning for craniomaxillofacial surgery. In a sense, traditional cephalometrics needs an "update" to recognize this fact. It also should be noted that while CT scans provide an excellent understanding of anatomical relationships, the surgeon still must make a mental extrapolation from surgical plan to implementation. Computer-based modeling may simplify surgical planning, and CAS surgical navigation for craniomaxillofacial surgery, which is still developmental, may provide direct intraoperative guidance. It is reasonable to make this entire process quantitative by applying principles learned from traditional cephalometrics.

CAS surgical navigation workstations already contain a variety of software tools that may be applied to CAS cephalometrics. Obviously, the specific details for these tools differ among the various CAS systems; however, most systems have some or all of these features. Even systems in which these tools are not readily apparent may have the capability of offering these tools, but the software interfaces used in the clinical applications are not offered in these particular systems.

CAS software tools facilitate a variety of functions:

Image review: CT data in the three orthogonal planes (namely axial, coronal, and sagittal planes) through a given point may be reviewed (Figure 21.1). Users can use the scroll buttons to sequentially review contiguous images.

Coordinate systems: Points within the imaging volume are assigned x,y,z coordinates (Figure 21.1). Such coordinates may be used to identify precisely and reproducibly a point within the image data set volume.

3D modeling: Three-dimensional models can be constructed from the raw

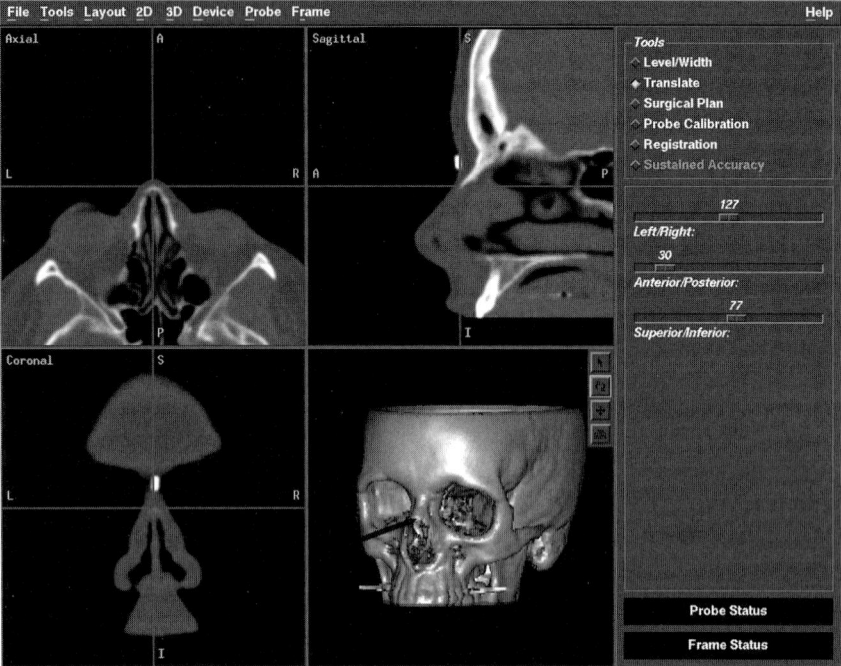

FIGURE 21.1 The surgical planning mode of the StealthStation 2.6.4 (Medtronic Surgical Navigation Technologies, Louisville, CO) includes the x,y,z coordinate system. The x-coordinate corresponds to "Left/Right," the y-coordinate corresponds to "Superior/Inferior," and the z-coordinate corresponds to "Anterior-Posterior." In this way, each point in the imaging volume has a unique x,y,z value. For cephalometrics, this facilitates the reproducible identification of specific points during the quantitative assessment of images. Other CAS software packages offer similar features. (From Ref. 15.)

thin-cut CT data (Figure 21.2). Users can manipulate the resultant models for review. Such manipulations may include simple rotations or even complex fly-by maneuvers.

Distance measuring: The distance between two points in the preoperative imaging data set volume can be calculated with this tool (Figure 21.3).

Special views: Another optional tool permits the reconstruction of special cut views that present planar data through a specific line in the imaging data set volume (Figure 21.4).

Together these tools provide a means for the quantitative assessment of CT images on a computer workstation. In this way, cephalometric principles may be applied to answer questions about three-dimensional anatomical relationships.

Software-Enabled Cephalometrics

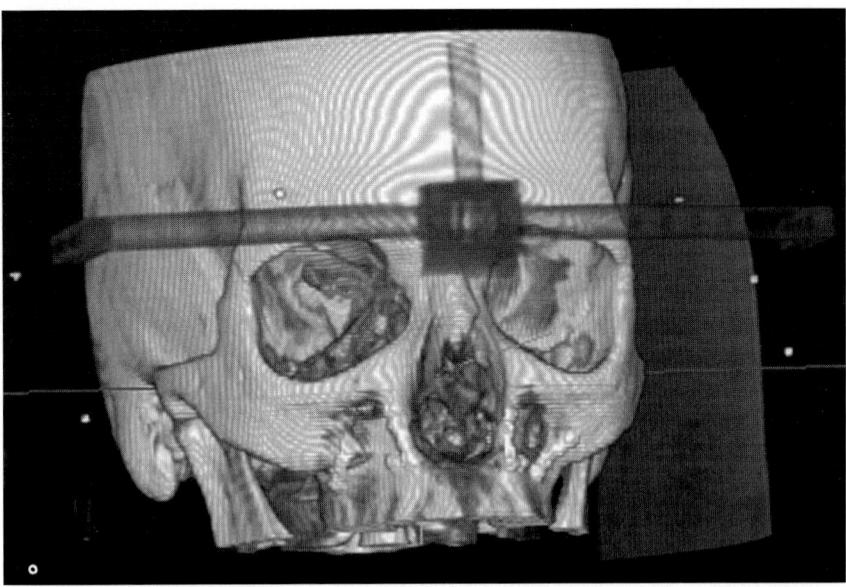

FIGURE 21.2 Technological improvements over the past 10–15 years have dramatically simplified the creation of 3D models from planar CT data. This process demands relatively sophisticated computer software and hardware; however, increasingly powerful microprocessors and memory at relatively low cost are now available so that 3D models can be made quickly and easily. This model, created in a semi-automated fashion on the SAVANT 2.0 (CBYON, Palo Alto, CA) from 1 mm axial CT scan images, is typical. (During the scan, the patient wore a headset that housed a fiducial system for automatic registration for surgical navigation. This headset is seen in the reconstructed skeletal image.) Other CAS systems function similarly.

In addition, prototype CAS software provides advanced surgical planning tools. These applications permit computer-based modeling of surgical procedures. Through these virtual models, surgeons may plan complex manipulations (such as osteotomies for the correction of craniofacial anomalies). The software provides predictive information about the impact of these manipulations of the craniofacial skeleton.

21.6 EARLY APPLICATIONS OF CAS CEPHALOMETRICS

The quantitative assessment of anatomical relationships based on computer-enabled review of CT imaging data (i.e., CAS cephalometrics) has not been stan-

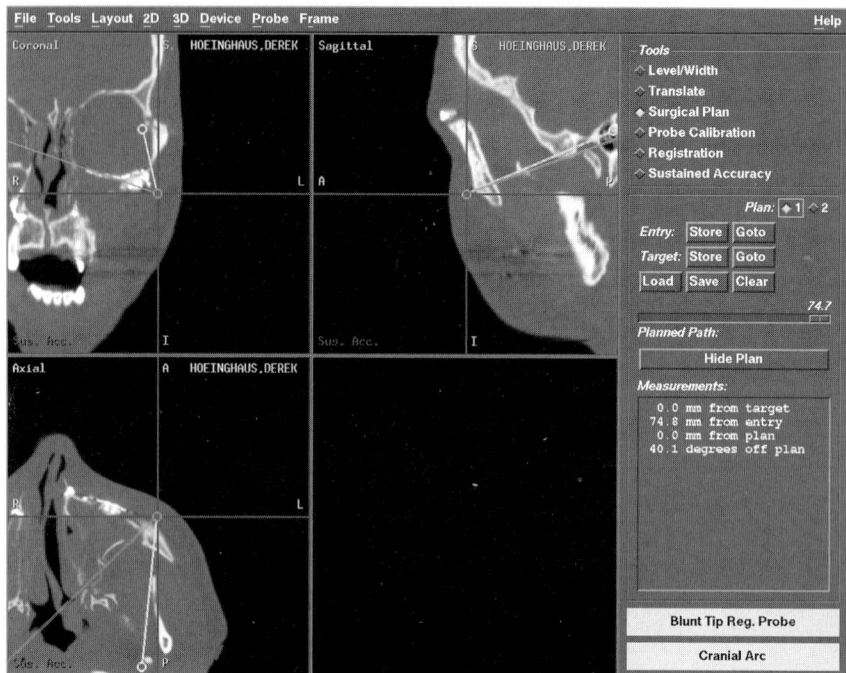

FIGURE 21.3 The LandMarX 2. 6.4 (Medtronic Xomed, Jacksonville, FL) has a distance measuring tool. In this example, distances from the right and left internal auditory canal transverse crests to a fixed point on the malar surface were calculated; in this way, the prereduction and postreduction position of the malar fragment could be monitored during its operative reduction. It should be noted that the trajectories depicted in the axial, coronal, and sagittal images represent only the vector component for that plane, not the true trajectory. As a result, the trajectory may seem inappropriately displaced on each of the planar images. This distance-measuring tool can be used to determine the distance between any two points in the imaging volume. Other CAS software packages include similar software tools.

dardized. Furthermore, the software used for this application has not been optimized for this purpose. As a result, all observations of this area are truly preliminary; it may be anticipated that significant changes will occur.

At first glance, it may seem obvious that software-derived measurements of distance between points on a CT scan correlate well to actual direct measurements in the real world; however, this may not necessarily be true. First, identification of the landmarks on the CT scan images may be imprecise, since difficult user interfaces may confuse even expert users, computer display systems may

Software-Enabled Cephalometrics

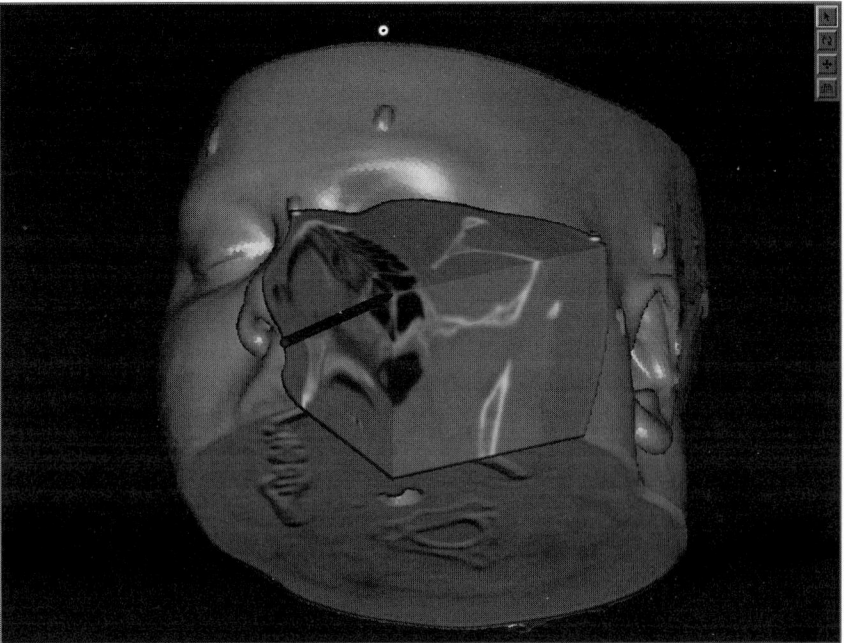

FIGURE 21.4 CAS software offers special views that may be manipulated at the computer workstation. This cut-view from the StealthStation 3 (Medtronic Surgical Navigation Technologies, Louisville, CO) is typical. Other systems offer similar capabilities.

poorly project images (due to a lack of sufficient resolution), and finally users may be unfamiliar with the identification of anatomical landmarks via a computer workstation. Furthermore, CT modeling protocols that the software utilizes may introduce errors. These problems reflect the limitations of traditional cephalometrics and the limitations of software for traditional cephalometrics. Fortunately, CAS-based measurements of distance between points on a CT scan correlate well with actual physical measurements. Using a cadaveric skull model, we examined this issue by comparing linear measurements obtained with scientific grade microcalipers with the corresponding linear measurements obtained with the distance-measuring tools of the Stealth Cranial CAS software (Medtronic Surgical Navigation Technology, Louisville, CO); differences between corresponding measurements were not statistically significant.[11]

The choice of parameters for CAS cephalometrics is also problematic. The direct use of parameters from traditional cephalometrics may be considered; however, practical considerations eliminate this option, since one cannot directly extrapolate from hand tracing on a lateral x-ray to CT-based, three-dimensional modeling on a computer workstation. For this reason, a new set of parameters for CAS cephalometrics is necessary.

It is important to consider the potential clinical ramifications of such parameters. Craniomaxillofacial surgeons are concerned with facial skeleton projection and symmetry (or asymmetry) as well as the resultant soft-tissue contours. The ideal system would provide information about projection. Comparison of relative projection between sides would form a measure of symmetry/asymmetry. To the extent that soft-tissue contours are a function of the underlying bony skeleton, a series of projection measurements from a fixed reference to multiple points along the bony contour would also provide information about the soft-tissue cover's projection. To the extent that soft-tissue contours reflect the intrinsic properties of the soft tissue, other modeling approaches that include virtual modeling of these mechanical proprieties would be necessary for a complete model of soft-tissue contours.

Linear projection measurements require two points that define the trajectory of the measurement, which runs from a fixed reference point to a target point. Each point must be easily recognized and reliably identified. Symmetry/asymmetry concerns can be addressed in two ways. In the first alternative, a midline reference point can serve as a frame of reference; measurements to targets on each side from the midline reference point provide quantitative information about projection and symmetry/asymmetry. The second alternative involves the selection of a reference point on each side; measurements to the ipsilateral and contralateral target points provide projection and symmetry/asymmetry data.

We have developed two systems for CAS cephalometrics. The first system focuses upon skull base length and width. In this paradigm, distances between the right and left palatine foramina and the distance between the right and left foramina spinosa serve as measures of skull base width, while the distance from the posterior foramen magnum point (the reference point) and the midpoint of a line between the right and left palatine foramina (the target point) serves as a measure of skull base anteroposterior projection (Figure 21.5) [11]. Admittedly, the clinical impact of this approach is probably limited to specific skull base procedures. The real issue here is the proof of concept; that is, computer-enabled review of CT data provides a means of assessing skull base projection.

Our second system is more directly tailored toward issues of malar contour and projection; as a result, this approach can probably be adapted for other craniomaxillofacial parameters. According to his paradigm, the reference points, which are called skull base reference points (SBR), are the left and right internal auditory canal transverse crests (Figure 21.6). Importantly, the SBRs are not part of the facial or maxillomandibular skeletons; therefore, they are unlikely to be altered by congenital and/or traumatic anomalies that affect the maxillofacial skeleton. Nonetheless, the SBRs provide a suitable reference frame for further measurements. The target points for malar projection (known as the malar points, or MPs)

Software-Enabled Cephalometrics

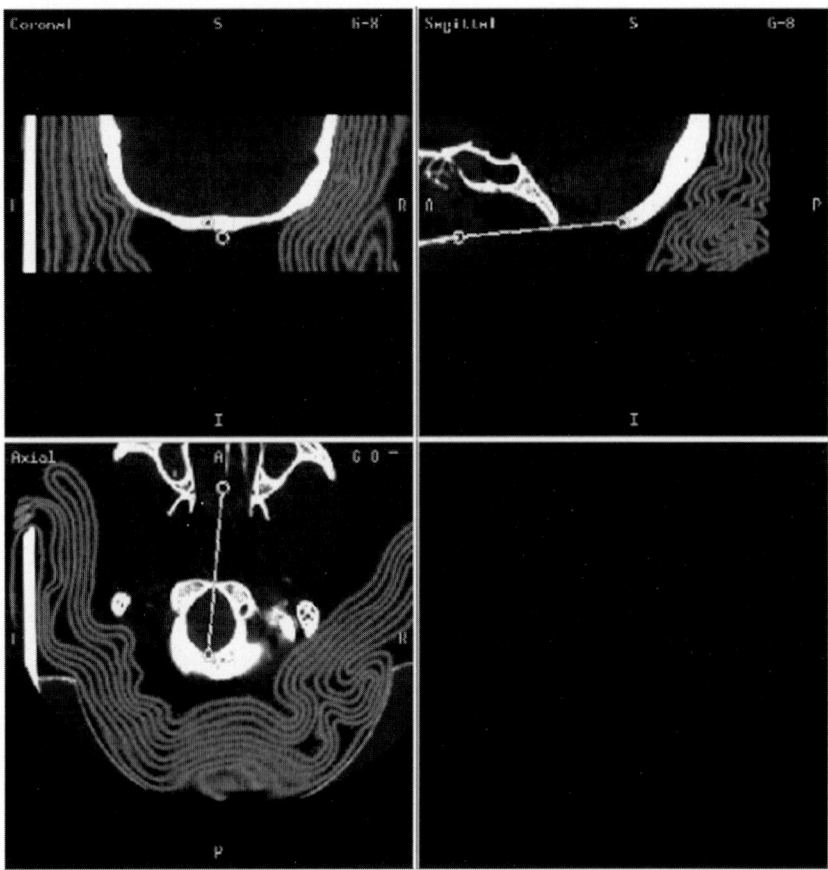

FIGURE 21.5 The straight line in these planar CT images, which are oriented in the orthogonal planes through a point along the posterior foramen magnum, shows the skull base length dimension in our paradigm [11]. The StealthStation 2.6.4 (Medtronic Surgical Navigation Technologies, Louisville, CO) distance-measuring tool was used for this project. The reference point was defined as the midline posterior foramen magnum, and the target point was defined as the midpoint along a vector between the right and left palatine foramen. The target point was established by calculating half the distance between the right and left palatine foramen using the same distance measuring tool. It should be noted that the trajectories depicted in the axial, coronal, and sagittal images represent only the vector component for that plane, not the true trajectory. As a result, the trajectory may seem inappropriately displaced on each on the planar images.

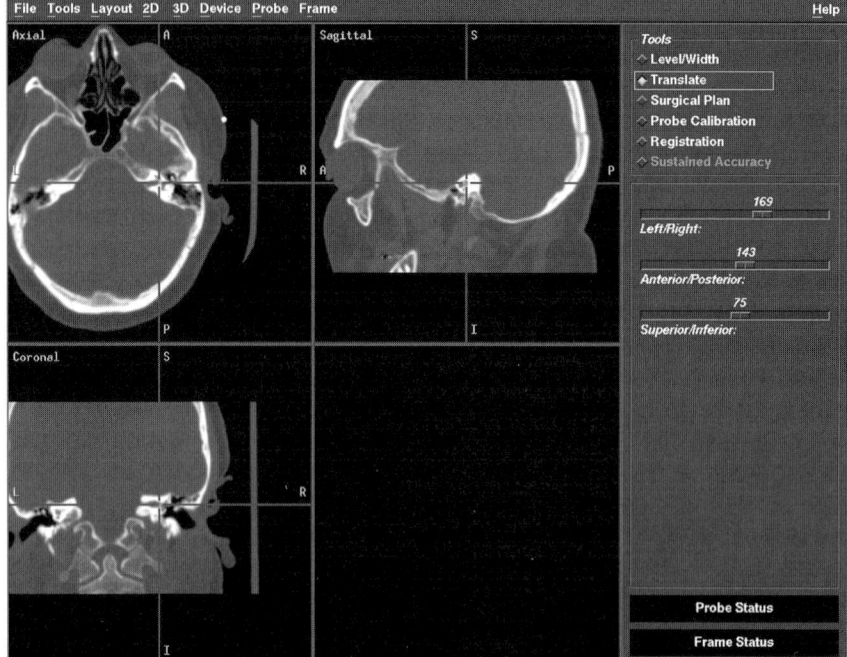

FIGURE 21.6 The right skull base reference (SBR), shown here on images obtained on the StealthStation 2.6.4 (Medtronic Surgical Navigation Technologies, Louisville, CO), was defined as the transverse crest of the internal auditory canal. The SBR serves as a reference point for the assessment of malar projection.

are the points of greatest curvature on the malar bony contour. In sum, the four points (namely the left and right SBRs and the left and right MPs) define a variety of measurements between each SBR and the ipsilateral and contralateral MP. The potential linear measurements are as follows: the right SBR to the ipsilateral MP (R SBR-iMP), the right SBR to the contralateral MP (R SBR-cMP), the left SBR to the ipsilateral MP (L SBR-iMP), and the left SBR to the contralateral MP (L SBR-cMP). Together these measurements summarize malar projection. Furthermore, R SBR-iMP and L SBR-cMP represent right malar projection, and L SBR-iMP and R SBR-cMP represent left malar projection. Symmetry/asymmetry determinations are reflected in the relative measurements for each side (Figure 21.7).

Our work on the SBR-MP system for CAS cephalometrics has focused on several related projects. In our first project, normative data were developed by performing the SBR-MP measurements on a series of CT scans obtained for

Software-Enabled Cephalometrics

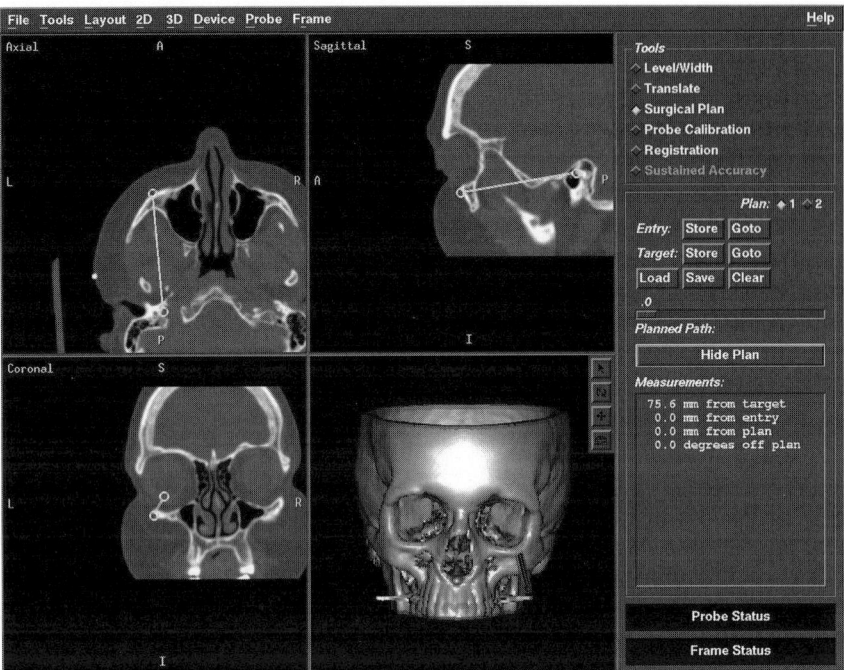

FIGURE 21.7 The StealthStation 2.6.4 (Medtronic Surgical Navigation Technologies, Louisville, CO) distance-measuring tool was used to measure the distance from the left skull base reference point (L SBR) to the ipsilateral malar point (iMP). This distance, known as L SBR-iMP, summarizes information about the position and contour of the left malar bone. It should be noted that the trajectories depicted in the axial, coronal, and sagittal images represent only the vector component for that plane, not the true trajectory. As a result, the trajectory may seem inappropriately displaced on each of the planar images.

surgical navigation during computer-aided transsphenoidal hypophysectomy [12]. In a clinical case report, the SBR-MP measurements were used intraoperatively for computer-aided malar fracture reduction [13]. This initial clinical experience led to a project, in which zygomatic fractures were created in cadaveric skulls and then repaired under CAS guidance [14]. (For a further discussion of computer-aided maxillofacial fracture repair, please see Chapter 24.)

We have also proposed a paradigm for the assessment of the bony nasal pyramid [15]. In this report, the CAS distance-measuring software tools were used to determine the thickness of the nasal bones at the level of the rhinion on thin cut axial CT data. We also proposed a technique for the measurement of bony nasal pyramid projection, which can be operationally defined by the rhinion nasal projection and the nasion nasal projection. The rhinion nasal projection is the distance from the nasomaxillary suture to the rhinion in the axial plane through the rhinion (Figure 21.8). A line that is perpendicular to the axial plane and passes through the nasomaxillary suture in the axial plane of the rhinion provides the reference frame for the nasion nasal projection. The nasion nasal projection is more complex; this parameter is the distance from the nasion to that perpendicular imaginary line in the axial plane through the nasion (Figure 21.9). The right and left measurements for the nasion and the right and left measurements for the rhinion summarize nasal projection.

Surprisingly, the nasion nasal projection values were consistently greater than the rhinion nasal projection values. At first glance, the nasion nasal projection and rhinion nasal projection both describe purely anteroposterior vectors; however, in reality, the nasion nasal projection parameters reflects an anteroposte-

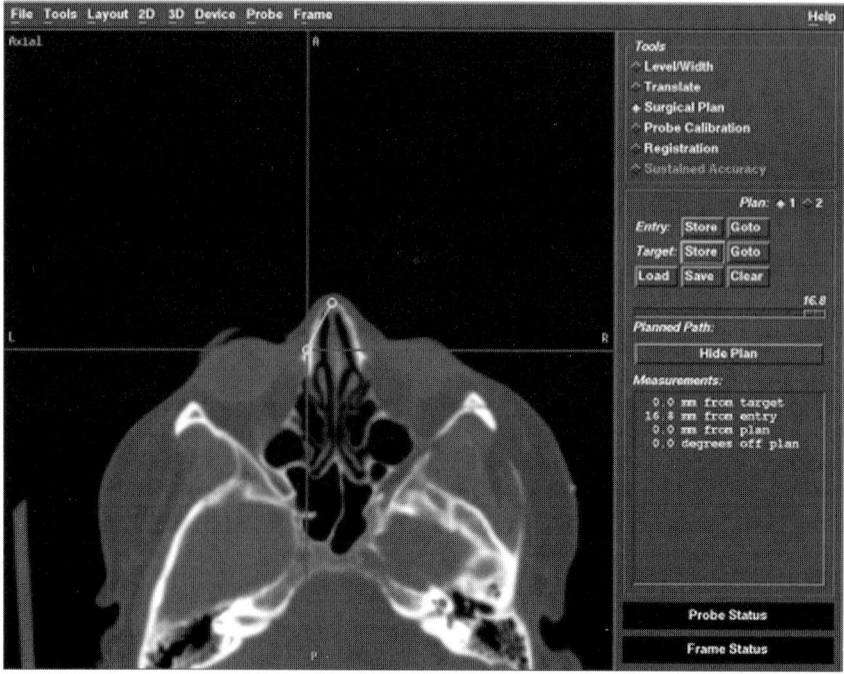

FIGURE 21.8 This axial image shows the rhinion nasal projection. The StealthStation 2.6.4 (Medtronic Surgical Navigation Technologies, Louisville, CO) distance-measuring tool was used to determine this parameter. The rhinion nasal projection is defined as the distance from the nasomaxillary suture to the rhinion in the axial plane through the rhinion. (From Ref. 15.)

Software-Enabled Cephalometrics

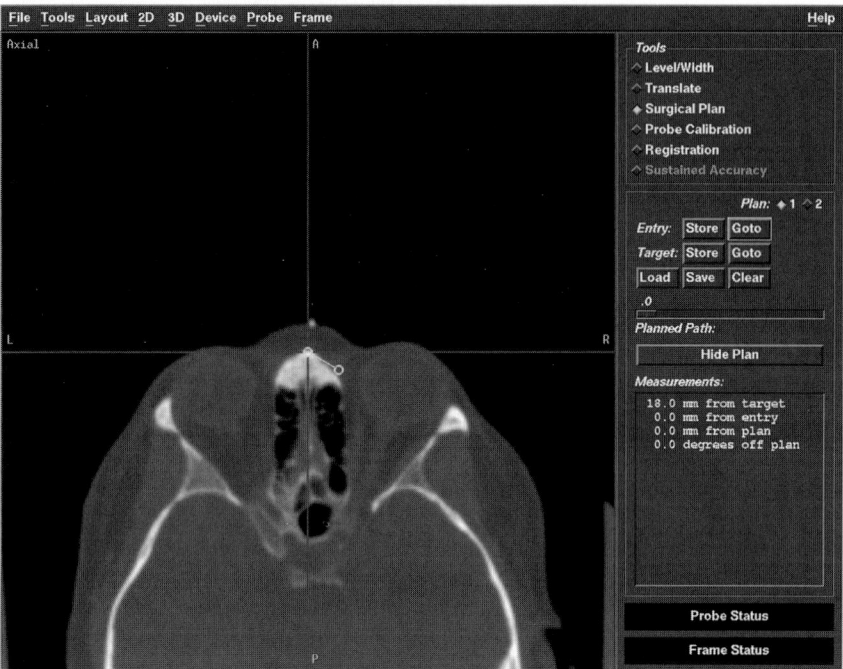

FIGURE 21.9 This axial image shows the nasion nasal projection. The StealthStation 2.6.4 (Medtronic Surgical Navigation Technology, Louisville, CO) distance-measuring tool was used to determine this parameter. The nasion nasal projection was defined as the distance from the nasion to a perpendicular reference line through the point defined by the nasomaxillary suture in the axial plane. This reference line runs perpendicular to the axial plane. (From Ref. 15.)

rior vector and nasal bone length, which is an oblique vector. As a result, rhinion projection values are smaller than corresponding nasion projection values.

The rhinion nasal projection and nasion nasal projection also represent asymmetries of the nasal bones. The right and left measurements for each of these parameters would be equal in perfectly symmetrical bony nasal pyramid. To the extent that the corresponding left and right measurements differ, the bony nasal pyramid will be deviated to the side of the lower measurement. This approach may be useful for the characterization of traumatic and congenital bony pyramid deformities. In addition, objective data for the results of rhinoplastic procedures are also possible.

Other applications of computer-aided assessment of the bony nasal pyramid are also feasible. Close monitoring of nasofacial growth and development is desirable in certain cases of congenital and acquired craniofacial anomalies. Our paradigm for measurement of the bony nasal pyramid can provide objective data for that monitoring. The paradigm also may provide guidance for the preoperative planning of craniofacial surgical procedures. The derived measurements may ultimately guide the design of nasal augmentation and reduction.

21.7 CAS CEPHALOMETRICS CHALLENGES

The objective data provided by CAS cephalometrics requires high-quality thin-cut CT scan images. Poor image quality from any cause whatsoever will limit the accuracy of the measurements. For this reason, specific protocols that ensure the quality of the scans are necessary. Casual adherence to these protocols must be discouraged.

CAS cephalometrics requires the relative orientation of the subject in the image volume be maintained throughout image acquisition. For all of our protocols, axial CT plane was parallel to the Frankfort line, and the subject was not rotated within in this plane. Failure to maintain an appropriate orientation needlessly complicates the review of the resultant images. Furthermore, this deficiency will also lead to inaccurate measurements, since the definitions of the various parameters assume that the subject orientation is consistently in the ideal position.

It should be added that the above comments about orientation really apply only to currently available software. In theory, it may be possible to standardize the orientation via software manipulations. Future software may permit the imposition of a virtual frame to the CT data set. In this concept, the axial CT data would be used to reconstruct coronal and sagittal planar data as well as the three-dimensional model, and the selection of specific anatomical points would serve to orient the virtual frame, which the software uses as a reference for reformatting the images. The reformatted images would represent the true axial plane, which would be parallel to the Frankfort plane, as well as the orthogonal coronal and sagittal planes. Because of the extent of the image manipulations, the raw CT data would need to be very high quality—probably, 1 mm contiguous slices would be necessary. Conceivably, overlapping slices would enhance the image reformatting.

The application of a standardized external frame, whose purpose and function would be similar to those of a traditional cephalostat, also may provide important orientation data. In this approach, the patient/subject would wear the frame during CT scan acquisition. The frame provides an external reference for CT image analysis. In this way, the frame functions mimics the function of the frames used in framed stereotaxy procedures. After the CT images have been transferred to the computer workstation, the software could maintain orientation relative to the frame (Figure 21.10).

The ultimate clinical utility of the information offered by CAS cephalomet-

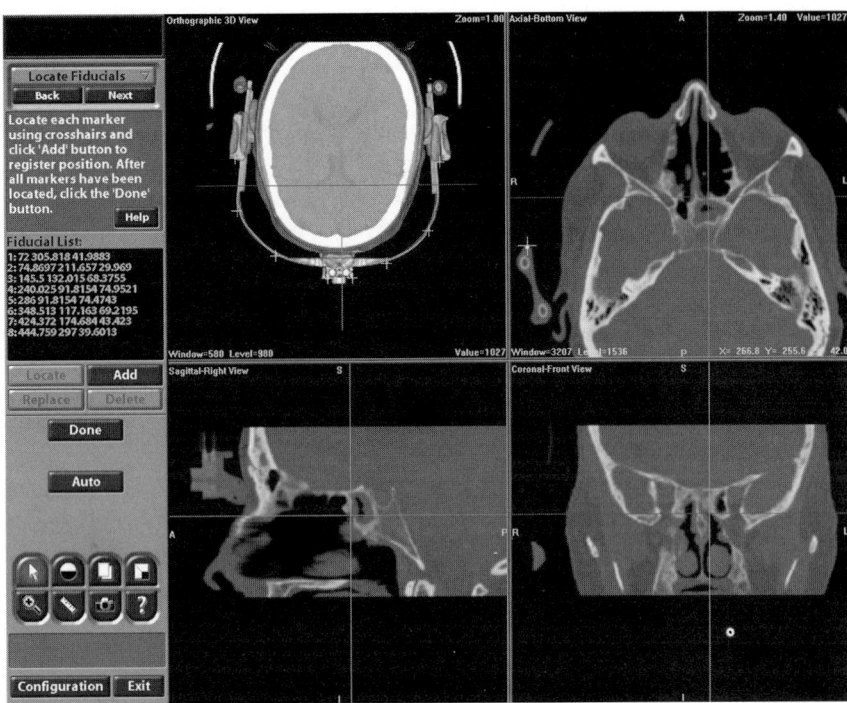

FIGURE 21.10 The SAVANT (CBYON, Palo Alto, CA) prototype head frame supports semiautomatic registration for sinus surgery. This screen capture shows the head frame in the reconstructed three-dimensional model. The SAVANT software can automatically recognize the positions of fiducial markers that are built into the headset. Because this head frame is designed so that it can be reproducibly placed on the patient's head, it has a unique position relative to the underlying craniomaxillofacial skeleton. As a result, it may serve as reference parameters for the proper orientation of CT images. In this theoretical approach, CAS software may construct a virtual cephalostat for computer-aided cephalometrics.

rics cannot be readily determined. Intuitively, CAS cephalometrics can provide significant information; however, many issues need to be resolved. The exact parameters that depict useful anatomical relationships have not been established. In fact, specific items, such as SBR or MP, may eventually be replaced by other parameters that carry more clinical significance. The current proposal needs firm validation; as clinical experience with this technology, it is likely that the described approaches will undergo revision.

To date, CAS cephalometrics has been greatly influenced by the limitations of the current CAS software, which was designed for surgical navigation and preoperative planning. The software clearly has not been optimized for quantitative image analysis that cephalometrics requires. Despite this obvious problem, the current CAS software tools offer remarkable capabilities for quantitative studies of the craniomaxillofacial skeleton. It may be anticipated that future versions of the software will be better adapted for cephalometric-type analysis.

REFERENCES

1. Zide B, Grayson B, McCarthy JG. Cephalometric analysis: part I. Plast Reconstr Surg 1981; 68:816–823.
2. Zide B, Grayson B, McCarthy JG. Cephalometric analysis for upper and lower midface surgery: part II. Plast Reconstr Surg 1981; 68:961–968.
3. Zide B, Grayson B, McCarthy JG. Cephalometric analysis for mandibular surgery: part III. Plast Reconstr Surg 1982; 69:155–164.
4. Thurow RC. Cephalometric methods in research and private practice. Angle Orthod 1951; 21:104–116.
5. Hall DL, Bollen A-M. A comparison of sonically derived and traditional cephalometric values. Angle Orthod 1996; 67:365–372.
6. Richardson A. An investigation into the reproducibility of some points, planes and lines used in cephalometric analysis. Am J Orthod 1966; 52:637–651.
7. Baumrind S, Frantz RC. The reliability of head film measurements: 1. landmark identification. Am J Orthod 1971; 60:111–127.
8. Baumrind S, Frantz RC. The reliability of head film measurements: 2. conventional angular and linear measurements. Am J Orthod 1971; 60:505–517.
9. Gerbo LR, Poulton DR, Covell DA. A comparison of a computer-based orthognatic surgery prediction system to postsurgical results. Int J Adult Orthod Orthognathic Surg 1997; 12:55–63.
10. Aharon PA, Eisig S, Cisneros GJ. Surgical prediction reliability: a comparision of two computer software systems. Int J Adult Orthod Orthognathic Surg 1997; 12:65–78.
11. Citardi MJ, Herrmann B, Hollenbeak C, et al. Comparison of scientific calipers and computer-enabled CT review for the measurement of skull-base and craniomaxillofacial dimensions. Skull Base Surgery 2001; 34:111–122.
12. Hardeman S, Kokoska MS, Bucholz R, et al. Computer-based CT scan analysis of craniomaxillofacial relationships. American Academy of Otolaryngology–Head and Neck Surgery Annual Meeting, Washington, DC, September 24–27, 2000.
13. Hardeman S, Citardi MJ, Stack BS, et al. Computer-aided reduction of zygomatic fractures. American Academy of Facial Plastic and Reconstructive Surgery Annual Meeting, New Orleans, LA, September 22–24, 1999.
14. Kokoska MS, Hardeman S, Bucholz R, et al. Computer-aided sequential reduction of frontozygomaticomaxillary fractures. American Academy of Facial Plastic and Reconstructive Surgery spring meeting, Orlando, FL, May 13, 2000.
15. Citardi MJ, Hardeman S, Hollenbeak C, et al. Computer-aided assessment of bony nasal pyramid dimensions. Arch Otolaryngol Head Neck Surg 2000; 126:979–984.

22
Computer-Aided Craniofacial Surgery

Alex A. Kane, M.D.
Washington University School of Medicine, St. Louis, Missouri

Lun-Jou Lo, M.D.
Chang Gung Memorial Hospital and Chang Gung Medical College, Taipei, Taiwan

Jeffrey L. Marsh, M.D.
Washington University School of Medicine and St. Louis Children's Hospital, St. Louis, Missouri

22.1 INTRODUCTION

Before discussing the subject of computer-aided craniofacial surgery, it seems appropriate to address the need for a discrete chapter on craniofacial surgery within a text whose focus is otorhinolaryngology–head and neck surgery. The term "craniofacial surgery" has come to connote reconstruction of major congenital or acquired deformities of the skull and face, including orthognathic surgery, as opposed to surgery for infectious or neoplastic head and neck disorders. In the mid-1960s, Tessier introduced craniofacial surgery as a discipline when he described the first intra/extracranial correction of orbital hypertelorism. Subsequently, the domain of craniofacial surgery has been regionalized into anatomical zones based upon skeletal subunits and their associated soft tissues: the calvaria, the upper face (orbits, zygomas, and brows), the midface (maxillae and zygomas), and the lower face (mandible). A set of technical intraoperative maneuvers has come to also characterize craniofacial surgery; these technical features include the use of concealed incisions (coronal, conjunctival, intraoral), the intra/extracranial approach to the upper and midface, and deconstruction/reconstruction of the craniofacial skeleton [1]. The anatomical complexity of these types of operations and the absence of easy anatomical locators for mobilized osseous segments (such as the teeth for orthognathic surgery) has made craniofacial surgeons dependent upon medical imaging since the inception of the discipline. The addition of the computer to such imaging has facilitated understanding aberrant anatomy, increased operative safety, and improved operative results.

Computer-aided craniofacial surgery is a broad term, which has been applied to a variety of frequently overlapping activities. These related disciplines include visualization and mensuration of craniofacial anatomy, preoperative planning of surgical interventions, intraoperative image-based guidance of surgical therapy, and postoperative evaluation of therapy and growth. The computer has become an indispensable tool for the craniofacial surgeon. It allows the practitioner to more effectively understand the patient's clinical problem, to share this understanding with both patient and colleague, to plan and execute an operation, and to obtain feedback regarding the outcome. The purpose of this chapter is to survey the current use of the computer-aided surgery (CAS) technology in all of these aspects of craniofacial surgery.

22.2 VISUALIZATION AND MENSURATION OF CRANIOFACIAL ANATOMY

22.2.1 Data Acquisition and Processing

Surgeons have traditionally interacted with anatomy through the direct experiences of physical examination, intraoperative observation, and postmortem dissection. Contemporary computer-aided medical imaging has greatly expanded in vivo anatomical study through its conversion of the physical body into a digital data set. The processing of this raw 3D image data is essential to all of the applications of computers in craniofacial surgery. It is important to consider understanding how such data is acquired and assembled before its use by the craniofacial surgeon

The unique assistance lent to the craniofacial surgeon by the computer comes from its power to provide infinite custom anatomical images that are unlimited by restrictive point of view, by preservation of essential structures, by tissue density, and/or by destruction of tissue (such as actual cutting of living flesh or a corpse). Furthermore, the ability of contemporary computers to process image data rapidly has facilitated their incorporation into clinical practice.

The main source of in vivo anatomical data for the craniofacial surgeon has been the computed tomography (CT) scanner, although magnetic resonance imaging (MRI) is increasingly in use. The basic concepts of data assembly and segmentation are similar regardless of the source of the three-dimensional (3D) data.

Computer-Aided Craniofacial Surgery

To create the images, the CT scanner passes a beam of x-rays through tissue, then assigns a gray-scale value, called a Hounsfield value or CT intensity, to small quantities of tissue. Each of these small quantities are called pixels. Each image is composed of a fine grid of pixels. Many modern CT scanners create images consisting of a 512 × 512 pixel matrix. Each square pixel contains the Hounsfield number of a small quantity of the patient's tissue. Hounsfield intensities range from approximately −1000 for air to about 3000 for dense bone. Water is always defined as having 0 intensity. The exact Hounsfield range differs slightly for each scanner.

22.2.2 Three-Dimensional Image Volume Assembly

Initially CT and, later, MRI data were presented as "slice" images, which resembled the cross-sectional anatomy seen in the pathology laboratory. The triple presentation of whole body slice, CT scan slice, and MRI slice used to study and display the "visible" man and woman documents the basic "slice" display modality. However, since surgeons, anthropologists, anatomists, and dysmorphologists usually interact with humans as surfaces and volumes, display of CT data as either surfaces or volumes has facilitated their incorporation into clinical and research roles. Such reformatted data has come to be known as 3D CT (or 3D MRI, if the data source is the MRI scanner).

It is important to clarify the term "3D" in computer-aided medical imaging. In this context, 3D refers to the data and not the presentation of that data. Data with x,y,z coordinates are 3D data, but that same data displayed on a computer screen are a two-dimensional (2D) representation of that data. This distinction is more than semantic and is easily communicated with an example. An artist, when depicting a space-filling subject, can do so by a drawing or by sculpture. A sketch is a 2D representation of a 3D surface, while a sculpture is a 3D representation of a 3D surface. A photograph of a drawing is a 2D representation of a 2D surface, while the photograph of the sculpture of the same model is a 2D representation of a 3D surface. Whereas a drawing needs to be redone every time the artist wants to render the subject from a different viewing position, the sculptor need only change the position of the sculpture to get the new effect. CT and MRI scanners capture 3D data, and software can be used to render these data from any viewpoint. These 2D renderings are analogous to having the ability to photograph a sculpture from an arbitrary viewpoint without the geometric distortion that photography introduces. CT and MRI image data can also be presented three-dimensionally using visualization technology such as holography or stereoimages or, more conveniently, as life-sized models.

The first task in CT and MRI image data postprocessing (image data manipulation after initial acquisition and storage of planar scan images) is to prepare a 3D volume of data from the set of standard 2D image data that a scanner routinely outputs. In our institutions, CT scans are acquired according to a standardized protocol, where contiguous, nonoverlapping, chin to vertex images are taken, each in a plane that is parallel to the orbitomeatal plane. The actual number of images per scan varies proportionately with patient size, the matrix size in which the data are stored, and the amount that the scanner table moves between each newly acquired image. For patients who are older than 6 months, images are taken every 2 mm, while younger infants have images taken with every 1 mm advance of the table. Using this protocol, a typical head CT scan contains 80–180 images. The data for the images in the series are stored in files on the hard drive of the computer that controls the scanner.

Previously, the exact format in which the images were stored varied tremendously, not only among scanners made by different manufacturers, but also by generations of the same manufacturer. This inconsistency caused considerable logistical difficulties for postprocessing. Now with the nearly universal acceptance of the DICOM data format [2], most software packages can read the image data generated by even different equipment makers. Once acquired, the image data are transferred to the postprocessing computer workstation, which runs a software package to manipulate the data. Data transfer from the acquisition site in the radiology department to the postprocessing site is today usually achieved over a network. The transfer task has been greatly facilitated by the installation of image archiving systems (PACS systems) at many hospitals, which can route DICOM data automatically or semi-automatically [3]. A number of commercial 3D surface and volumetric CT/MR imaging software packages exist. Although each of these applications offers varying capabilities, all of these software packages are similar in that they take as their input the raw image data that are the output of the scanner. Until recently, many of the software packages available for manipulating images only could be run on expensive, specialized, UNIX-based computer workstations. This situation has changed dramatically in the past few years as the power of personal computers has increased as has the number of imaging packages for these less expensive platforms.

The key concept for understanding the creation of a 3D volume from a set of 2D images is the pixel-to-voxel transition. A voxel is a cube of tissue, rather than a square of tissue like the pixel. The computer uses a mathematical algorithm called trilinear interpolation to add a third dimension to pixels, thereby expanding them to create cubic voxels. Thus, the paradigm shifts from a Hounsfield value in a two-dimensional square to a Hounsfield value in a three-dimensional cube. Schematically, 2D images are transformed into 3D image slabs, which are then stacked in order to assemble the 3D image volume.

The assembly of the 3D image volume allows it to be displayed using any one of a number of rendering algorithms. These algorithms differ somewhat between software packages but can be divided into two general types: volume-rendering algorithms and surface-rendering algorithms. In volume rendering, a subset of voxels determined by the user is displayed by projecting these images into 2D pixel space, using a ray-casting algorithm. In volume rendering, the more external layers of selected voxels can be made to appear translucent by altering their opacity, visualizing the external and internal structure of an object of interest simultaneously. In surface rendering, the volumetric data must first be converted into geometric contours or wire-frame polygon meshes of the outer surface of the object of interest. This technique assumes that the voxels that compose the object of interest have already been identified. This process of identifying an object of interest is called *segmentation*, which will be discussed further below. These polygon meshes or contours are then rendered for display using conventional geometric rendering techniques and shaded using one of a variety of reflectance models (e.g., Phong, Gourand).

Each of these techniques has advantages and disadvantages. In surface rendering, the conversion step to the polygonal mesh surface can be computationally intensive. Such conversion steps are prone to sampling artifacts, due to decisions made in the algorithm regarding polygon placement, which secondarily may lose detail. However, once it is segmented and converted, the surface is fast to render, because only surface points are considered. In addition, surface rendering is often performed with the assistance of specialized hardware cards rather than in a purely software algorithm. In contrast, since the entire set of image data is considered at all times in volume rendering, the computer needs to consistently interact with all of the data during each new rendering. In volume rendering, no segmentation needs to be done prior to rendering, and any part, including internal structures, may be rendered and is always available for viewing.

Once the 3D volume has been assembled and visualized, several display tools are available to work with it. The simplest tool is rotation. The volume can be turned about any combination of the three coordinate axes. Clipping is another simple tool allowing the user to visualize a portion of the 3D volume constrained by a set of planes specified by the user. Volume reslicing can also be performed, allowing the user to visualize the data in slices parallel to any arbitrary user-specified plane.

22.2.3 Segmentation

One of the most common manipulations of the data is isolation of anatomical subunits for closer study or independent display. These subunits usually are specific bones or soft tissues, such as the mandible or the orbital contents. This process, called segmentation, divides the volume into subset collections of voxels, which are called objects.

One of the simplest tools for segmentation is thresholding. This is a method of instructing the computer to display only those voxels that contain Hounsfield numbers that meet user specified criteria. For example, in CT data, it is a fact that all soft tissues in the head have Hounsfield values less than a certain critical value, which is necessarily less than the Hounsfield value of bone. If we assume, for purposes of illustration, that this critical value is 90, then one can display only the bone by applying a threshold criterion requiring voxels to contain Hounsfield values greater than 90 in order to be retained and displayed. Thus, thresholding is a simple and efficient way of segmenting bone on the basis of similar gray-scale intensities of the desired object.

While segmentation of anatomical objects of interest can be done in many ways [4], three of the most common techniques will be reviewed: slice-by-slice region of interest outlining using cursor and mouse; coring out full-thickness pieces of the volume; and segmentation by connecting adjacent voxels. The first technique for segmentation is slice-by-slice outlining, in which a mouse is used to edit each slice of the volume in order to isolate the object of interest. This is the most time-consuming of the techniques, requiring repetitive user interaction with a series of slices that contain the object of interest. The second segmentation method is coring, which takes full-thickness pieces of the volume, based upon a user-defined trace upon a volume-rendered image, and assigns the cored piece to a new object, much like coring an apple. The coring procedure is repeated, outlining the object more closely from multiple different viewpoints and trimming away unwanted voxels. The third segmentation technique, called seeding, exploits the computer's ability to connect all voxels attached to a "seed voxel" that have nonzero Hounsfield values within them. The computer has the ability to connect all voxels that are adjacent to an arbitrary seed voxel. This technique exploits the spatial arrangement of voxels that are contained within the object of interest.

Once the objects of interest have been segmented using these techniques, several tools are available for measuring quantities of interest pertaining to them. The volume of any object can be calculated by the computer. Since the volume of a single cubic voxel is known and the number of voxels in the object is known, calculating the volume is simply the product of the unit voxel volume times the number of voxels in the object. Since every voxel has known x,y,z coordinates, the computer can also calculate the distance between any two voxels or the angle formed by lines connecting any three voxels. The computer can also calculate 2D or 3D distances on any object. Although these distances may seem similar, 2D and 3D distances are not the same measurements. A 3D distance is analogous to what one would get by using a caliper on the 3D volume or by using a caliper on a sculpture. The 3D distance is the same no matter what perspective the object is rendered from, much as a fixed distance between two points on a sculpture is insensitive to how the sculpture is rotated on its pedestal. The 2D distance is different in that it is a projection of a 3D distance onto a 2D surface, and as such it is sensitive to the viewpoint from which it is rendered. (If one photographed a sculpture from two different angles and measured the distance between two points on the pictures, the distances between the points would vary.)

Object segmentation is the basis for many of the applications of computers in craniofacial surgery. Objects of interest within the 3D image volume can be moved arbitrarily within the volume while maintaining the rest of the volume stationary. This type of procedure is particularly useful in surgical planning, which will be described in detail later in this chapter. There is no limit to the number of segmentations that can be performed on a single 3D dataset, nor are there limits to the ways in which such segmentations can be usefully displayed with different coloring and opacities applied. It is often challenging to find methods of segmentation that can be performed rapidly and with some automated assistance from the computer, rather than having to perform a manual slice-by-slice segmentation. Considerable work is being undertaken to find image-processing methods for automated and semiautomated segmentation of the anatomy of interest to craniofacial surgeons, as few surgeons are able to spend the time necessary to master the process of segmentation, although these tasks are becoming more simplified as the technology improves.

22.3 PREOPERATIVE MODELING, PLANNING AND SIMULATION

22.3.1 Rapid Prototyping Modeling Technologies and Applications

Computers have greatly facilitated the rapid creation of high-quality three-dimensional physical models. These models precisely reproduce the anatomy of interest to the craniofacial surgeon. The models may be used to plan osteotomies and hardware placement (e.g., prebending of reconstructive plates), during mock surgery or surgical simulation. Proponents of these models believe that the ability to simulate and practice the surgery may lead to decreased operative times and superior results, although it is difficult to support such claims quantitatively. The other use for such models is in the creation of prefabricated implants for reconstruction [5]. Implants can be directly created, in which case the model produced by the prototyping machine serves as the implant. In this instance, the implant may be made from glass fiber nylon or acrylic. Alternatively, the prototyping machine can produce a reverse model (a form or mold) into which semisolid biocompatible hydroxyapatite can be placed in order to give the desired shape to the implant.

In general, rapid prototyping technologies can reproduce any object that that can be analyzed through segmentation. In this way, the model is derived from base imaging data, which typically is a high-resolution CT scan. There is no doubt that bone may be easily segmented from CT data through simple thresholding operation. Nevertheless, soft tissue can also be modeled using these techniques, and independently segmented soft tissue (e.g., tumor) and bony objects can be created and fit together into a unified model (Figure 22.1). Base data collected from multiple modalities (e.g., CT and MRI) can also be fused, allowing the construction of more complex models. ''Mirroring'' can also be used to reproduce a reversed symmetric model, which is sometimes useful in cases where a unilateral defect is being reconstructed to match the contralateral undamaged appearance.

The procedure for the construction of these models varies and can follow one of several paradigms. Often the companies that produce these models sell them to the surgeon. In this approach, the surgeon specifies the characteristics of the desired model and then sends the base scan data to the company. The data may be sent electronically. Alternatively, digital storage media (such as optical disks that store the CT data) may be shipped to the manufacturer (either electronically or by physical media transfer). The model manufacturer does all segmentation and data manipulation. It is important for the surgeon to understand that the anatomical fidelity of the final model is sensitively dependent upon the expertise of the individual performing the data manipulation and segmentation. In the situation where the manufacturer performs a complex segmentation at a site distant from the surgeon, it behooves the surgeon who ordered the model to confirm that the segmentation was done in a way that matches the surgeon's understanding of the underlying anatomy and pathology and that the segmentation is consistent with the goals for the model's use.

It also may be possible for the surgeon to perform the segmentation and then export the segmented data for model creation. Nonetheless, many companies still prefer to do the segmentation, since the data manipulation may be cumbersome and dependent upon proprietary algorithms and data formats. Objects segmented from a volumetric data set must be converted into the expected input format of the prototyping machine. The specific steps of this process vary and may make it inefficient or impossible for the surgeon to perform the segmentation.

Some companies sell the rapid prototyping equipment directly to the medical institution. In this case the surgeon has greater control of the segmentation and model production. However, the costs of such systems are still beyond the means of craniofacial surgeons in most settings.

Regardless of the location of model production, the per model cost of production of these models currently is almost prohibitively high. However, costs may decrease as other manufacturers enter the marketplace and produce competition for price and services. When used in the clinical setting, medical insurers usually will not pay the full price of prototype production, but sometimes third-

Computer-Aided Craniofacial Surgery

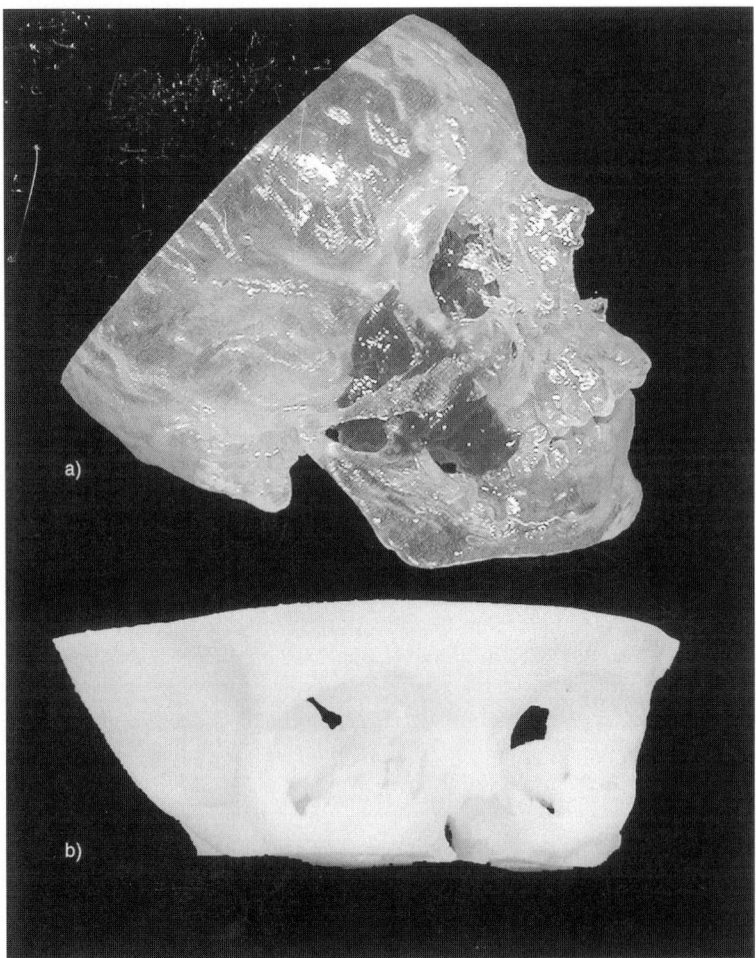

FIGURE 22.1 Rapid prototyping technologies for creation of 3D solid models. (a) Stereolithographic model of a skull with a shaded tumor (Courtesy ProtoMED CT Bone Models). (b) Fused deposition model (Courtesy of Stratasys, Inc.).

party payers will partially subsidize the cost of model manufacture. Unfortunately, economic considerations have probably significantly inhibited the clinical use of such models.

Several different rapid prototyping technologies are capable of producing high-quality anatomical models:

Stereolithography: Stereolithography builds the model through the sequential addition of multiple layers that are added by a computer-guided ultraviolet laser, which polymerizes a photosensitive resin made of acrylic or epoxy [6]. New layers are formed at the liquid/surface interface of the resin bath. After a layer is completed and hardened by the laser at the surface, the model is then submerged in the bath of liquid resin on a precisely controlled movable platform. The process then repeats, and the next layer is then solidified at the surface. The resin is translucent when dry. The process may be time-consuming, taking a full day to produce a model. Postprocessing is also required to remove the supports that were placed to prevent sagging of overhanging structures. Stereolithography has been the most commonly used technology in the production of medical models. This type of model is most often custom-ordered from a private company by the surgeon.

Fused Deposition Modeling: Fusion deposition modeling generates physical models by depositing extruded molten plastic in layers, which then solidify as they cool. Equipment for the production of these models can fit on a desktop and may be sold to institutions that may control the production of models locally. The costs of such equipment could only be justified if the institution requires a sufficiently high volume of models. This technique also produces supports, which are generated by the machine to prevent sagging of overhanging structures during the model-building process and need to be removed prior to model completion.

Selective Laser Sintering: Selective laser sintering uses a flat sheet of powder, which is heated to close to its melting point. A carbon dioxide laser beam scans over the powder and heats the grains so that they melt on the outside and stick together (*sinter*). The base plate then moves down slightly, and the next layer of powder is spread across the surface by a rotating roller. The object is supported as it is made by the tightly packed unsintered powder, so it does not need extra supporting structures. At the end of the build process, the entire cake of powder, sintered and nonsintered, is allowed to cool down and lifted out of the machine. Then the loose powder is shaken off and the sintered object is freed. The finished objects have a matte, powdery surface. These models can be made in wax, sand or steel powder as well as nylon.

22.3.2 Assessment of Anatomical Deformities and Planning of Surgical Interventions

Surgical simulation necessitates a surgical plan. The appropriateness, accuracy, and safety of the surgical plan depend on comprehension of the relevant anatomy. Reformatted CT data, displayed both as two-dimensional slice and three-dimensional volume-rendered images, provide the simulator with the information necessary for comprehension of that anatomy.

Segmentation of bone is done by thresholding. Simultaneous display of specific soft tissues, such as ocular globes, is accomplished by editing the soft tissue on two-dimensional slices or by using other segmentation techniques such as region growing. The edited soft tissue is then saved as an independent object or subvolume that can be displayed with or without the associated osseous structures. Following segmentation, which is the most time-consuming task in the surgical planning process, the resulting composite volume data set can be freely manipulated in six degrees of freedom and their surfaces deformed and reintegrated into a new whole. Of particular concern are quantitative and qualitative definitions of the specific anatomical relationships. As a result, the surgeon, during surgical planning, should focus on the brain and the orbits, the nasal cavity, the orbits and the maxilla (including the maxillary dentition and the infraorbital nerve foramina), the maxilla and the mandible.

While a variety of software packages are capable of performing at least a portion of the imaging tasks requisite for this type of surgical simulation, we have heavily relied upon the ANALYZE software package (Mayo Biomedical Imaging Resource, Rochester, MN) for these tasks. The software's modules support all image processing in a flexible, but cohesive application environment. Furthermore, this software now runs well on a standard personal computer using the Windows operating system (Microsoft Corporation, Bellevue, WA).

Once the anomalous anatomy has been defined, a surgical plan can be synthesized. Initially, the plan is based on the dysmorphology, which will be surgically altered; then the plan is individualized for the patient specific pathology, the age of the patient, and the extent of correction desired by the patient and/or responsible adult(s). Generation of a surgical plan implies definition of a desired end result. If the patient truly has a unilateral deformity (such as a localized osseous or soft tissue hyper- or hypoplasia), the unaffected contralateral side can be used as a template for the reconstruction of the affected side. Usually, the side that is contralateral to the major pathology has secondary deformation owing to skewed growth. Unicoronal synostosis (discussed later in this chapter) exemplifies this problem. Often, the actual pathology is bilateral.

Traditional craniofacial reconstructive surgical planning has been based upon data from a variety of sources: standardized life-sized lateral and AP skull x-rays (cephalometry), direct surface measurements (anthropometry), and replicas of the dentition (dental study models or casts). Such planning began with orthognathic surgery, where direct assessment of the occlusion (dental models) and indirect assessment of the jaws (cephalometry) usually yielded a surgically reliable plan. Reconstruction for grossly asymmetric jaw deformities and for upper face and calvarial deformities independent of the dentition was much more difficult to plan from conventional 2D radiographic images and dental models.

Nonetheless, an extensive and published normative database has been derived from cephalometry and dental study models. Although the cephalometric data are two-dimensional, they have been adapted for three-dimensional use [7,8]. The efficacy of such adaptation remains debatable. Data for select skull measurements have been derived from two-dimensional axial CT scan images without digital registration to anatomical fiducial points of individual subjects. Such data would be more reliable if they had been obtained within the three-dimensional CT digital data itself [9].

Regarding the orbital region, anthropometric data are available for standard surface measurements of the upper face [10], including the ocular globes [11], and conventional radiographic data are available for the interorbital space [12]. The discordant change in both intraorbital (the globe, extraocular muscles, and periorbital fat) and periorbital (eyelids and medial and lateral canthi) soft tissues compared with change in subjacent bone compromises the utility of such data since accurate soft-tissue outcome predictions in the orbital region are not currently possible. In short, true three-dimensional normative craniofacial data that are age, gender, and race specific are not available at this time. We have acquired and use a small set of normative data from infants and children with normal craniofacial structures who required CT scan for evaluation of neurological or traumatic disorders. A similar approach has been presented by the Australian group [13].

Three principles guide the planning of craniofacial interventions:

Calvaria. The calvaria are operated upon to release premature osseous fusion (craniosynostosis), to release intracranial constraint, to normalize dysmorphic shape, and to repair osseous defects. The extent of the calvarectomy required for both surgical safety (i.e., surgical exposure) and reconstruction varies depending upon the specific pathology. Nonetheless, attention is primarily focused on normalization of the frontal region; frontal deformation directly affects appearance because the region is not hidden by hair. Reconstruction of the superior orbital rim or rims is often a component of frontal reconstruction.

Globe-Orbit Relationship. Orbital region dysmorphology may consist of malrelationships between the orbits in the axial (horizontal), coronal (cephalad-caudad), or sagittal (anterior-posterior) planes; malrelationships between the ocular globe and the orbit with proptosis/exorbitism (too much ventral projection of the globe) or enophthalmos (posterior displacement of the globe); deformation of the orbit; abnormal size of the globe; or combinations thereof. Correction of such dysmorphology requires an anatomically exact understanding of the relationship between the ocular globe and its orbit. That relationship is a composite of the size of the orbit, the shape of the orbit, the position of the orbit relative to the rest of the skull, the size of the globe, and the volume of the extraocular orbital contents. The size and shape of the orbit and its position relative to adjacent bones can be altered purposefully with surgery. Such alterations are part of the surgical plan. The volume of the extraocular orbital contents often is inadvertently altered during periorbital surgery; this alteration cannot be planned predictably.

Maxillary-Mandibular and Dental Occlusal Relationships. Orthognathic surgery may be indicated for improvement of a compromised upper airway, protection of the globes (through enlargement of the inferior orbits), improved mastication, and correction of speech distortions. Cephalometric data and dental study models are time-proven effective planning tools for jaw surgery in dentoskeletally mature patients with essentially symmetrical malocclusions. Such patients usually do not require the sophisticated three-dimensional surgical planning discussed in this article. Planning of correction of major jaw asymmetries in mature patients and upper or lower jaw operations in young patients, however, is facilitated with three-dimensional computer-aided planning.

22.3.3 Philosophy for Surgical Simulation

Ideally, craniofacial surgical simulation should begin with the desired appearance and function and end with the hard and soft tissue operative plan to achieve that result. This process can be conceptualized as the following steps:

1. Preoperative skin surface three-dimensional image of the patient with documentation of functional limitations
2. Simulated desired skin surface three-dimensional image
3. Simulation of functional correction
4. Simulated hard and soft tissue three-dimensional imaging of the head coincident with the desired skin surface image and function
5. Blueprint of hard and soft tissue changes necessary to convert the real preoperative configuration to that simulated in step 4

This ideal is yet to be realized.

Nonetheless, the technology needed for the implementation of this ideal sequence is beginning to emerge [14,15]. The process begins with generation of polygonal surface meshes representing both the osseous and facial skin surfaces. The osseous surface is segmented from CT data, while the facial surface is extracted from a laser scan of the face. These two meshes are then registered anatomically to each other. The elastic and mechanical properties of the skin are modeled by mathematically treating the soft tissue as behaving like springs. These springs represent several physical properties of skin, including turgor, and gravity. The spring model is used to estimate the soft tissue deformation that would be caused by the specified bone repositioning (Figure 22.2). The output of this method [14] is a photorealistic three-dimensional representation of the external appearance of the patient. This representation allows dynamic views of the face (e.g., prediction of soft tissue deformation with jaw motion).

The actual process of surgical simulation we routinely use today for complex craniofacial operations, whether done conventionally or with computer assistance, consists of the acquisition preoperative osseous images (plus dental models if relevant) and then planning/simulation for osseous normalization [16]. It is hoped that normalization of the bony skeleton will produce normalization of overall appearance and function; that is, the soft tissues will assume the desired position/appearance after correction of the targeted bony abnormalities/anomalies. Regretfully, this is not always the case. As we discuss skeletally based surgical planning and simulation subsequently, it is important to remember that appearance and function are the goals of surgery rather than the achievement of specific skeletal measurements. It is hoped that increasing sophistication of computer-assisted surgery will facilitate the attainment of these goals.

22.3.4 Techniques for Computer-Aided Surgical Planning

Having transferred the CT data to the graphics workstation in a suitable format, the simulator produces a series of three-dimensional osseous surface volume–rendered images of the skull in standard projections. The planned osteotomies and ostectomies are drawn on these images in anatomically correct locations. Each bone segment to be altered is defined as a separate object by ''cutting'' the proposed sites, as if using a saw. Bone segments, such as an orbit, can be moved in all six degrees of freedom: anteroposterior, right-left, cephalad-caudad, and the rotations about each of their axes. ''Bending'' of a bone segment, a common technique for contouring of the calvaria and supraorbital bandeau in infants, can be achieved by creating multiple objects out of the bone segment. These component segments are moved or warped or both to reshape their contour, according to the plan. Bone grafts are simulated by creation of de novo objects.

If the operation includes alteration of the globe-orbit relationship, the globes and optic nerves are visualized as independent objects and then embedded into the three-dimensional osseous surface images. When globe position is expected to remain constant with respect to the majority of the skull (as in the correction of the orbital deformity of unicoronal synostosis), the mobilized bone segments are moved until the desired globe-orbit relationship is achieved. If the purpose of the operation is to reposition the globe(s) (as in hypertelorism correction), either a new composite object consisting of the globe and its orbit is created to be moved as a single unit during the simulation or the globe and its orbit can be moved independently to achieve a best-fit appearance.

Computer-Aided Craniofacial Surgery

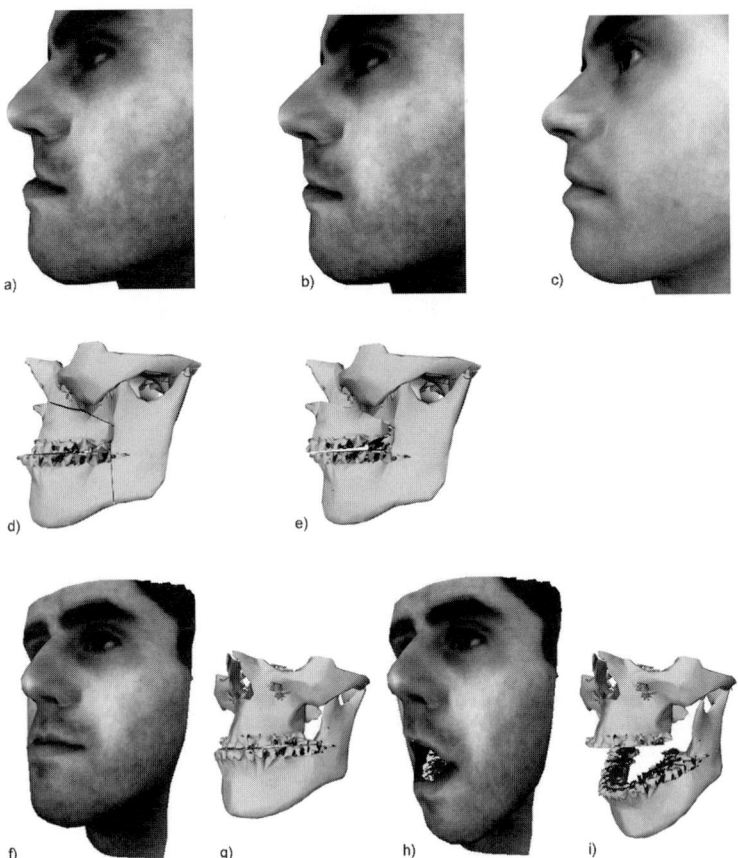

FIGURE 22.2 Simulation of soft tissue deformation in craniofacial surgery. (a) Preoperative appearance. (b) Simulated postoperative appearance. (c) Postoperative appearance. (d) Preoperative bone structure. (e) Simulated postoperative bone structure. (f, g) Soft tissue and bony appearance before simulated jaw motion (h, i) Soft tissue and bony appearance with simulated jaw motion. (Courtesy of Matthias Teschner, Telecommunications Laboratory, University of Erlangen-Nuremberg, Erlangen, Germany.)

The completed simulation is examined for correspondence with the desired outcome. If the coincidence is not satisfactory, the plan is altered, the simulation repeated, and the result rechecked. This process is reiterated until a satisfactory simulation is achieved. At that time, the movement of each defined object is recorded in voxels of the translation in the x,y,z coordinates and as degree of rotation around the x-, y-, and z-axes, relative to the object's original position. Voxels are then converted into metric measurements for intraoperative use. The spatial relationship between a displaced bone segment and unaltered reference points also can be obtained. Such reference surgical landmarks help determine the designated position while relocating a bony segment during the operation. A number of experimental and commercial intraoperative navigation systems have been used to make relocation of osseous segments more exact (see below). Nonetheless, intraoperative execution of the simulated "blueprint" remains a surgical challenge. Dental occlusion serves as the guide for maxilla-mandible movement, as was the case before computer-assisted surgery.

22.3.5 Computer-Aided Surgical Simulation Case Reports

22.3.5.1 Case 1: Nonsyndromic Bicoronal Syntosis

A 2-month-old female baby was evaluated for brachycephaly without acral anomalies. Her family history did not include craniofacial deformities. Preoperative three-dimensional CT reformations documented bilaterally fused coronal sutures, a broad flat forehead, nasion recession with an obtuse nasofrontal angle, recessed supraorbital rimes, vertical elongation of the orbits, and bilateral superior proptosis. The surgical plan included bilateral coronal extended suturectomy, bilateral frontal bone recontouring, and supraorbital bar recontouring and advancement. The orbital aspect of the plan was quantified by assessing the position of the superior-inferior orbital rim tangent relative to the corneal plane and was found to be 10 mm dorsal to this plane (normal = ± 2 mm).

Surgical simulation (Figure 22.3) began with bifrontal osteotomy including

FIGURE 22.3 This case summary illustrates simulation and verification of correction of the fronto-orbital deformities of nonsyndromic bicoronal synostosis in a 2-month-old girl. (Top row) Preoperative reformations. Note frontal and supraorbital recession with proptosis. (Second row) Surgical simulation. The frontal bones (blue) and the supraorbital bandeau (yellow) have been advanced and recontoured as independent objects based upon desired frontonasal contour and superior orbital rim-globe relation (see CD-ROM for color image). (Third row) Actual perioperative result (CT scan 4 days postoperatively). These images differ from the simulation in frontonasal contour and the presence of calvarial grafts at the pterions. (Bottom row) Three-dimensional longitudinal orbital projection to show the orbit-globe relationship in preoperative scan (left) for planning the supraorbital bandeau movement, simulated image (middle) demonstrating normalization of the relationship, and the actual perioperative result (right). Note the normalization of the superior-inferior orbital rim tangent to corneal plane distance: a change of 10 mm in both the simulation and the actual operation.

Computer-Aided Craniofacial Surgery

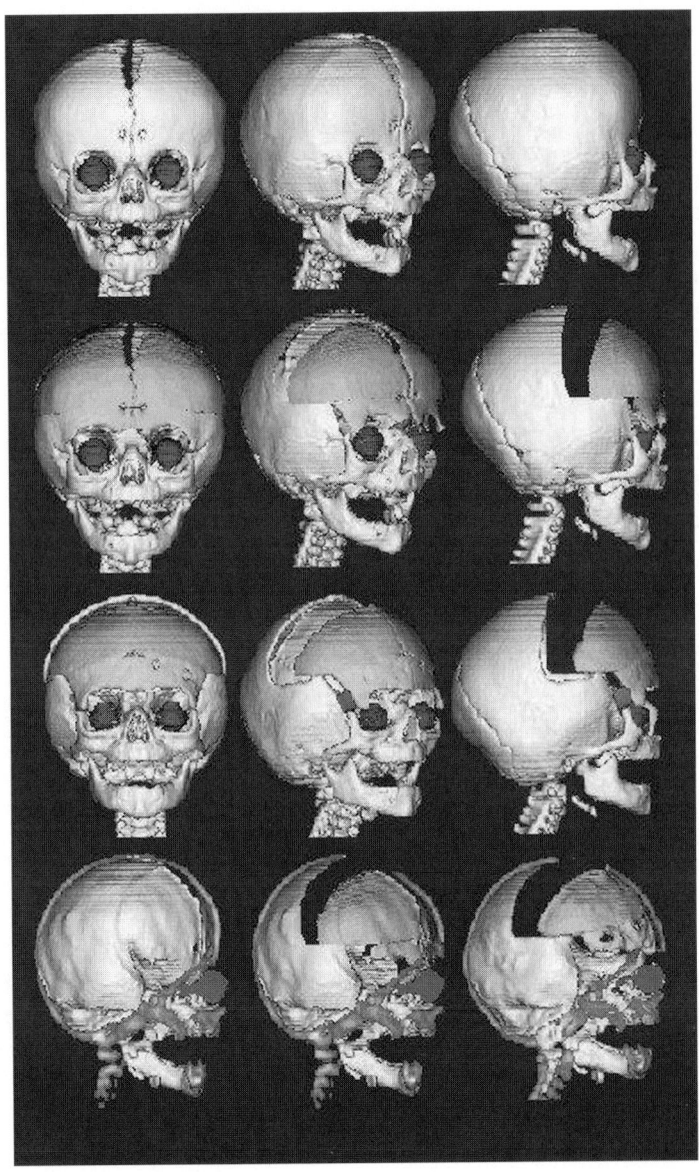

the fused coronal sutures, leaving 1 cm height of supraorbital bandeau in situ. The supraorbital bandeau was separated from the orbits and displaced ventrally by 10 mm at each midorbit region. The fused sutures were excised from the frontal bone flap. The remaining frontal bone was replaced to produce an appropriate frontal contour. Following simulation, the superior-inferior orbital rim tangent was coincident with the corneal plane, a normal relationship. The quantitative movements to achieve these results, relative to initial position were as follows: supraorbital bar moved 10.2 mm ventral and 2.4 mm cephalad and rotated 13 degrees about the x-axis; frontal bone moved 3.6 mm ventral and 1.8 mm cephalad and rotated 12 degrees about the x-axis.

The simulation approximated the actual operative results well. The two differed in the amount of rotation of the supraorbital bandeau and the curvature of the frontal bone–bandeau unit.

22.3.5.2 Case 2: Nonsyndromic Unicoronal Synostosis

A 4-month-old boy was evaluated for plagiocephaly with clinical stigmata of right unicoronal synostosis. Preoperative three-dimensional CT reformations documented a fused right coronal suture, skewing of the anterior fontanel to the left of the midsagittal plane, right frontal bone and superior orbital rim recession with hypoplasia of the zygomatic process of the frontal bone, left frontal bone prominence, verticalization of the right orbit, widening of the left orbit, and deviation of the base of the nasal pyramid to the left. Quantitative measurements were performed. The right orbital rim height and width were 30.9 mm and 26.4 mm, respectively, while the left orbital rim height and width were 27.9 mm and 30.5 mm, respectively. A mild degree of relative proptosis was noted on the right, with 22.7% of the globe volume outside of the orbital cavity, as compared with

FIGURE 22.4 This case summary illustrates simulation and verification of correction of the fronto-orbital deformities of right unilateral coronal synostosis in a 4-month-old boy. (Top row) Preoperative reformations. Note frontal and orbital asymmetries. (Second row) Surgical simulation. Following extended bilateral coronal suturectomies, the frontal bones (blue) were recontoured and repositioned. The right superolateral orbit (yellow) was recontoured and moved ventrally and caudally to equalize orbital rim shape. A bone graft (gray) was inserted to maintain the advancement at the pterion. The mesial left supraorbital bandeau (green) was recontoured (see CD-ROM for color image). (Third row) Actual perioperative result (CT scan 6 days postoperatively.) The corresponding bone segments are labeled with the same colors as for the simulation. (Bottom row) Outcome 1 year postoperatively. Note reintegration of the right orbit with symmetric normalization of the fronto-orbital region. (Please see the text for quantitative pre- and postoperative comparisons.)

Computer-Aided Craniofacial Surgery

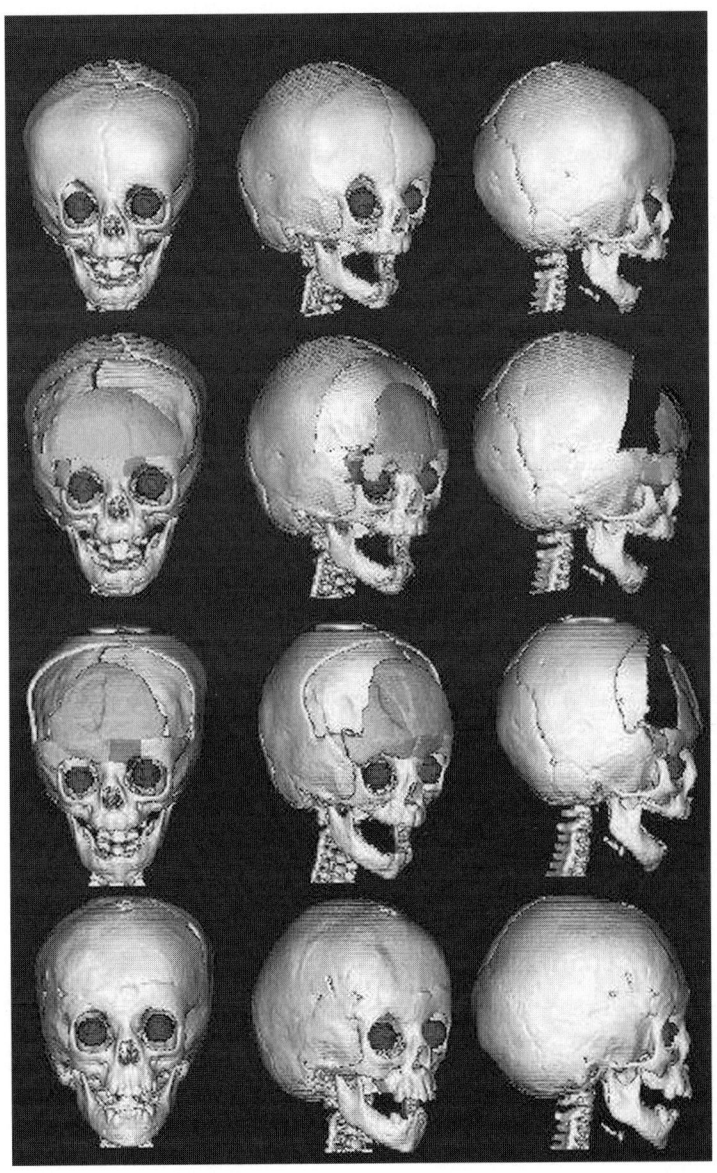

11.3% on the left. The volume of the right orbital cavity was 93% of the corresponding volume on the left side.

The surgical plan included removal of the fused suture, right frontal bone advancement and recontouring, left frontal bone recession and recontouring, right superior orbital rim recontouring and movement ventrally and caudally, mesial left supraorbital bandeau recontouring, and bone graft placement at the pterion to maintain the advancement of the right superolateral orbital rim.

Surgical simulation (Figure 22.4) began with bifrontal osteotomy including both coronal sutures, leaving 1 cm height of supraorbital bandeau in situ. The right superior orbital rim was separated from the right orbit and recontoured so that its shape was changed to make the mesial segment rotate 22 degrees ventrally, the middle segment 16 degrees ventrally, and the lateral segment 10 degrees dorsally along the z-axis for a net relocation of the rim dorsally 6 degrees in the midportion and 26 degrees at the lateral portion. The recontoured right superior orbital rim was then displaced ventrally, 10 mm at the midorbit and caudally, 3 mm medially and laterally. The resultant gap at the pterion was filled with a 10 mm wide calvarial self-retained bone graft. The medial aspect of the left supraorbital bandeau was bent ventrally (6 degrees in z-axis). The fused suture was excised from the frontal bone, and partial craniectomy was performed. The remaining frontal was replaced to produce a new frontal contour.

The simulation approximated the actual operative results well. The two differed in the amount of rotation of the supraorbital bandeau and the curvature of the frontal bone–bandeau unit. One year postoperatively the volume of the right orbit was 96% of that of the left orbit, and the volume of the right globe outside the orbit was 14.0%, as compared to 13.3% on the left (Figure 22.4). The preoperative orbital asymmetry had been normalized both in the simulation and in reality.

22.3.5.3 Case 3: Craniofrontanasal Dysplasia with Unilateral Cleft Lip/Palate (Tessier Cleft No. 3-11)

A 9-year-old boy was evaluated for asymmetric hypertelorism and residual cleft lip/palate deformities. Coronal strip craniectomy and partial cleft repair had been performed elsewhere. His craniofacial physical examination was remarkable for brachycephaly, hypertelorism, left proptosis, strabismus, maxillary left lateral lingual crossbite, anterior open bite, residual cleft lip and nasal deformities, and an anterior palatal fistula. The medial canthus to midsagittal line was 35 mm on the left and 25 mm on the right. The interpupillary distance in central conjugate gaze was 80 mm. Preoperative three-dimensional CT reformations documented partially reossified coronal craniectomies, a broad flat forehead, nasion recession with an obtuse nasofrontal angle, recessed supraorbital rims, hypertelorism, laterally rotated orbits, left proptosis, an anterior maxillary cleft, medial displacement

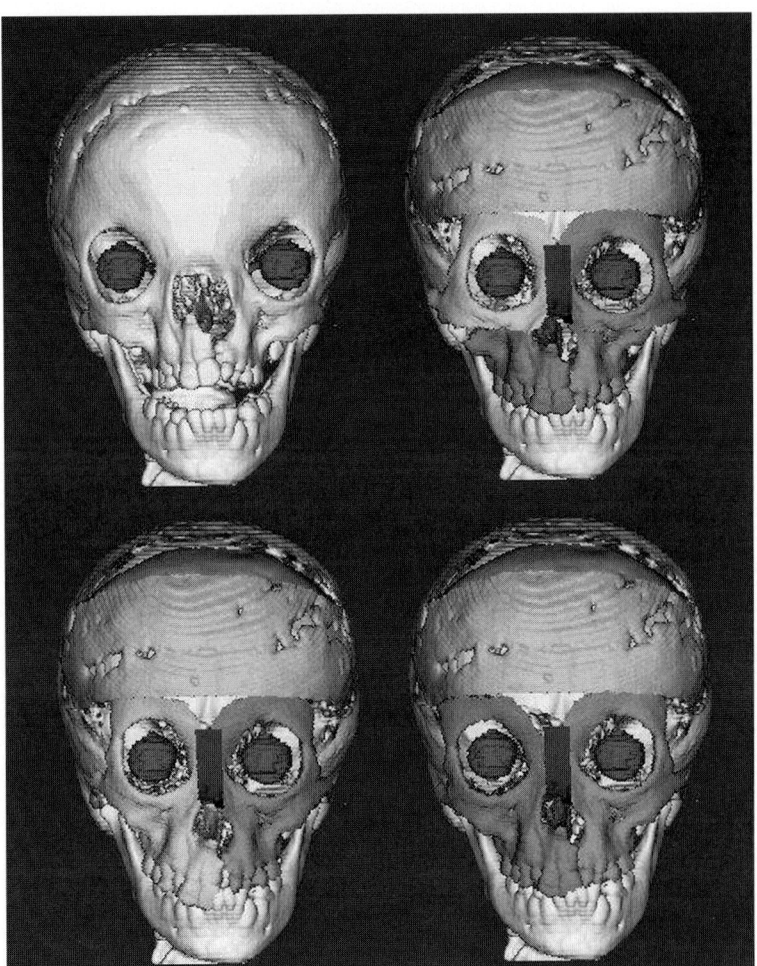

FIGURE 22.5 This case summary illustrates simulation of three possible surgical solutions for hypertelorism and unilateral facial cleft in a 9-year-old boy. (Top left) Preoperative reformation. Note anterior open bite and maxillary arch collapse in addition to asymmetric hypertelorism with malrotated orbits. (Top right) Preferred surgical simulation and actual operation performed with independent movement of each orbit and hemimaxilla. (Bottom left) Facial bipartition optimized for orbital position. Note unsatisfactory occlusion. (Bottom right) Facial bipartition optimized for occlusion. Note unsatisfactory position and rotation of the right orbit with persistent asymmetric hypertelorism.

of the left hemimaxilla, and premature contact of the molars, producing an anterior open bite. The preoperative bony interorbital distance was 41 mm, compared with a mean normal of 22.2 mm for age.

The classical solution for this constellation of anomalies is a facial bipartition [17,18]. This was attempted by surgical simulation (Figure 22.5). It was not possible to optimize both the orbital position and the dental occlusion. If the orbits were optimized, the right hemimaxilla would be displaced caudally and laterally with respect to the mandibular teeth. If the occlusion were optimized, the right orbit would be displaced and rotated laterally. Therefore, it was decided to move each orbit and each hemimaxilla independently to achieve optimal positioning of each.

The selected surgical plan included bilateral frontal craniotomy, arcuate segmentation of the frontal bone with anterior-posterior exchange of the segments, nasion craniectomy, bilateral independent "useful" orbit osteotomies, [19] bilateral independent high LeFort I type maxillary osteotomies, expansion and rotation of the maxillary alveolar arch with closure of the cleft gap, posterior maxillary impaction to close the anterior open bite, and nasal dorsum bone grafting (Figure 22.6).

The simulation well approximated the actual operative results. The interorbital distance on the postoperative scan was 21.7 mm, which compares favorably with 21.6 mm in the simulation. The most striking difference between the simulation and the actual postoperative result is the location of the ocular globes within the orbits. Whereas the simulation produced centrally located globes equidistant from all orbital walls, the actual globes were against the lateral rims with increased space between the globe and the medial and superior orbital rims.

22.4 INTRAOPERATIVE NAVIGATION

While the architect's blueprint specifies the builder's goal, there is nothing intrinsic to this specification that will assure that this goal is realized. Analogously, the ability to precisely plan surgery using computer-aided techniques does not confer a concomitant ability to execute the plan in the operating room. Computers can facilitate the transfer of the plan to the operative field.

Systems based upon frameless stereotaxy (i.e., surgical navigation systems) are increasingly used in craniofacial surgery. There are several applications for these guidance systems. Prominent among these is visualization of abnormal anatomy in areas where surgical exposure is limited such as in intraorbital dissection or decompression of the optic nerve [20]. These systems also are used to localize structures that need to be resected, as in the case of access to cranial base tumors and the removal of osteomyelitic bone. Similarly, these systems can also guide the identification of embedded foreign bodies. These systems have also been used to optimize the position of the globe during procedures that alter the intraorbital

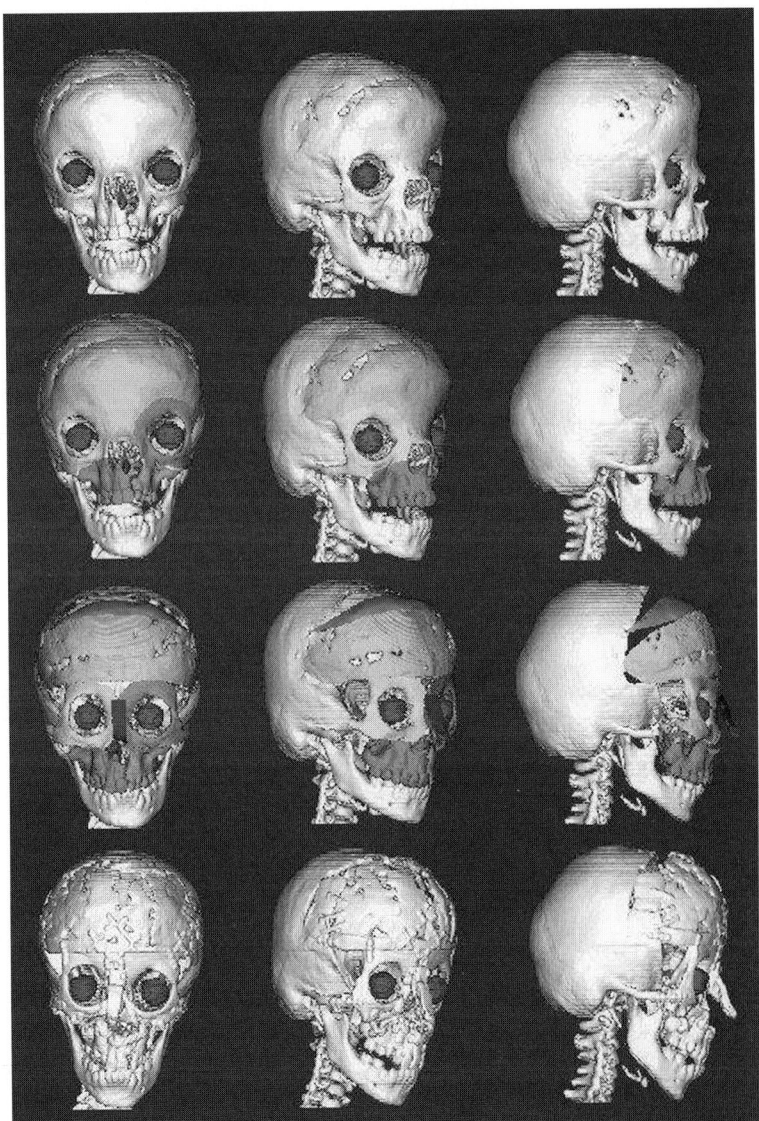

FIGURE 22.6 This case summary illustrates simulation and verification of correction of the frontal, orbital, and maxillary deformities. (Top row) Preoperative reformations. Note left proptosis. The interorbital distance is 41 mm. (Second row) Surgical plan. Independent frontal, orbital, and maxillary units are selected for simulated movement. (Third row) Surgical simulation of the preferred plan. Note correction of hypertelorism, orbital symmetry, and normalization of the occlusion. A nasal bone graft is indicated. (Bottom row) Actual postoperative result (CT scan 3 months postoperatively). Although there is good skeletal congruence between the simulation and the actual outcome, the true globe position is asymmetric with lateral displacement within both orbits.

volume in order to obtain symmetry with the undisturbed side. Unfortunately, increased operative time has been reported with these systems.

Frameless stereotaxy systems utilize a preoperatively acquired three-dimensional image volume, which is then correlated with the patient position on the operating table and with the position of a probe within the operative field. A computer, typically located on a cart in the operating room, is loaded with the patient's preoperative images and linked to position-sensing equipment that is able to map the movement of a probe to the patient's preoperative images in real time. Several technologies accomplish the positional sensing. Each technological approach has its advantages and disadvantages. In electromechanical tracking, the system incorporates a multijointed articulated arm that is rigidly attached to the operating table. A surgical probe is attached to the end of the articulated arm, which allows six degrees of freedom in motion. Some authors have concluded that the arm can be a hindrance to the range of the surgeon's motion [21]. An alternative technology involves the use of infrared light-emitting diodes (LEDs) mounted to the probe instrument. These optical systems require the maintenance of a clear line of sight between the LED arrays and the overhead camera apparatus so that the camera can "see" the LEDs and provide positional information. Some authors have noted that the overhead camera apparatus, which is mounted on a boom, can be cumbersome, especially in a crowded operating room. Also, in certain circumstances in which the surgery is within a narrow cavity, the wound itself may block the LEDs and prevent instrument tracking [20].

In all surgical navigation systems, the probe must be registered to the position of the patient's head and then correlated to the images on the computer. This process, known as registration, requires point mapping between known points on the patient's head and the corresponding points in the preoperative imaging volume [22]. Surface fiducial markers may be glued onto the patient's skin before the scan. These same points can then be used in the OR for registration. Obviously, it is critical that these markers not be moved or removed before surgery. Bone-anchored fiducial markers are the most accurate registration point, but they are obviously cumbersome. Alternatively, anatomical landmarks may also serve as fiducial points. Finally, in contour-map registration, the computer calculates a surface contour from a series of random points on the patient's face and head and then matches this contour to the surface of preoperative imaging volume. Automatic registration, which requires a special headset at the time of the preoperative imaging and during surgery, is less useful for craniofacial surgery since the headset can interfere with access to the craniofacial skeleton and the patient's underlying craniofacial anomaly may interfere with the accurate placement of these headset devices.

All available frameless stereotaxy systems are based upon preoperative images; therefore, the accuracy of the system degrades as the surgical procedure alters the patient's anatomy. In the realm of craniofacial surgery, where multiple osteotomies are often made, with resulting large shifts in the segments, such degradation becomes particularly relevant. Until it becomes possible to update the preoperative CT data intraoperatively, standard localization still requires the surgeon to have a depth of anatomical and surgical experience to allow safe interpolation between the preoperative images and the intraoperative alterations. Intraoperative CT scanners may permit the acquisition of updated CT images for use during intraoperative surgical navigation.

In order to track the position of mobile bone fragments, a minimum of three noncollinear fiducial markers must be placed on each mobile fragment. If these markers were placed before the segment is mobilized, then the fiducial markers can be reliably tracked in order to provide information about the translations and rotations necessary to accomplish a preoperatively determined goal position for the fragment. One such system utilizes custom infrared LEDs that are affixed to the osteotomized bone segment with Kirschner wires [23].

22.5 FINAL COMMENTS

Craniofacial surgery and computer-aided surgery technology have matured in parallel. In order to reduce the stigmata and functional compromise of craniofacial deformities, craniofacial surgeons must first deconstruct and then reconstruct the hard and soft tissues of the head. This process requires detailed anatomical information. Postprocessing of digital CT scan data, which yields 3D surface-rendered and volume-rendered images, provides such anatomical detail in formats that surgeons may readily interpret and apply. The resultant images facilitate diagnosis, surgical planning, operative execution, and postoperative evaluation as well as physician and patient education. The surgical challenges for the craniofacial surgeon do not have animal models and occur infrequently in humans. It currently almost takes a surgeon's career to develop the depth of knowledge and experience to perform such operations safely, efficiently, and accurately. Computer-aided surgical education offers the promise of easing the learning curve through computerized anatomical libraries and surgical simulators.

REFERENCES

1. Salyer KE, Bardach J. Atlas of Craniofacial Surgery. Philadelphia: Lippincott-Raven, 1999.
2. Association NEM. Digital Imaging and Communications in Medicine (DICOM). 1996.
3. Deibel S, Greenes R. Radiology systems architecture. Radiol Clin North Am 1996; 34(3):681–696.
4. Robb RA. Biomedical Imaging, Visualization, and Analysis. New York: John Wiley & Sons, 1999.
5. Chang SC, Liao YF, Hung LM, Tseng CS, Hsu JH, Chen JK. Prefabricated implants or grafts with reverse models of three-dimensional mirror-image templates for recon-

struction of craniofacial abnormalities. Plast Reconstr Surg 1999; 104(5):1413–1418.
6. Petzold R, Zeilhofer H, Kalender W. Rapid prototyping technology in medicine-basics and applications. Comput Med Imaging Graphics 1999; 23(5):277–284.
7. Cutting C, Bookstein FL, Grayson B, Fellingham L, McCarthy JG. Three-dimensional computer-assisted design of craniofacial surgical procedures: optimization and interaction with cephalometric and CT-based models. Plast Reconstr Surg 1986; 77(6):877–887.
8. Altobelli DE, Kikinis R, Mulliken JB, Cline H, Lorensen W, Jolesz F. Computer-assisted three-dimensional planning in craniofacial surgery. Plast Reconstr Surg 1993; 92(4):576–585; discussion 586–587.
9. Waitzman AA, Posnick JC, Armstrong DC. Craniofacial skeletal measurements based on computed tomography: Part II. Normal values and growth trends. Cleft Palate J 1992; 29:118.
10. Farkas LG. Anthropometry of the Head and Face in Medicine. New York: Elsevier, 1981.
11. Feingold M, Bossert WH. Normal values for selected physical parameters: An aid to syndrome delineation. Birth Defects 1974; 5(13).
12. Hansman CF. Growth of interorbital distance and skull thickness as observed in roentgenographic measurements. Radiology 1966; 86:87.
13. Abbott AH, Netherway DJ, Moore MH, David DJ. Normal Intracranial Volume. VIIIth International Congress of the International Society of Craniofacial Surgery, Taipei, Taiwan, 1999.
14. Teschner M, Girod S, Girod B. Optimization approaches for soft-tissue prediction in craniofacial surgery simulation. In: Taylor C, Colchester A, eds. MICCAI '99. Cambridge, UK: Springer, 1999:1183–1190.
15. Schutyser F, Van Cleynenbreugel J, Schoenaers J, Marchal G, Suetens P. A simulation environment for maxillofacial surgery including soft tissue implications. In: Taylor C, Colchester A, eds. MICCAI '99. Cambridge, UK: Springer, 1999:1211–1217.
16. Lo LJ, Marsh JL, Vannier MW, Patel VV. Craniofacial computer-assisted surgical planning and simulation. Clin Plast Surg. 1994; 21(4):501–516.
17. Tessier P. Facial bipartition: a concept more than a procedure. In: Marchac D, ed. Berlin: Springer-Verlag, 1987:217–245.
18. Van der Muelen JC. Medial faciotomy. Br J Plast Surg. 1979; 32:339.
19. Tessier P, Guiot G, Derome P. Orbital hypertelorism. Scand J Plast Surg. 1973; 7:39.
20. Demianczuk AN, Antonyshyn OM. Application of a three-dimensional intraoperative navigational system in craniofacial surgery. J Craniofac Surg 1997; 8(4):290–297.
21. Hassfeld S, Muhling J. Navigation in maxillofacial and craniofacial surgery. Comput Aided Surg 1998; 3(4):183–187.
22. Hassfeld S, Muehling J, Wirtz CR, Knauth M, Lutze T, Schulz HJ. Intraoperative guidance in maxillofacial and craniofacial surgery. Proc Inst Mech Eng [H] 1997; 211(4):277–283.
23. Cutting C, Grayson B, McCarthy JG, et al. A virtual reality system for bone fragment positioning in multisegment craniofacial surgical procedures. Plast Reconstr Surg 1998; 102(7):2436–2443.

23

Computer-Aided Soft Tissue Surgery

Joseph M. Rosen, M.D.
*Dartmouth-Hitchcock Medical Center, Lebanon,
and Dartmouth College, Hanover, New Hampshire*

Marcus K. Simpson
Dartmouth College, Hanover, New Hampshire

23.1 INTRODUCTION

Plastic surgery is a field of medicine that is especially dependent on the ability of the surgeon to plan for his cases. The earliest efforts to create models for soft tissue surgery began several centuries ago. Although it is a common procedure today, nasal reconstruction was one of the most complicated surgical procedures performed during the early days of surgery. In India a leaf was used as a template for the forehead flap that was designed for the reconstruction of the nose. Eventually, surgeons moved to clay as the choice of material for modeling the nose, and the Russian surgeon Limberg created an advanced model for nasal reconstruction during the first half of the twentieth century [1]. Limberg's templates contained multiple types of materials; his paper templates were used to geometrically model the flap and to study the three-dimensional distortion caused by the removal of the forehead flap tissue. By attempting to incorporate mathematical models into plastic and reconstructive surgery, Limberg stands as one of the first surgeons to attempt to simulate the consequences of geometric manipulation on living tissue. However, Limberg found that the few available materials could not accurately simulate the properties of skin and underlying tissue. He perhaps envisioned a time when modeling techniques and applications would ubiquitously assist physicians in planning and simulating their more complex procedures. Though many hurdles have yet to be overcome, we are closer today than ever before to realizing Limberg's vision in soft tissue surgery. The development of complex modeling, data fusion, and virtual reality systems will empower today's and tomorrow's physicians.

In this chapter we will explore the present state of computer-aided surgery (CAS) applications in soft tissue surgery and project potential future developments. Section 23.2 will address the specific challenges of CAS in soft-tissue surgery. Section 23.3 will explore the benefits of CAS in this field and will detail state-of-the-art applications and techniques. Patient-specific models have been used in our institution, Dartmouth Hitchcock Medical Center, for a variety of applications. We have chosen three different etiologies and facial areas for examples in this chapter. We have used these patient-specific models to help plan surgeries for defects created by congenital anomalies, tumors, and trauma. In Section 23.4 we will present our vision for CAS in the future by detailing key forthcoming technologies.

23.2 SURGICAL CHALLENGES AND CAS SOLUTIONS

Shortly after the introduction of the computer, physicians recognized the applications of modeling human tissues. Up until the past decade, while computational power may have been adequate for complex modeling, the mathematical models describing the motion and properties of human tissue had not yet been developed. Additionally, the equations defining skin and soft tissue were too large for all but the most powerful of machines. Recently, both of these impediments are dwindling, and today we are closer than ever before to creating simulations that accurately behave like human skin, muscle, and bone. The field of surgical simulation is a vast one with applications in medical training, preoperative planning, telesurgery, and many other areas. The ultimate progression of surgical simulation technology will incorporate enhanced visualization and proprioception of a completely immersed virtual reality display. Wearing a pair of electronic gloves and a specialized helmet called a head-mounted display (HMD), the surgeon of tomorrow will be able to see and feel the reconstructed nose described above. He will decide among multiple options by performing the reconstruction in a virtual operating environment and studying the results of tissue change. Figure 23.1 presents this technology as it would be applied to a nasal reconstruction.

Improvements in decision making and simulation technologies in medicine have moved together throughout the development of the most modern CAS techniques. The computer has long been used as an expert system to aid the physician

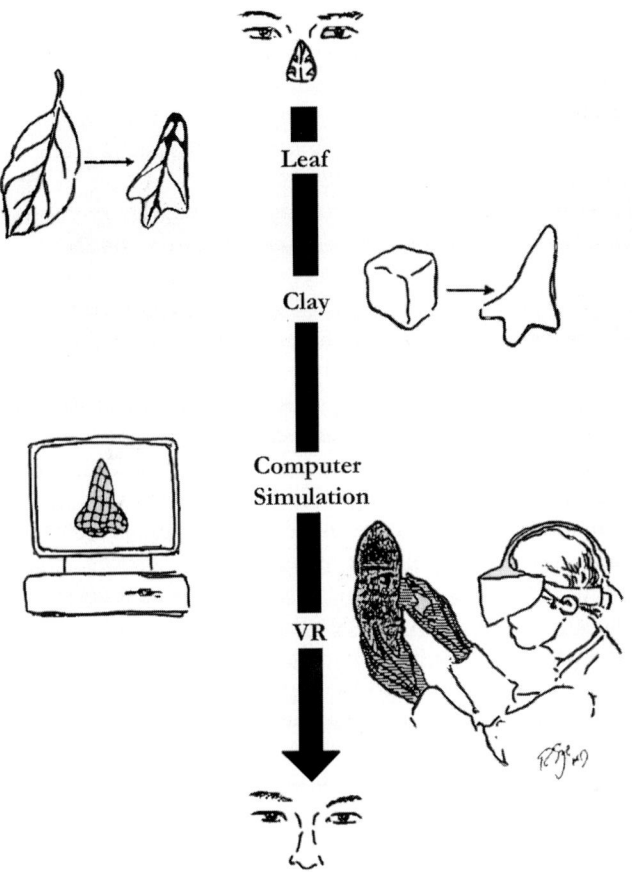

FIGURE 23.1 The history of planning for nasal reconstruction begins with a leaf template, progresses through clay modeling and computer-based simulation, and ultimately ends with virtual reality. (From Ref. 32.)

in decision making. An expert system is an algorithm or flowchart that summarizes an expert's approach to a certain problem. The computer then takes the form of an interactive textbook by providing multiple approaches to specific problems. The computer will present predetermined case histories, and the outcomes to these cases can be compared. The user is able to select from a menu of possible actions and images. Based on the entered information the system will present a prediction of the outcome on the chosen procedure. Importantly, the expert system can be almost infinite in its knowledge databases through the use of networking technologies. Outcomes of all cases with the same initial conditions can be stored in its databases. The rhinoplasty simulator developed by Constantian et al. is an elegant example of an expert system [2]. Movement of tissue in this program affects a down-line of responses on associated tissues. The system presents known case histories and images that apply and suggest a number of possible outcomes. From this information, the surgeon is more equipped to make the best decision for the patient.

Expert systems are currently used for a variety of different applications, including rhinoplasties, mid-face advancements, and mandibular osteotomies, among others [3]. The computer herein displays two-dimensional (2D) images that have been digitally retouched or painted by the surgeon or operator. This graphical system has no incorporated data on the physical properties of the tissue. Such systems rely on the ability of the surgeon to predict the outcome of his planned procedure through photo retouching. One can recognize the insufficiencies of systems that fail to incorporate models of tissue change.

A major accomplishment in the field of CAS was the development of reformatted CT/MR data. By this method, CT/MR imaging scans are digitized and reformatted by a computer using graphic rendering techniques to construct three-dimensional (3D) models. What is significant here is the fact that the models are patient-specific; the total model incorporates combined data. First-generation models of this sort were rigid and limited. Though good for procedures like bone reconstruction, these models lacked wide utility [2]. What soft tissue modeling needed was the ability to position tissue in one area and observe the response from another area. To accomplish this goal, the computer requires a model of the physical properties of tissues involved. To analyze relative mechanical responses to certain surgical procedures, the patient model must be designed to accurately account for patient tissue at each location of the body.

Current medical imaging technologies, including computed tomography (CT), magnetic resonance imaging (MRI), and positron emission tomography (PET), are all encoded volumetrically such that the spatial reference frame of the scan is independent of the patient. However, these imaging technologies fail to incorporate information as to how each element of tissue connects and interacts with other elements of tissue; herein lies the shortcoming of these scans. A partial solution to this problem was developed by Pieper and Chen, who designed a simulation system for soft tissue plastic surgery [4–10]. Recognizing the need of the surgeon to approximate responses to change and also properties of skin, muscle, and bone, they created CAPS, a software package for computer-aided plastic surgery. This system is based upon the formation of a finite element mesh (FEM) in which each segment of the face is divided into regions called elements. These complex geometric elements are linked such that their movements together approximate that of the original tissue. Each element is defined by the boundaries that it shares with other elements representing tissues.

CAPS uses a 3D model of the human face with FEM overlaid soft tissue to estimate the results of tissue ablation and rearrangement. First, a video scan of the face is performed that records skin color and cylindrical coordinates. The program converts the cylindrical coordinates to rectangular coordinates, which allows the surgeon to manipulate the image from any external point. A FEM is then constructed and the surface is color mapped accordingly. A skin stiffness matrix is referenced to integrate the strain and distortion this reconstruction produces on the skin soft tissue. An algorithm for the displacement data then constructs the CAPS predicted outcome. The surgeon views the 3D model on a computer screen and is able to cut, excise, create flaps, and rearrange tissues as the procedure requires. The computer incorporates the changes to the model and using the FEM shows the results on the tissue overall. The surgeon is able to visualize how excision of the lesion affects all areas of the face. The user designates simple approximation or a double Z-plasty rhomboid-to-W closure [5–11].

CAPS and other systems like it have great utility in facial plastic and reconstructive surgery. In addition to planning and simulating multiple types of tissue rearrangements, several other goals are achieved. Notably, the surgeon can choose among several types of flaps and incision plans to least affect the patient's appearance and expressions. The patient is able to see how the surgery may change his appearance, which may reduce miscommunication and patient anxiety. Future CAPS systems may incorporate algorithms for tissue aging to yield more true results several years postoperatively. Though these algorithms have a long way to go before adequacy, CAPS is one of the best examples of soft-tissue patient-specific modeling systems available. Eventually, we envision this type of system to be used preoperatively and postoperatively for surgical planning and analysis.

Several state-of-the-art augmented reality (AR) systems allow for the joining of real and virtual data in the operating room. In AR, virtual patient information is fused with real patient data via a process called "data fusion." There are numerous potential applications of AR systems in otolaryngology. In the clinical setting (such as the operating room), the surgeon employing AR must wear special glasses or a HMD so that the CT and MRI data appear superimposed on the area of interest. This type of system has been used to visualize a fetus in a woman's abdomen prior to operation. Novice surgeons may have difficulty visualizing organs in 3D, and this technology adds dimensionality and a frame of reference to different types of visualization [12].

A plastic surgeon may choose to superimpose a nasal reconstruction procedure plan directly onto the patient's skin. The computer software incorporates general principles of tissue change, including elasticity of different tissues, and then it can project how movement of a particular tissue area on the face will affect other tissue areas. In this way, the computer may offer guidance to the physician in his surgical plan. The ability of the computer to compute mathematical relationships of tissue movement will enhance the surgeon's abilities. An AR system for neurosurgeons allows for CT or MRI imaging of a brain tumor to be transformed into a 3D image and superimposed on the patient's head to help plan the skin incision and bone flap approach. The surgeon may then use the program in the operating room as a reference map to help assess the surgical margins.

In 1993, Performance Machines, an integrated approach for the AR in the operating room, was introduced. The Performance Machines system superimposed the patient-specific imaging data on the living patient in real time in the operating room. The registration of patient and dataset were done through an optical tracking system. When using this device, the surgeon must wear a HMD virtual reality helmet, or a display may be mounted upon a boom within the view of the surgeon. A combination of real patient images, mathematical models, and patient-specific imaging data, as well as procedure-specific cues and flags, would be projected within the surgeon's perspective. During a tumor resection, Performance Machines gives the surgeon the ability to see through a tumor. This would allow the surgeon during a tumor resection to look through the tumor to see critical structures behind the tumor, such as a carotid artery, optic nerve, etc., and to avoid them. The patient-specific model is dynamic so that if the soft tissue moved, then the tumor within the soft tissue can be readjusted to predict its new position. Functional outcomes, including the motion of the jaw, may be predicted during the actual procedure.

Several medical robotic systems that are currently available are likely to gain additional applications in many new areas. Robotics are useful for calibration and the elimination of tremor. Surgical robotics also may perform tasks that are beyond the capabilities of human hands. Plastic and reconstructive surgeons will use robotic technologies to enhance and broaden their skills in numerous surgical procedures. ORTHODOC is a hip replacement surgery robotic system that helps the surgeon plan the operation in three dimensions [13]. The computer system takes a special CT of the hip after implanting three bone screws as reference points. ORTHODOC then gives instructions to a robot that forms the cavity using the screws for guidance. This system drills consistently with more precision that any human hand can. The surgeon may stop the robot at any point and revert to customary procedure as the operative field is in full view. Traditionally, the size and type of implants for hip replacement have been determined by overlaying templates on x-ray scans [14]. ORTHODOC and robotic systems like it reduce the margin of error in determining orthopedic implant sizing and types. The concept behind ORTHODOC may be applied to other surgical challenges. The reconstructive surgeon is frequently confronted by cases involving complex traumatic fractures of the craniomaxillofacial skeleton. For surgical reduction of these fractures, the surgeon must not only determine how to reconstruct a particular bone structure, but also choose among available fragments and donor sites. Robotic

Computer-Aided Soft Tissue Surgery

systems will enhance the ability of plastic surgeons to reattach bone fragments, and in more delicate procedures robots themselves may perform procedures semi-autonomously or even autonomously. Undeniably, robots will enhance the abilities of surgeons by performing actions outside the abilities of human hands.

Otorhinolaryngology–head and neck surgery is unique in that it encompasses a wide range of medical fields, including trauma, complex reconstructive surgery, elective surgery, complex tissue rearrangement, and other fields. Soft tissue surgery is an area of medicine that is especially enhanced by the ability of the surgeon to plan his cases. Reconstructive plastic surgeons are often faced with highly complex cases. The remedies for these cases require the collaborative efforts of surgeons from multiple specialties for the determination of the best course of treatment for the patient. It is crucially important that surgeons have the capacity to plan for these cases. Ideally, surgical planning would include surgical simulation. The various CAS technologies described in this section represent typical examples of CAS-based solutions for critical surgical challenges.

The goal of this technology is the prediction of surgical outcomes. As mathematical models improve, they should be better able to predict the response of skin, soft tissue, muscle, and joints to various procedures. Virtual reality simulators can now predict the mechanical outcomes of some musculoskeletal procedures. Similar computer-based information systems for other procedures involving the head and neck region would also be desirable.

23.3 CAS APPLICATIONS

At Dartmouth Hitchcock Medical Center, we have used patient-specific models for a variety of applications. We have chosen three unique cases, which have distinct etiologies for the facial deformity. In addition, each case focuses upon a specific facial area. We shall discuss how state-of-the-art modeling and simulation technologies in congenital anomalies, tumors, and trauma have helped us to plan for complex surgical cases. For each case, we will discuss how CAS enhanced traditional preoperative planning. These cases illustrate that CAS can help surgeons achieve specific goals in soft tissue surgery with more precision and confidence than previously possible.

23.3.1 Congenital Anomalies

In the case of congenital anomalies, we have used patient-specific modeling for microtia, cleft lip repair, and other more rare anomalies (such as craniosynostosis). In these cases, it was possible to predict the outcomes of surgery using complex mathematical models. The patient-specific models allow the surgeon to compare several different lip repairs in a given patient before the actual surgical procedure commences.

Microtia, which is a particularly interesting congenital anomaly, demonstrates computer-based modeling technologies in a direct clinical application. The technique developed over the years has been to use rib cartilage to create a framework that is placed under the skin in the first stage. The framework and skin are then elevated at the second stage. The lobule and concha reconstruction are either done at additional stages or combined with the first two.

Traditionally, a cast of the opposite ear has served as a planning guide for the reconstruction. Unfortunately, this technique is often inadequate for the reconstruction of a mirror image of the normal ear. Recently, a computer-based system has been used to scan the normal ear; this data may then serve to create a model of the intact, normal ear. Then the computer software may segment the cartilage independently from the skin in this model and subsequently create a true mirror image. This gives us a far more exact model of the ear we wish to create. The data set comprising the 3D model may guide the manufacture of a physical model of the missing ear and a physical model of the cartilage framework of that ear (Figure 23.2). In the past, surgeons would have carved a balsa wood model of the missing framework and then used this wood model to guide the construction of a rib cartilage framework. Obviously, these models—whether carved balsa wood or machine-milled material—serve the same purpose, that is, to approximate the creation of the cartilaginous framework from rib cartilage. Of course, the machine-milled models are more precise than other alternatives.

23.3.2 Tumors

Computer-aided soft tissue surgery using patient-specific models also has applications in the reconstruction of defects that result from the surgical excision of benign and malignant neoplasms as well as trauma. In this case, the CAS-derived approach was used to form the reconstruction of bone and soft tissue defects caused by the removal of a recurrent dermatofibrosarcoma protuberans.

In this case the tumor involved the left side of the forehead, the eyebrow, and the glabella area. The model helped to predict the size of the defect after the resection of the tumor, and during the subsequent reconstruction it was possible to compare the tumor side with contralateral, normal side (Figure 23.3). Since this was a recurrent lesion, the ipsilateral side was distorted by both the recurrent neoplasm and the first surgical excision. The contralateral side formed a template for the reconstruction. The computer simply created a mirror image of the unaffected side.

With the aid of the patient-specific anatomically mapped model, one may predict the size of the defect and plan the best donor site for a free tissue transfer. Often these procedures must be staged. In this example, the initial reconstruction

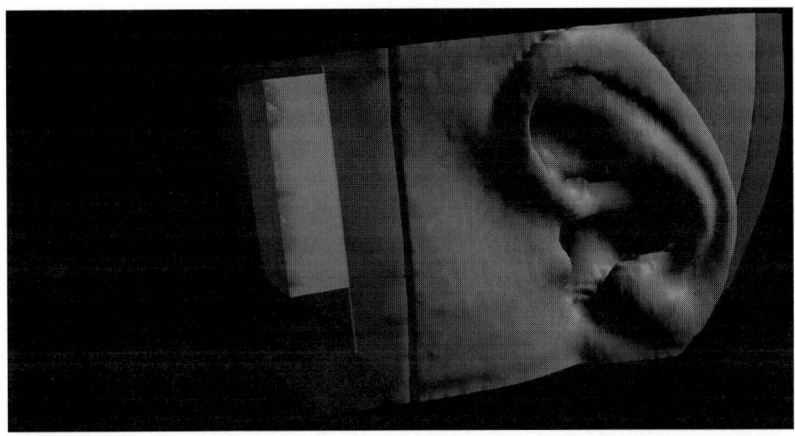

(A)

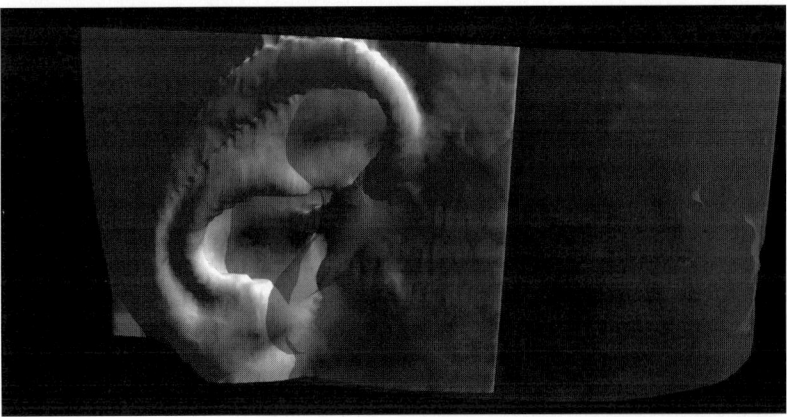

(B)

FIGURE 23.2 Computer-based imaging technology may be used to reconstruct an external auricle for the correction of microtia. (A) A patient-specific 3D model of the normal ear is shown. (B) The mirror image of the normal ear has been created by the computer from the imaging data from the normal side. (Copyright 2000 Medical Media Systems, Inc. with permission.)

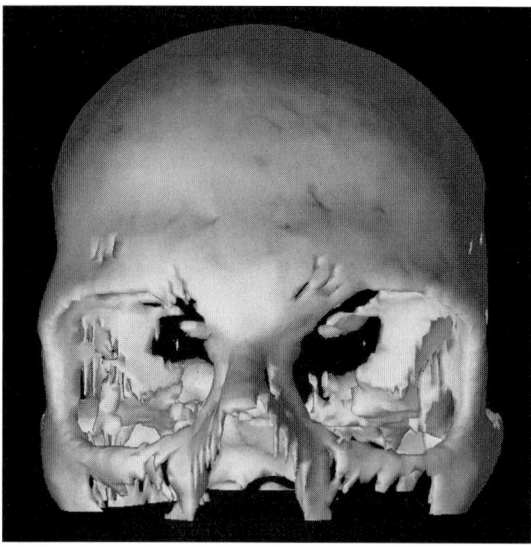

(A)

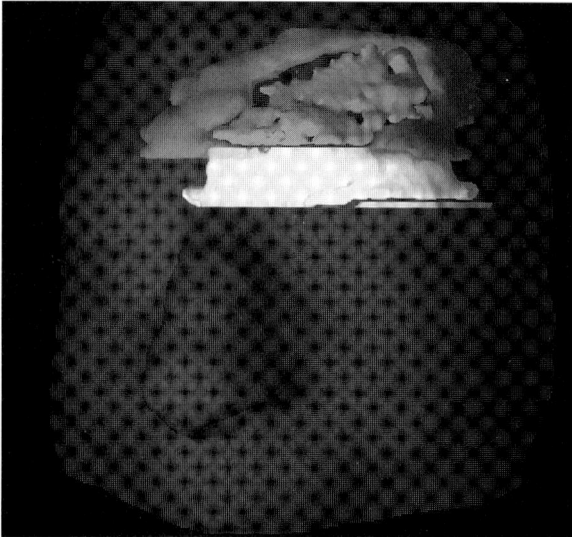

(B)

FIGURE 23.3 Preoperative modeling of tumor boundaries as well as adjacent tissues may guide intraoperative tumor resection and reconstruction. (A) The skull model depicts the underlying bony anatomy. (B) The imaging data was reformatted by the computer to present the tumor, resection margins, and the patient's overlying soft tissue. (Copyright 2000 Medical Media Systems, Inc. with permission.)

used a lateral arm flap; later an eyebrow reconstruction, which involved tissue transfer from the contralateral brow was performed.

23.3.3 Trauma

The deformities that result from head and neck trauma are among the most challenging. In this example, a patient sustained a facial gunshot wound, which caused extensive destruction of the tissues of the left cheek, skin, muscle, body of mandible, and mucosal lining, as well as secondary ankylosis of the ipsilateral temporo-mandibular. A 3D model was created at the CAS workstation for surgical planning (Figure 23.4).

The reconstruction of this type of defect requires a composite flap encompassing bone, muscle, soft tissue bulk, and skin. A vascularized free tissue transfer of iliac crest bone with adjacent muscle and soft tissue can make possible the appropriate combination of tissue types for successful reconstruction. A computer-generated, patient-specific model can help the preoperative planning of this reconstruction.

This complex reconstruction may be termed a multiplex flap, since multiple tissue types share a single blood supply through a single vascular connection (see Ref. 15). In this case, the multiplex flap provides intraoral lining, bony reconstruction, soft tissue bulk, and facial motor function. The flap also serves to release the temporomandibular ankylosis. The bony part of the reconstruction can even support the placement of osteo-integrated dental appliances, whose introduction requires a second delayed procedure. From a soft-tissue perspective, the flap's soft tissue must replace the entire ipsilateral cheek cosmetic unit. A computer-generated mirror image based upon the contralateral side can provide information about what is missing on the traumatized side.

23.4 FUTURE DEVELOPMENTS

The changes in medicine afforded by computer technologies over the next decade will be nothing short of revolutionary. Herein, we will present a vision for the future of CAS. The applications of virtual reality and its associated components in medicine are numerous and not specific to head and neck surgery. We will describe how these technologies will enhance the surgeon's ability with respect to the cases previously discussed. Presently, computational power is great enough to handle the tasks of accurately modeling change in human skin, muscle, and bone. Virtual reality (VR) encompasses a number of surgical research topics, including computer graphics, imaging, visualization, simulation, datafusion, and telemedicine. All of these areas are essential for our proposed vision.

Imagine a patient who requires a complex operation for the removal of a cancerous mass in the left cheek. The surgeon faces more than several critical

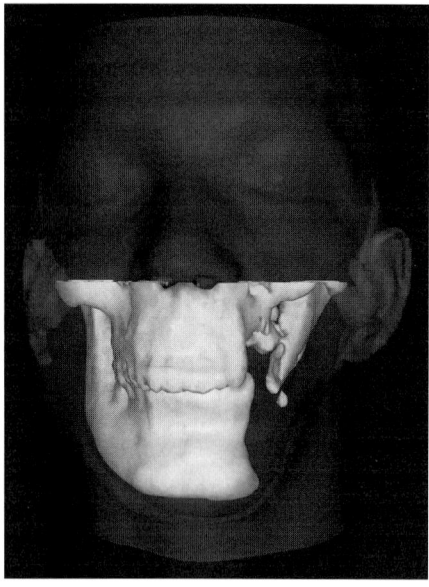

(A)

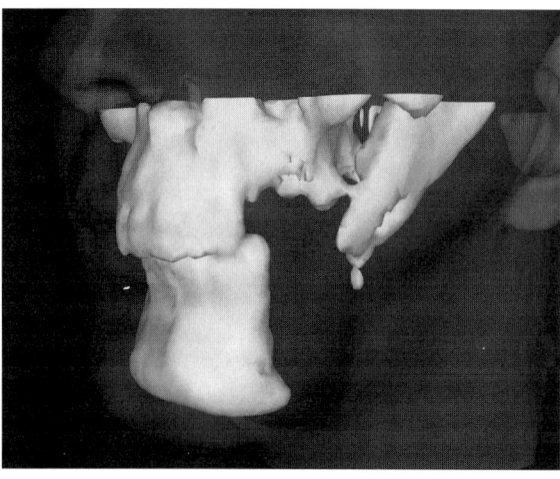

(B)

FIGURE 23.4 Computer-aided modeling can present three-dimensional information about complex traumatic deformities. (A) The model highlights the missing mandibular segment. (B) The model has been manipulated so that a close-up view of the defect is shown. (Copyright 2000 Medical Media Systems, Inc. with permission.)

decisions. Reconstruction options include the choice of donor site, tissue types (i.e., bone, muscle, skin, etc.), postoperative rehabilitation, and follow-up protocols. Of course, the surgeon wishes to select the ideal option at each treatment point so that the optimal outcome is assured for the patient. Thus, for a surgery involving multiple decisions, numerous outcomes, all of which have a great personal impact on the patient, are possible. A better approach is necessary. A potential solution stems from work done by Mann in the 1960s [16].

Mann's vision was to create a virtual patient-specific model of the patient, procedure, prostheses, and rehabilitation. Operating within a virtual environment, the physician would pursue several different alternatives approaches. The patient would then undergo rehabilitation for a period of several years. The physician would subsequently analyze the model to determine which surgical procedure would lead to the best outcome. Once this was accomplished, the surgeon could choose which complex procedure should be performed in reality and carry it out [17]. The first steps toward this vision have been realized. Further research needs to be done in a number of areas that will be described below.

To realize the above vision, several hurdles need to be crossed. Most importantly, a precise and specific patient model needs to be developed so that it accurately represents the anatomy and physiology of the particular patient. While current patient-specific models may be used for sizing and preoperative and intraoperative planning, these models cannot presently demonstrate tissue change over time. The ideal virtual model needs to incorporate a wealth of data about the patient, including both normal anatomy and pathology as well. If the patient suffers from a degenerative disease, the model must also incorporate information about how surrounding tissues are changing irrespective of the course of operations chosen. It is even more difficult to predict wound healing and subsequent rehabilitation. Software presently exists that simulates some of these processes; additional mathematically based modeling paradigms need to be developed so that outcomes in all of these parameters can be predicted.

At a minimum, surgical simulators must fulfill three specifications [18]. Following from the above, the first need is for an accurate and comprehensive virtual human model. Ultrasonography (USG), CT, and MRI provide two-dimensional imaging that may be manipulated by volumetric mathematical computation to provide an anatomically accurate patient-specific 3D model; however, even this is not enough. A fourth dimension, showing function and predicted healing operative parameters, must be added. More than simply accurate enhanced visualization, true simulation requires solving the hard questions of tissue change, function, healing, etc. Second, surgeons require accurate and convincing virtual instrumentation and tools. True reproduction of the sense of touch is an incredibly difficult task, since touch encompasses proprioception, vibration, texture, temperature, kinesthesia, and pressure. To perform surgery in a virtual environment the surgeon must have accurate feedback for incising and detecting abnormal tissue. Additionally, virtual instrumentation and tracking are required as well. The third requirement is that the virtual environment have demonstrable effectiveness in terms of outcomes, surgeon's acceptance, and physician teaching in a cost-effective way. A virtual environment system consists of the operator, the display interface, and the computer simulator. The user must feel completely immersed within the computer representation for acceptance in the medical fields. True surgical simulators must reflect all of these features.

In order to anticipate future developments, it is important to assess the current situation. Patient-specific, anatomically mapped models provide our departure point. To expand the utility of these models, they need to incorporate the parameters of tissue change. Currently, the surgeon can visualize patient-specific morphology in three dimensions. In addition, there is some ability to fuse imaging data intraoperatively with real tissues through data fusion protocols. Yet what is ultimately needed is the ability to simulate soft tissue change over time before, during, and after the procedure. Work at several institutions has begun to provide solutions for this challenge.

The National Library of Medicine (NLM) has sponsored The Visible Human Project, which has yielded complete, anatomically detailed, three-dimensional representations of the normal male and female human bodies. In this effort, transverse CT and MRI were performed on a representative male and a representative female cadaver, which were then cryo-sectioned at 1 mm and 1/3 mm intervals, respectively [19,20]. These data support the reconstruction of models that are the most accurate of all available models.

The VR human model requires accurate patient-specific data to be mapped to the tissue, organ, system, and body region from CT, MRI, and USG imaging. This requires volumetric encoding with reference to an absolute reference frame independent and exterior to the patient. Mathematical algorithms can define a finite element mesh. This allows a computer to model how distortion of one set of elements will affect a second. The behavior of tissues and organ systems over time is an important future research question [21]. This information must then be incorporated into the mathematical algorithms that underlie FEM.

Surgeons require precise virtual instrumentation for VR to be widely applied to medicine. Many of the virtual tools for the user interface are available today. Current systems include the MIT Newman Laboratory joystick, which simulates forces on an instrument while held in the user's hand [22]. However, the conversion of texture from the 3D virtual model to actual touch perception is presently a research challenge. Microelectromechanical systems (MEMS) employ computer chip fabrication technology with mechanical components to create miniature sensors for pressure, acceleration, and fluid flow. By combining computer chip technology with sensors and actuators, MEMS promises future progress as more mechanical functions can be matched to advances in mirocomputing.

This should be expected to impact future haptic research [23]. These force feedback devices transform information from the virtual patient model into a realistic sense of touch to the surgeon. Alhough these devices have improved recently, they lack the resolution needed for a surgeon to fully experience and learn from operating in a virtual world.

Many instruments in the operating room need to be tracked by the virtual environment. These instruments can then provide accurate guidance during the actual surgical procedure. For instance, a surgical probe may show a green indicator light when the tip of the probe has reached its intended target, but the indicator light would shine a red signal at all other times. Similarly, this system could also show trajectory information. If the angle or position of the probe shifted from the planned trajectory, the probe would not display the green indicator light. This approach can also work to signal to the surgeon the proximity of certain structures. For example, during tumor ablation procedures, the instrument's indicator would show a red light as the boundaries of the planned ablation are approached. In this way, adjacent normal tissues may be spared unnecessary trauma. In addition, the instrument may be attached to a robotic arm that is programmed to increase resistance to movement as certain predefined boundaries are approached.

Tracking of instruments may be done with real-time imaging and processing (such as x-ray fluoroscopy or USG); alternatively, external sensors may be attached to instruments. Optical, electromagnetic, and ultrasonic sensors can provide continuous spatial localization. This technology is useful in compensating for human limitations of hand positioning (approximately 200 µm), intention tremor, and eye saccade motion [24]. The Hunter telepresence system for ophthamological surgery tracts the motion of the eye such that 1 cm of hand motion equals 10 µm of laser movement. Video images magnify retinal vessels to the size of fingers and digital signal processing and filtering remove hand tremor. By using these techniques, the accuracy is improved from 200 to 10 µm. The ophthalmologist will calibrate his movements such that he can target single retinal cells. Additionally, because the patient-specific data is accurately represented in a virtual environment, any sort of data, including but not limited to added visualization keys, surgical plans, and various operative data, can be fused in that environment.

Finally, the need for true-to-life virtual operating environments must be addressed. The University of Illinois has developed the CAVE system in which 3D images are projected in an 8 foot cubic room that permits physicians to walk between images. Holographic imaging is another area of investigation [25]. In theory, this type of environment may serve as a virtual meeting place in which surgeons from multiple locations may join in virtual space to perform a difficult operation. Although this approach is now possible, the resolution of these sense of touch and vision is still limited. It must be emphasized that the detail necessary in touch is unique to surgery. On the other hand, the vision component is being actively addressed in other industrial fields. Additionally, the resolution of HMDs is currently nearing television-like quality [2]. Several institutions are researching alternative visual systems. Moreover, other research efforts are pursuing a virtual operating tray, from which a surgeon can choose virtual instruments used to manipulate and repair soft tissue and bone trauma [26].

Initial efforts in the construction of models focused on accurate reproduction of structures of interest. Even virtual models emphasize this type of accuracy. However, all of these models are merely static. True virtual reality in medicine must be four dimensional; that is, the models must also incorporate tissues changes as function of time. Current haptic interface technologies primarily sense pressure; for virtual reality, they must also convey greater dimensionality. Furthermore, the user interfaces for these systems must be optimized so that surgeons may effectively employ them in the clinical setting. Finally, virtual environments should also support collaboration among multiple physicians, even if they are separated by great distances.

The technological advances that are driving CAS are also changing the means of communication among physicians. By using electronic information and communication technologies, surgeons can practice at a distance from the patient [21]. Local practitioners may be able to coordinate care with distant clinicians to improve decision making for patients. In addition, long-distance medicine and VR will change the way that surgeons maintain their credentials and obtain new skills.

A surgeon may use telemedicine capabilities in numerous ways. Telesurgical clinics in remote or poor areas may consult with colleagues anywhere in the world via a global communication network. Currently, this system includes a high-resolution digital camera and a desktop personal communicator. Local physicians can then summarize relevant clinical information, including images, and send this clinical report to consultants via e-mail worldwide. The consultation is routed to the appropriate physician, who then initiates correspondence and provides expert advice on how to treat the patient. In this way, physicians may draw upon clinical resources that are not locally available. Although many institutions have constructed high bandwidth networks for telemedicine, such network capacity is limited in more remote areas. As a result, real-time video transmission is not practical. Similarly, operating remotely via robotic surgery systems is not yet possible, since the available bandwidth (cable or satellite) is not fast enough to accommodate the delay from the movement of the surgeon's hand to the robotic arm operating on the patient. Consequently, the low bandwidth solution, based on sequential asynchronous e-mails, has emerged as a viable alternative. E-mail communications, coupled with digital photography, create a means for low-cost telementoring and teleconsultation and can improve decision making. In this way the expertise of a tertiary referral center can influence the quality of care on a worldwide scale.

Eventually, telesurgery will allow surgeons from multiple locations to reunite in one virtual operating space. Consider the case of a patient with a large lesion that covers almost all of her left cheek. The operative team removes the lesion quickly and then reconstructs the defect. A real model, based on high-resolution preoperative imaging, will support preoperative planning. Such models ultimately will permit the visualization of blood vessels and tissue flaps in virtual space, although that objective has not yet been realized. The creation of multiple surgical plans will yield the optimal choice for the specific case. Postoperative results will also be predicted with complex mathematical algorithms, which model complex tissue interactions over time. During the procedure, the operating surgeon may call upon several experts from remote sites for consultation via live video. Eventually, consultants at distant sites may join the operative team in a virtual operating environment. The presence of the consultant surgeon will be manifest through robotic arms that exactly carry out movements initiated by the consultant at a distant location. In this manner, technology will enable surgeons to operate in multiple spaces at one time.

A number of U.S. clinics make use of real-time video transmission for telementoring. An experienced plastic surgeon may remotely telementor a colleague through a complex trauma case requiring immediate attention. Surgeons have evaluated and certified skills of a student surgeon for laparoscopic hernia repairs and other teaching situations [27]. The future of VR for training and procedural testing starts with the categorization of surgical procedures into the components of skills, knowledge items, tasks and subtasks. VR can make this educational process lifelike, variable, and real time capable.

The application of VR in the clinical setting faces some important limitations. First, it is too difficult to simulate the complexity of an entire surgical procedure. The specific situations where VR is most helpful have not been defined. Many questions regarding licensing requirements for practicing medicine with telesurgery technologies, have not been answered. Technological failures and crashes are inevitable, and backup plans must consider possible communication breakdown. The performance of surgery from sites remote from the operating room is limited by current technological capacity, since data transmission over 200 miles via cable or over 50 miles via wireless systems produces sufficient lag-time delays that produce unacceptable effects on coordination. Similarly, satellite transmission produces similar lag-time effects and cannot be used for this specific application.

VR is predicted to very soon play a critical role in credentialing surgeons [27,28]. With its power to allow training and testing in any procedure, it will serve as an objective tool to measure competence, just as it is used in the airline industry. It will offer the additional advantage of avoiding the use of animal laboratories or patients to improve surgical skills [29]. VR for teaching and credentialing is an important area for further research. Flight simulators are cost-effective and proven means to train pilots and maintain skills. This technology is now aiding medicine and surgery to train and assess professional skills [30]. There has been mounting concern that traditional continuing medical education (CME) courses that utilize didactic lectures do not improve physician performance. Interactive CME, alone, or combined with traditional didactic instruction, allows an opportunity to practice skills and can change physician performance [31]. VR will become the natural progression of these methods for teaching and CME. With the SRI System (SRI International, Menlo Park, CA), the surgeon views a 3D image from a minimally invasive procedure, which portrays organs and instruments as if the operative field was fully open. The surgeon sits at a console, in or outside the operating suite, while an assistant stays with the patient and receives tactile feedback from the instrument tips. A number of animal procedures have also been demonstrated; they include gastrostomy and closure, gastric resection, bowel anastomosis, liver laceration suture, liver lobe resection, splenectomy, aortic graft replacement, and arteriotomy repair [21]. Thus, it is clear that VR will play a critical role in various medical applications.

Younger surgeons will be more adept at learning these technologies than their more senior colleagues. Learning laparoscopic or endoscopic surgery requires a decoupling of the oculo-vestibular axis from the tactile-proprioceptive axis so that the surgeon may manipulate the controls or instruments. Younger surgeons tend to be more capable of making this switch due to their experiences with video games and computers.

23.5. CONCLUSION

The critical steps to realizing the vision presented in this chapter involve significant development in the fields of human models, interface devices, and system verification. Human modeling poses the greatest challenge, since it will require several generations of improved computer mathematical algorithms to accurately represent normal tissues and pathological conditions as well as the changes in normal and pathological tissues as a function of time. Interface tools, whether haptic or visual, will continue to evolve with the help of many industries that also require improving this technology. For system verification, the ability of VR systems to reproduce the perception of true reality must be conclusively demonstrated and the positive impact of CAS-based surgical planning and VR-derived educational experiences must be objectively confirmed. System verification is, of course, necessary for widespread adoption of these technologies by practicing surgeons.

Mathematical modeling of complex tissue interactions will dramatically alter the practice of medicine over the next 50 years. The software that results from better computational paradigms that can predict tissue interactions and outcomes will improve the diagnostic processes and therapeutic processes of health care. A generalized approach that creates a flexible model of the human body will let us superimpose information from various sources on a model of a specific patient. Ultimately, we will attain a higher standard of patient care through these advanced technologies.

The specific applications of CAS presented in this chapter are just the beginning. In the not-so-distant future, surgeons will be able to predict the outcome of therapies for a given patient, rather than predict the outcome based upon accumulated data from other patients in the population. This approach will ultimately lead to patient-specific therapies that provide a greater likelihood of success with a lower risk of morbidity.

Note: Although we have illustrated these cases with a few figures, the true beauty of these methods is the ability to manipulate the patient data set on a computer in an interactive way. We can provide to interested readers these data sets on a CD that supports interaction between the data and user (contact Joseph.Rosen@hitchcock.org). In this way, readers can better understand the value of this approach.

REFERENCES

1. Limberg AA. The Planning of Local Plastic Operations on the Body Surface: Theory and Practice. DC Heath and Company, Lexington, MA, 1984.
2. Constantian MB, Entrenpries, C., Sheen JH. The expert teaching system: a new method for learning rhinoplasty using interactive computer graphics. *Plast Reconstr Surg* 79:278, 1987.
3. Mattison RC. Facial video image processing: standard facial image capturing, software modification, development of a surgical plan, and comparison of pre-surgical and post surgical results. Ann Plast Surg 29:385, 1992.
4. Chen DT, Zelter D. Pump it up: computer animation of a biomechanically based model of muscle using the finite element method. Comput Graphics 26:89–98, 1992.
5. Pieper S. More than skin deep. Unpublished master's thesis. Massachusetts Institute of Technology, Cambridge, MA, 1989.
6. Pieper S. CAPS: computer aided plastic surgery. Unpublished thesis. Massachusetts Institute of Technology, Cambridge, MA, 1992.
7. Pieper S, Rosen J, Zeltzer D. Interactive graphics for plastic surgery: a task-level analysis and implementation. In 1992 Symposium on Interactive 3D Graphics. ACM, New York, 1992.
8. Pieper S, Chen D, et al. Surgical simulation: from computer-aided design to computer aided surgery. In Proceedings of Imaging. Monaco, OCM, 1992.
9. Pieper S, McKenna M, Chen D. Computer animation for minimally invasive surgery:

computer system requirements and preferred implementations. In SSPIE: Stereoscopic Displays and Virtual Reality Systems—The Engineering Reality of Virtual Reality. SPIE, Bellingham, WA, 1994.
10. Pieper SD, Laub DR, Jr, Rosen JM. A finite-element facial model for simulating plastic surgery. Plast Reconstr Surg, 96(5):1100–1105, 1995.
11. Pieper SD, Delp S, Rosen JM, Fisher S. A virtual environment system for simulation of leg surgery. In SPIE—The International Society for Optical Engineering, Stereoscopic Displays and Applications II. SPIE, Bellingham, WA, 1991.
12. Fuchs H, Livingston MA, Raskar R, et al. Augmented reality visualization for laparoscopic surgery. In First International Conference on Medical Image Computing and Computer-Assisted Intervention (MICCAI '98). Massachusetts Institute of Technology, Cambridge, MA, 1998.
13. DiGioia AJ, Jaramaz B, Colgan BD. Computer assisted orthopedic surgery. Clin Orthop, 354(Sept):8–16, 1998.
14. DiGioia AJ, Jaramaz B, Colgan BD. Computer assisted orthopedic surgery. Clin Orthop 354(Sept):8–16, 1998.
15. Rosen JM. Advanced surgical techniques for plastic and reconstructive surgery. Comput Otolaryngol 31(2):357–367, 1998.
16. Mann R. The evaluation and simulation of mobility aids for the blind. In Rotterdam Mobility Research Conference. American Foundation for the Blind, New York, 1965.
17. Mann R. Computer-aided surgery. In Proceedings of RESNA 8th Annual Conference. Rehabilitation Engineering Society of North America, Bethesda, MD, 1985.
18. Delp S. Surgery simulation: Using computer graphics models to study the biomechanical consequences of musculoskeletal reconstructions. In Proceedings of NSF Workshop on Computer-Assisted Surgery. National Science Foundation, Biomedical Engineering Section and the Robotics and Machine Intelligence Program. Washington, DC, 1993.
19. The Visible Human Project. National Library of Medicine, 1999. http://www.nlm.nih.gov/research/visible/visible_human.html.
20. Ackerman M. Accessing the visible human project of the National Library of Medicine. D-Lib Magazine, 1995.
21. Satava R. Cybersurgery: Advanced Technologies for Surgical Practice. Wiley-Liss, Inc., New York, 1998.
22. Adelstein BR, Rosen JM. Design and implementation of a force reflecting manipulandum for manual control research. In ASME 1992: Advances in Robotics, DSC, 1992, pp. 1–12.
23. Madhani A, Niemeyer G, Salisbury JK. The Black Falcon: a teleoperated surgical instrument for minimally invasive surgery. In Int. Conf. on Intelligent Robots and Systems (IROS), Victoria, B.C., Canada, 1998.
24. Satava RM. Virtual reality surgical simulator: the first steps. Surg Endosc, 7(3):203–205, 1993.
25. Fakespace Systems announces industry first: a fully reconfigurable display system for immersive visualization. 1999. http://www.fakespace.com/press/101599.html.
26. Madhani A. Design of teleoperated surgical instruments for minimally invasive surgery. In Mechanical Engineering. Massachusetts Institute of Technology, Cambridge, MA, 1997.

27. Krummel TM. Surgical simulation and virtual reality: the coming revolution [editorial]. Ann Surg, 228(5):635–637, 1998
28. Raibert M. Surgical certification using virtual reality. 1996
29. Bodily K. Surgeons and technology: presidential address. Am J Surg 177(5):351–353, 1999.
30. Isenberg SB, McGaghie WC, Hart IR, et al. Simulation technology for health care professional skills training and assessment. JAMA, 282(9):861–866, 1999.
31. Davis D, Thomson O'Brien MA, Freemantle N, et al. Impact of formal continuing medical education. JAMA 282(9):867–874, 1999.
32. Rosen JM. Virtual reality and plastic surgery. Adv Plast Reconstr Surg 13:33–47, 1996.

24

Computer-Aided Reduction of Maxillofacial Fractures

Mimi S. Kokoska, M.D.
Indiana University School of Medicine, Indianapolis, Indiana

Martin J. Citardi, M.D., F.A.C.S.
Cleveland Clinic Foundation, Cleveland, Ohio

24.1 RATIONALE FOR COMPUTER-AIDED REDUCTION OF MAXILLOFACIAL FRACTURES

The goals of surgical reduction of maxillofacial fractures include restoration of skeletal structure, masticatory function, and craniomaxillofacial contour. During these procedures, the uninjured portion of the skeletal framework serves as a guide for the reduction. In addition, the surgeon's knowledge of normal anatomical relationships also provides critical information for the reduction. More complex fractures (i.e., bilateral fractures and/or those fractures with extensive comminution) often disrupt the craniomaxillofacial skeleton to the extent that the determination of normal craniomaxillofacial relationships is problematic. In these instances, the reconstructive surgeon must rely upon approximations that are little more than educated guesses.

Often access for surgical manipulation can be challenging. Recently, minimal access and endoscopic approaches have been developed to minimize soft tissue scarring [1,2]. These minimally invasive techniques are better suited for fractures that involve little bone loss and minimal comminution, since they rely heavily on normal adjacent facial skeleton for contouring. Traditional incisions and wide access approaches (such as bicoronal and gingivo-buccal incisions) allow visualization of a greater area of the facial skeleton in the immediate operative field; this enhanced access is essential to restoring contour in cases of segmental bone loss and/or severe comminution. Despite open access approaches in these complex cases, normal facial projection still may not be attained. Frequently, in cases of severe bilateral midface trauma, normal facial projection is not available for comparison, and even seasoned surgeons may note suboptimal outcomes in their patients, which may include varying degrees of hypesthesia, dystopia, enophthalmos, malocclusion, and asymmetrical malar projection [3]. Many of these unfavorable results are the result of poorly reduced or misaligned skeletal fragments. Failure to obtain optimal skeletal contour is likely due in part to the inability to confirm three-dimensional skeletal relationships and projection in relation to normal landmarks. In many instances, only a limited number of normal skeletal landmarks are available for reference. Even restoration of normal dental occlusion or normal ophthalmic projection does not necessarily ensure normal midface skeletal contour.

24.1.1 Characteristics of the Ideal Guidance System for Craniomaxillofacial Surgery

In patients with complicated fractures, additional guidance systems, which can guide and confirm the reduction, would greatly facilitate the restoration of normal skeletal anatomy. [It should be noted that the term ''guidance system'' does not refer specifically to computer-aided surgery (CAS); rather ''guidance systems'' include any technology, technique, and/or methodology that provides additional information about the operative reduction.] These guidances systems must accommodate traditional incisions and approaches as well as the newer minimally invasive techniques in order to be a practical alternative for intraoperative application. Guidance systems that are too cumbersome for efficient use of operative time or that prevent adequate access for reduction or instrumentation will not gain wide acceptance among practicing surgeons. It should be remembered that the reduction of skeletal segments frequently requires the exertion of strong forces on the bony fragments and skeleton. Of course, these forces can disrupt patient positioning. As a result, the guidance system must be able to maintain crucial system accuracy before, during, and after the application of external forces for reduction or osteotomies. Head-fixation devices, which may work well for sinus surgery or neurosurgery, may be rendered useless in craniomaxillofacial surgery, where stronger forces are frequently necessary to achieve surgical objectives.

This concept of a "guidance system" can reflect a variety of technologies and/or strategies. In this regard, craniomaxillofacial surgeons require additional means for assuring optimal surgical results. Over the past 10–15 years, CAS platforms have gained considerable acceptance for specific applications in sinus surgery, neurosurgery, and spine surgery. Although CAS has not been optimized for craniomaxillofacial applications, it holds tremendous promise in this area. The major limitation of today's CAS systems is that they provide information about the relative positions of the tips (functions that are useful during sinus surgery, neurosurgery and spine surgery); however, in craniomaxillofacial surgery, the objective of guidance systems is the verification of skeletal projection. The assessment of skeletal projection focuses upon the relative position of a given point, not its absolute position. To the extent that CAS does not provide this type of information, additional development is necessary. Nonetheless, CAS can provide useful information—even in its currently suboptimal form.

24.1.2 Computed Tomography Scan Issues in Computer-Aided Craniomaxillofacial Surgery

Recently, computed tomography scans have replaced plain film x-rays as the preoperative imaging modality of choice for midface fractures. Although two-dimensional plain x-rays are still obtained in the initial evaluation, CT scans with three-dimensional reconstruction are commonly obtained for preoperative planning. Three-dimensional CT scans offer more information regarding the degree of skeletal displacement and comminution and the volume of bone loss; such information is especially useful in cases of complex midface trauma [4]. Such bony detail is often lost in two-dimensional x-rays, in which the fractures or bone fragments may be superimposed (thereby obscuring skeletal relationships). Recently, helical CT scans have become readily available and are now preferred over earlier generations of scanners. Helical scanners, which generate images more quickly, decrease motion artifact in the resultant CT images. Minimal motion artifact is crucial in CT scans that will be utilized for three-dimensional image reconstruction. CAS systems also require optimal CT images with minimal artifact. In fact, any image artifact whatsoever may lead to erroneous image manipulation and reconstruction. Minor errors in interpretation of positional information could be exponentially multiplied if the CT scan data are artifactual.

Although CT scans provide detailed information about bony anatomy, CT scanners only offer stationary images that the surgeon still must interpret. During presurgical assessment and surgical planning, the surgeon must reconstruct the planar CT images into a mental three-dimensional model from which he or she extrapolates information to operative field. CAS can dramatically simplify this process. First, CAS permits three-dimensional image manipulation that was not available with traditional plain x-ray and CT films. In addition, the surgical navigation features of CAS permit a direct correlation of the preoperative imaging data with the intraoperative anatomy. The optimal setting for surgical navigation is a rigid structure—like the craniomaxillofacial skeleton. The firmness of skeletal bone permits localization of predetermined points on the bone with accuracy. Unlike soft tissues, which are easily deformed or stretched, the rigid skeleton is an ideal volume for surgical navigation for positional information and even projection information. In theory, specific modeling strategies can be crafted. For instance, virtual computer models can guide surgical planning, and intraoperative surgical navigation can guide the implementation of the resultant strategies. Similarly, computer-based systems can direct the creation of milled models that can be used during surgery. Virtual or milled models can be designed to achieve symmetry with the normal, untraumatized side (if available). In those instances where the injury is bilateral, archived normative data may guide the creation of these guides. Normative data also may be used for computer-aided cephalometric analysis (see Chapter 21).

24.2 CAS SYSTEMS

In general, CAS systems consist of a computer workstation, monitor, tracking system, and software tools. The workstation houses the patient's imaging data and facilitates data manipulation using specific software designed for this purpose. A high-resolution computer monitor displays the image and tracking data for use

---

24.1 Prior to intraoperative surgical navigation, registration, which functions as a calibration step, must be performed. Registration involves a correlation between corresponding points in the imaging data set and the operating field. In A, external fiducial markers, which have the appearance of small rings, were applied to the patient before her CT scan; during surgery, the surgeon touched each marker sequentially to complete the registration step (StealthStation, Medtronic Surgical Navigation Technologies, Louisville, CO). In this example, a Mayfield head holder secured the patient's head position, and the large cranial arc DRF (dynamic reference frame), which is attached to the Mayfield, provided a tracking reference for surgical navigation. This DRF, while appropriate for neurosurgical cases, is too cumbersome for craniomaxillofacial surgery. In B, the computer software has calculated a registration based upon the fiducial markers that were built into a special headset (SAVANT, CBYON, Palo Alto, CA). The computer then calculates localizations relative to this reference frame that was defined by the headset. Since the position of the frame relative to the patient is constant (that is, the frame only fits a patient's head in one way), these localizations show positions relative to the patient.

Computer-Aided Reduction of Maxillofacial Fractures

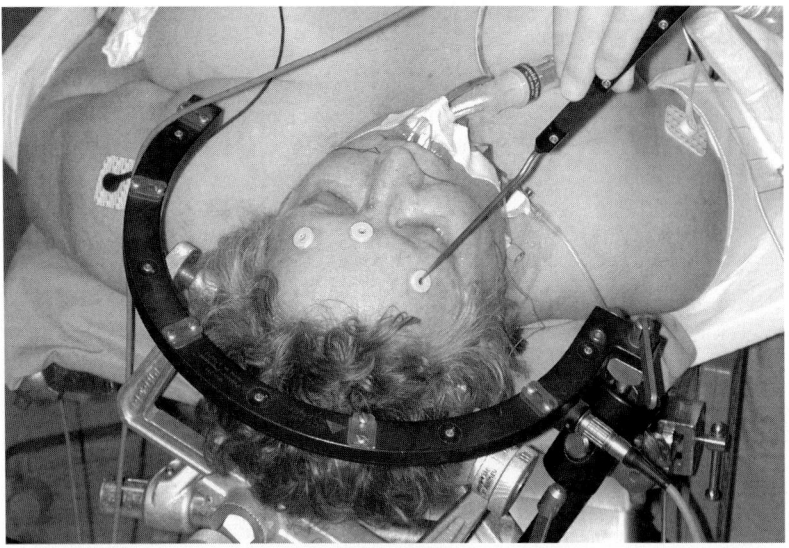

(A)

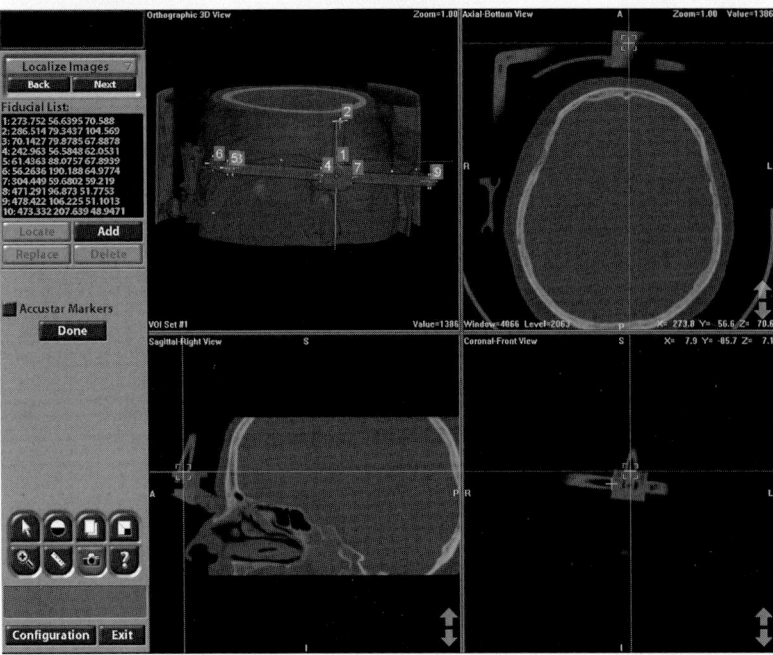

(B)

in the operating room. The tracking system allows the computer to track the position of the patient, fracture fragment(s), and surgical instruments in three-dimensional space.

Considerations of CAS usually focus upon the surgical navigation capabilities of these systems. After registration (a calibration step in which known points in the operative field are correlated with their corresponding points in the preoperative imaging data set volume) (Figure 24.1), the CAS computer provides specific localization information about the position of various surgical instruments in the operating field volume. Although this particular aspect of the technology is impressive, one must not overlook the other CAS features, which have potential uses in craniomaxillofacial surgery. The typical CAS computer processes a subject's thin-cut axial CT scans with coronal, sagittal, and three-dimensional reconstruction. The software tools assigns an x,y,z value to each unit volume in the preoperative imaging data set (Figure 24.2). The distance-measurement tools calculate the distance between specific points. The surgical planning tools project the instrument trajectory; during surgery, the actual trajectory of the instrument can be actively tracked and thereby compared to the planned trajectory. Three-

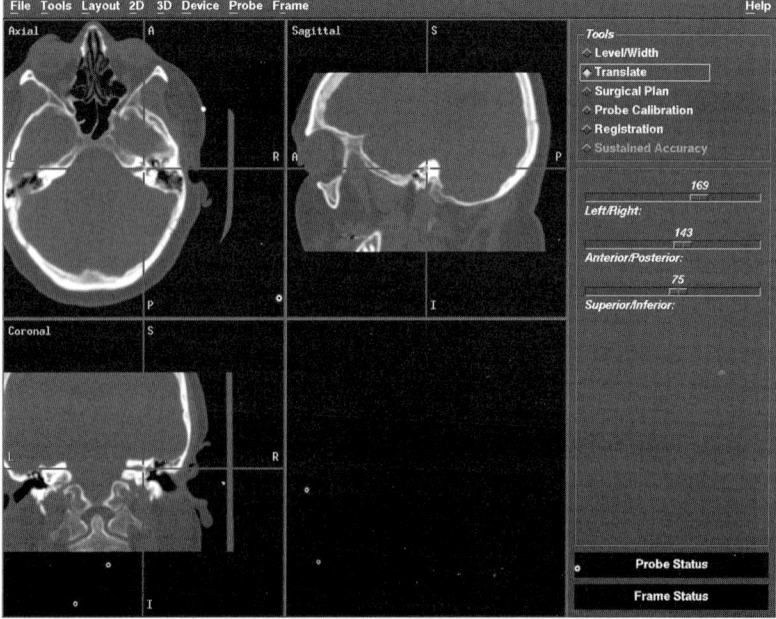

FIGURE 24.2 CAS systems assign x,y,z coordinates to points within the imaging data set volume. In the StealthStation 2.6.4 (Medtronic Surgical Navigation Technologies, Louisville, CO), these data are displayed as shown here.

Computer-Aided Reduction of Maxillofacial Fractures 449

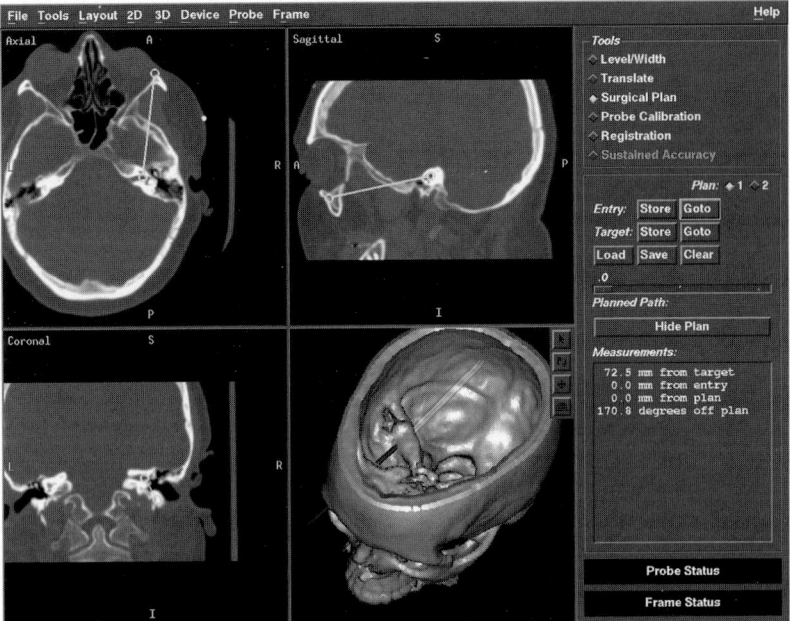

FIGURE 24.3 CAS surgical planning tools permit the calculation of distances between selected points as well as the calculation of a trajectory along these points. An example from the StealthStation 2.6.4 (Medtronic Surgical Navigation Technologies, Louisville, CO) is shown. It is important to realize that the trajectories depicted in each of the orthogonal CT scan views represent only the vector projection of the entire trajectory in that particular plane, not the actual trajectory. For instance, the trajectory shown on the axial CT is only the vector component of the total trajectory in the axial plane only. The sagittal and coronal images are similar.

dimensional models are created from preoperative imaging data. The intraoperative instrument guidance tool determines the position of the surgical instrument relative to the surgical plan. Finally, surgeons can simultaneously review images of the same relative point in all three orthogonal planes by scrolling through the image data set—providing maximal information about three-dimensional relationships from the image data (Figure 24.3). These features can be adapted to answer specific challenges in craniomaxillofacial surgery.

24.3 SPECIFIC TECHNIQUES

As described above, current CAS platforms have not been designed for craniomaxillofacial surgery, although they have been used during these procedures. In a similar fashion, prototype CAS systems have also been described for these procedures. As one reviews this area, it becomes apparent that these reports answer specific questions in the development of the ideal CAS system for craniomaxillofacial surgery, but that ideal system has not been developed yet. A brief summary of these efforts follows.

24.3.1 CAS-Based Comparison of Prereduction and Postreduction Projection

Only real clinical experiences can determine the true limitations of CAS for facial fracture reduction. As a result, CAS was used to measure prereduction and postreduction position of displaced frontozygomaticomaxillary fractures [5]. Although CAS surgical navigation has acceptable accuracy for sinus surgery, spine surgery, and neurosurgery, its practical accuracy during facial fracture reduction was unknown. Similarly, specific design limitations of CAS were also unknown.

Since maxillary or mandibular dentition is frequently available as a guide for adequate reduction of LeFort fractures and mandibular fractures, the need for CAS for these fractures is relatively small. Therefore, the application of CAS for these fractures is a lower priority. A displaced frontozygomaticomaxillary fracture was selected for this initial trial, since this fracture is representative of a displaced facial fracture in which the reduction relies on adjacent skeletal relationships, rather than dental occlusal relationships.

In this report, LandMarX 2.6.4 (Medtronic Xomed, Jacksonville, FL) was used to measure bilateral malar projection before and after reduction of a unilateral frontozygomaticomaxillary fracture. In this way, quantitative assessment of symmetry was achieved. Projection measurements were performed with the LandMarX distance-measuring tool, a standard software tool that is common in most CAS systems. In order to achieve meaningful measurements, a series of steps were necessary. First, the skull base reference points (SBRs) were defined as the right and left internal auditory canal transverse crest. The SBRs provide a frame of reference for all subsequent measurements. Next, a point on the malar surface was determined in the x,y,z coordinate system. Finally, the distance measuring tools were used to determine the distance between the right and left SBR and each malar surface point before and after fracture reduction. Comparisons before and after reduction provided information about the amount of reduction, and comparisons between sides provided information about symmetry. Transconjunctival, gingivobuccal, and frontozygomatic incisions were used for exposure at these sites during reduction. After initial fracture reduction was performed, the new coordinates for the malar points were recorded. In addition, the new distances from these new coordinates to the SBR points were measured. These measurements were then utilized to assess and adjust the fracture reduction. Then the measurements were repeated (Figure 24.4).

Computer-Aided Reduction of Maxillofacial Fractures 451

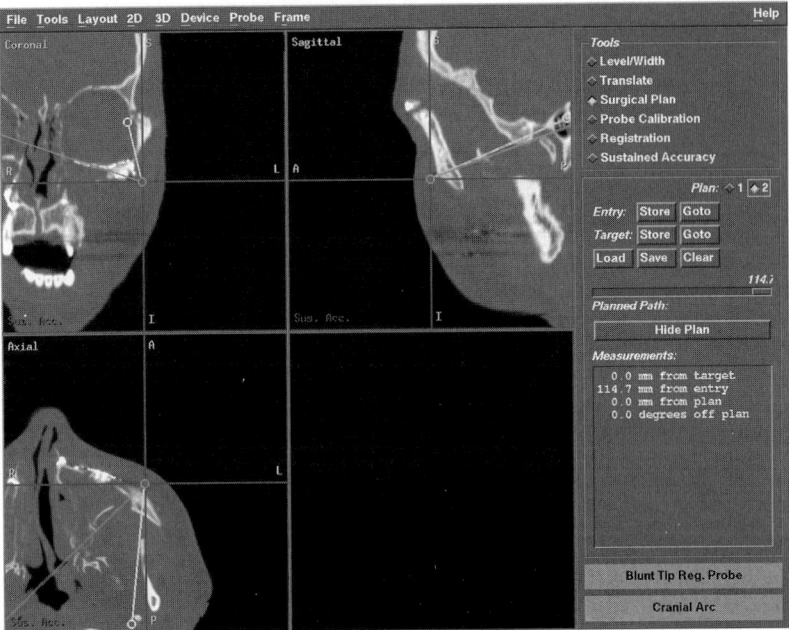

FIGURE 24.4 Intraoperatively CAS can track the projection of the bony midface by localization to specific points on the malar eminence outer surface and the subsequent calculation of distances from predefined skull base reference points. In this example from a revision reduction of a frontozygmaticomaxillary fracture, the surgical planning tools shows the trajectory and distance between the malar surface and the ipsilateral and contralateral skull base reference points, which were defined as the transverse crest at each internal auditory canal (LandMarX 2.6.4 Medtronic Xomed, Jacksonville, FL).

This project provided useful lessons in several regards. First, the LandMarX system was useful in confirming adequate malar projection in these subjects. In addition, it was observed that smaller dynamic reference frame (DRF) arrays can provide adequate spatial orientation for surgical navigation. In these cases, the smaller ENT or spine DRF was used in the place of the much larger cranial DRF (Figure 24.5). The smaller DRF is less bulky, but it gave a stable reference for optical tracking during the procedure. Since the DRF was screw-fixated to the outer calvarium via a small scalp incision, the surgical navigation was dynamic; that is, the tracking system automatically corrected for patient head movement, since the DRF was directly attached to the cranial skeleton. This DRF arrangement also minimized potential disruption of the DRF due to forces required for fracture reduction.

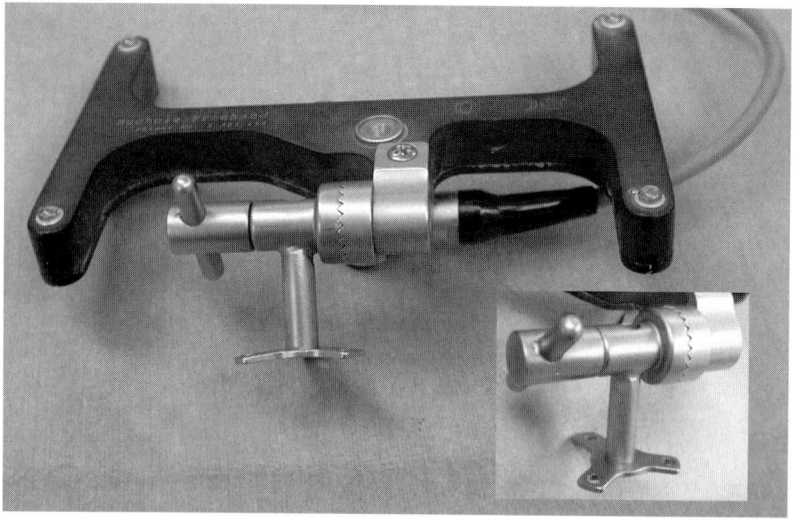

FIGURE 24.5 For surgical navigation, the CAS system must track the position of the operating field volume. This small dynamic reference frame (DRF) contains small light-emitting diodes (LEDs) that the CAS camera array recognizes (LandMarX 2.6.4 Medtronic Xomed, Jacksonville, FL). This DRF is attached to the skull base post (shown in the inset photo); during the surgery, the post is secured directly to patient's skull with monocortical bone screws.

24.3.2 Sequential Reduction of Frontozygomaticomaxillary Fractures

Since surgical navigation provides precise localization information, similar localization information may also guide fracture reduction. In this approach, preoperative modeling and planning determine the optimal positions of bone fragment(s), and intraoperatively, the bone fragment position is tracked as the fracture is reduced. Obviously, this strategy requires positioning of bone fragments, rather than the usual instruments. As already stated, current CAS systems do not provide information about projection and/or contour; however, relative projection and contour assessments may be derived from the point localizations. Furthermore, the CAS software distance-measuring tools can provide some quantitative data about projection from defined reference points (typically at the untraumatized skull base) through the localization points.

In order to test the applicability of these concepts, the sequential reduction of displaced frontozygomaticomaxillary fractures was performed on cadavers (Figure 24.6) [6]. The goals of this study included the development of techniques

Computer-Aided Reduction of Maxillofacial Fractures

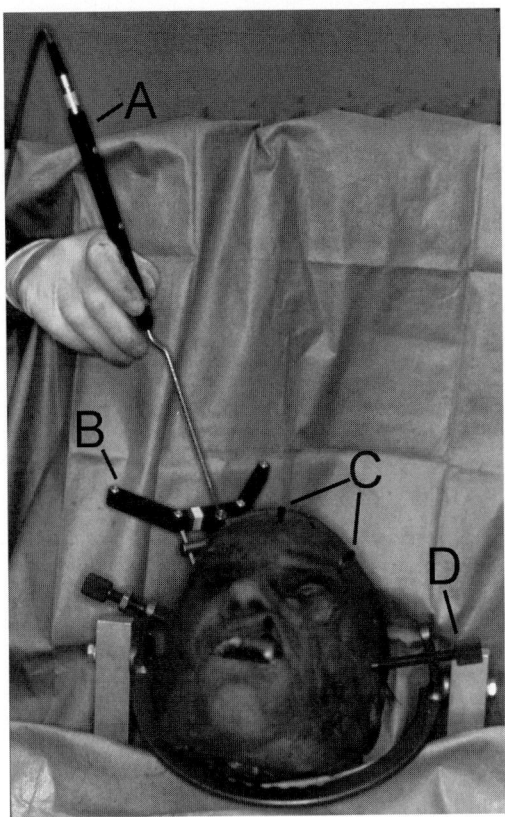

FIGURE 24.6 The photo summarizes the experimental setup for the sequential reduction of the frontozygomaticomaxillary fracture. The cadaver head was placed in a modified Mayfield head holder (D). The dynamic reference frame was secured directly to the skull. For probe calibration, the tracking probe or "localizer" (A) was placed in the calibration divot as shown. Registration was performed using bone-anchored fiducial screws (C), which were place prior to the CT scan. The probe and DRF (B) are from the Stealth-Station (Medtronic Surgical Navigation Technologies, Jacksonville, FL).

for fracture tracking during operative reduction as well as the confirmation of optimal fragment reduction. In addition, this project also served as a proof of concept for real-time CAS guidance during actual fracture reduction.

In this cadaveric study, frontozygomaticomaxillary fractures were created by blunt blows to the malar eminence. After a postfracture CT, operative reduction was performed under CAS guidance with StealthStation 2.6.4 (Medtronic Surgical Navigation, Louisville, CO). Again, the SBR points served as a reference system for CAS-derived measurements, and the point of maximal curvature on the malar eminence was selected to represent fragment position. As in the clinical study, the distance-measurement tools provided information about malar projection and position before, during, and after reduction. The StealthStation also includes a surgical guidance mode that tracks positioning of a surgical probe/instrument relative to planned trajectory. This surgical guidance mode was used during the reduction.

Analysis of the coordinate measurements at these intervals of fracture reduction (prereduction, intermediate reduction, and final reduction) confirmed that the surgical guidance mode can be used to direct and confirm the adequacy of fracture reduction. In addition, this study model closely simulated the actual intraoperative process, where sequential reduction is frequently done to find the "bestfit" result. In this project, the sequential reduction was performed with CAS guidance, which was felt to reduce the complexity of this task.

24.3.3 Pre-Operative Virtual Modeling and Simulation

Potentially, a computer workstation that has specific software for preoperative CT image manipulation could support the modeling of specific surgical maneuvers (i.e., implant placement and anticipated osteotomies for facial bone advancement or reduction) [7]. In this way, preoperative surgical plans could potentially be tested prior to entry into the operating room. Although this strategy has not been conclusively validated, these computer-based simulations should facilitate more effective and more efficient surgery with lower overall morbidity. The resultant shorter operative times would yield cost savings. Patient satisfaction should also improve. Surgical simulation could also introduce another teaching modality, which would allow trainees the opportunity to test and observe the results of surgical maneuvers without any patient morbidity. Unfortunately, the computer systems for this type of work has not been full developed. At least, such technology should be technically possible.

Preoperative virtual modeling and simulation can be directly applied during the actual procedure through the surgical navigation features of CAS. For example, after the surgical simulation has been performed on a computer workstation, the intraoperative position of fragments can be compared to this preoperative simulation [8]. Light-emitting diode (LED) markers, which can be tracked by an overhead camera array, permit intraoperative navigation, and permit comparisons between planned positions (from the preoperative simulation) and the positions in the operating field. In this report, the LED markers were attached to the patient's skull base (as a frame of reference) and a mobile, osteotomized bone fragment. Through surgical navigation, the surgeons monitored the position of this fragment relative to a preoperative surgical plan that was stored in the CAS computer. In this way, the optimal position of the osteomized fragment (determined by a preoperative surgical plan) could be recognized directly during the surgery. Before clinical use, laboratory testing of this technique was completed [9]. A similar system has been developed for orthognathic surgery [10].

24.3.4 Milled Model and Stereolithography

Replica models of reconstructed CT scan data may also be created. These models can be constructed through conventional milling techniques or through stereolithography. Stereolithography is a modeling method in which a laser polymerizes liquid resin to yield a three-dimensional model of the CT scan data. A computer system that processes the CT scan data set guides the laser as it polymerizes the liquid resin. In this way, an accurate and real model of the craniomaxillofacial skeleton (as visualized on the CT scan) is manufactured. Both conventional milling and stereolithography produce an actual model that is derived from the patient's preoperative CT scan.

Because conventional milling is less costly and less time-consuming, it probably deserves a greater role, except when the anatomical region of interest includes significant hollow areas and/or fine structures, where stereolithography is preferable [11]. For example, stereolithography is a better modeling method for the paranasal sinuses and skull base. Although stereolithography usually produces accurate models, some models may not always be entirely accurate [12]. Consequently, standard CT scan images should also be available for review and comparison in all cases. Clinical experience with stereolithography has grown considerably; the models manufactured with this technique have been found helpful for congenital anomaly assessment [13], orbital reconstruction [14], and maxillofacial surgery [15].

Real three-dimensional models can also be combined with CAS surgical navigation. A technique for intraoperative tracking of bone fragments during craniofacial surgery has been presented [16]. This method, called computer-assisted bone segment navigation, does not require standard intraoperative surgical navigation using preoperative CT and/or MR data. Instead, repair of the bony defect was performed using an actual milled model. The DRF, which was a simple LED array in this study, was applied to the mobile fragment as well as the larger, fixed segment. An overhead digitizer then tracked the movements of both DRFs. During the simulation, the surgical segment navigator (SSN) computer then calculates the movement vectors that are necessary to move the mobile segment into the desired position. Intraoperatively, the DRFs were applied to the mobile segment and the fixed segment in an identical fashion. The SSN computer tracked the actual surgical reduction and compared its vectors to the preoperative simulation.

24.3.5 Comparisons with Normal Projection

Computer-aided CT cephalometrics also can be incorporated into intraoperative surgical navigation for craniomaxillofacial surgery. (Computer-aided cephalometrics is discussed in Chapter 21.) After bone fragment repositioning, repeat measurements can be obtained. These measurements can be compared to the contralateral side for the confirmation of symmetry. Alternatively, such measurements can be compared to normative data as such data become available. Experience with this approach is limited; however, it has been applied with some success to orbitomaxillozygomatic fracture reduction [5].

24.4 Limitations of the Current Technology

Despite the impressive advances in preoperative imaging and surgical techniques, the operative repair of complex facial fractures is still less than optimal. Reduction of the fracture requires the positioning of the fragment or fragments in a precise, three-dimensional arrangement. Although preoperative CT scans facilitate the recognition of fracture patterns and secondary deformities, the scans themselves do not directly guide the operative reduction and fixation. Instead, the surgeon must extrapolate information from the preoperative images and intraoperative findings. The actual reduction is usually just an approximation that hopefully will restore function and cosmesis. Clearly, better methods must be sought. CAS may provide a means for better intraoperative reductions; however, the current systems really have not been optimized for these applications.

A variety of deficiencies in current CAS technology have been identified:

As already stated, commercially available CAS systems have been designed for neurosurgery, spine surgery, and rhinologic surgery, but not craniomaxillofacial surgery. Current reports on CAS for facial fracture reduction and related procedures typically describe a prototype system or an adaptation of a commercially available system.

Although CAS availability has improved considerably, it is still relatively expensive, especially when one considers that any hardware and software purchased now will shortly be obsolete. From a cost and marketing perspective, the ideal CAS system would contain software that is specific for use in other subspecialty applications (i.e., sinus surgery and neurosurgery) but also contain software that is particular to craniomaxillofacial surgery. The LED array or reference frame could be designed specifically for each subspecialty so that the designs accommodate the incisions, anatomy, patient positioning, and other issues that are considerations in specific procedures. In this way, the core CAS platform would be used by multiple surgical disciplines; this platform would then support various modules that would be optimized for specific applications.

Recent improvements have simplified CAS systems for routine use; nonetheless, CAS is still relatively complicated. Even surgeons who are familiar with computers and CAS may have difficulty with CAS applications for computer-aided reduction of facial fractures.

Computer-Aided Reduction of Maxillofacial Fractures

Preoperative CT scan data are frequently imperfect due to poor patient positioning, motion artifact and foreign body or implant artifact. In the worst cases, the CT scans must be repeated or CAS is of little value, since the accuracy of the system is poor. Even newer generation CAS systems cannot compensate for the effects of input artifact (Figure 24.7).

Craniomaxillofacial surgeons are most concerned about facial projection and contour, not absolute position information. CAS surgical navigation provides mostly positional systems in the currently available systems. This emphasis on position, rather than projection and contour, limits the applicability of CAS for facial fracture reduction.

Facial fracture reduction generates considerable forces that may disrupt patient position, even if the patient is immobilized with pins in a Mayfield head holder. This movement may cause drift in registration; as a result, surgical navigation may become unreliable unless registration is repeated. Considerable forces may be generated during fracture reduc-

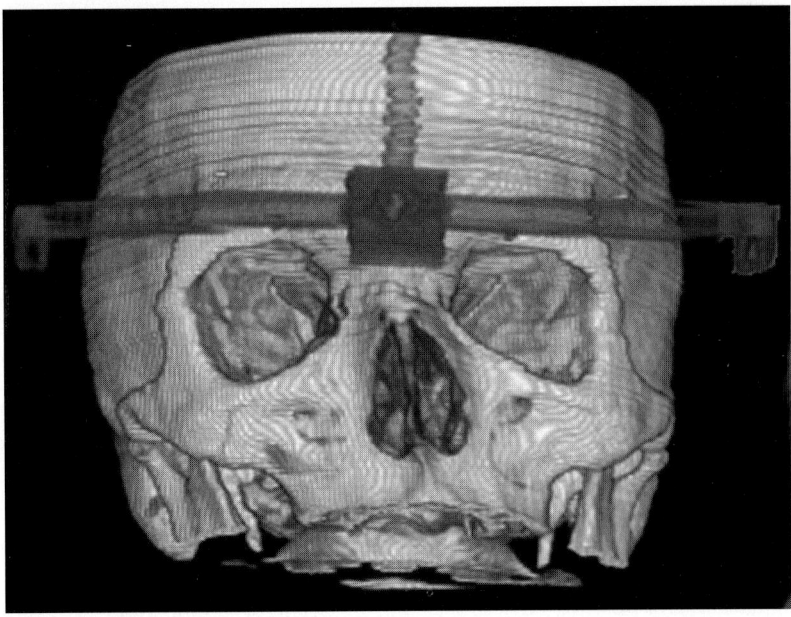

FIGURE 24.7 Poor preoperative CT image quality can adversely affect the quality of the reconstructed images. In this three-dimensional reconstruction from 1 mm direct axial CT scan images by SAVANT 2.0 (CBYON, Palo Alto, CA), obvious asymmetry and distortion are present, although the patient did not have a congenital or traumatic craniomaxillofacial anomaly. The inaccuracies present in the reconstructed images were ascribed to CT scanner calibration errors (i.e., a poor CT scan).

tion, an aspect absent in other subspecialty applications. If accuracy of the system is dependent on absolute patient immobility, then it is unlikely to be optimal for reconstruction of traumatic facial deformities.

Registration for CAS surgical navigation currently uses a variety of strategies, including anatomical fiducial points, bone-anchored fiducial points, external fiducial points, contour mapping, and fiducial headset reference frames. None of these alternatives are well suited for registration of the severely (or even moderately) traumatized head. New strategies for registration are needed.

Anatomical data, which can be directly applied in CAS measurements and ultimately fracture reduction, may not be readily available. Normative information regarding orbital volume and/or cross-sectional area or area would be useful in repositioning bone fragments and the intraoperative evaluation of fracture reduction of complex orbital fractures. Similarly, information about the relative angles of the orbital walls would also be helpful.

CAS instrumentation for facial fracture reduction is nonexistent, since the optimal way to use CAS for this purpose has not yet been defined. As a result, surgeons must use instruments designed for other procedures if they wish to use CAS during facial fracture reduction.

The use of current CAS systems often requires a considerable time commitment, since the introduction of additional hardware typically requires additional time for its appropriate use. For instance, surgical navigation requires specific tracking devices and patient positioning. Furthermore, the various measurements that the CAS software package supports must actually be performed. All of these steps take time. Of course, new technology may ultimately increase efficiency; however, this has not happened yet in CAS for facial fracture reduction. These somewhat time-consuming aspects of CAS may serve as a deterrent for any surgeon considering the use of CAS. On the other hand, greater efficiency can be anticipated as improved strategies for CAS are developed and implemented.

24.5 FUTURE DEVELOPMENTS

The use of CAS for facial fracture reduction is currently in its initial stages. Most craniomaxillofacial surgeons would welcome a method of intraoperative tracking and/or imaging of the craniomaxillofacial skeleton and overlying soft tissues. After additional refinement and innovation, CAS may meet the demanding criteria set by these surgeons, who are seeking a better alternative for their patients.

Obviously, further rapid developments in CAS can be anticipated. Rapid enhancements in microprocessor computing power, data storage capacity, network bandwidth, and image displays will like drive this growth. In addition, more surgeons are gaining experience with this technology in their clinical practices; this familiarity will likely encourage further technological adaptations. Collaborative efforts among surgical specialists, who share common and divergent interests and experiences, will also drive specific CAS adaptations.

The role of computers in the workplace will likely undergo substantial revision and modification. Standard CAS systems use a cathode ray tube (CRT) or liquid crystal display (LCD) computer monitor for the presentation of information for use by the operating surgeon. In this approach, the computer workstation tower is intrinsically separate from the actual operation. As an alternative to this arrangement, new display technologies, including integrated head-mounted displays worn by the surgical team, may create an "augmented reality," in which the surgeon can directly access all information [17,18].

As the systems grow more powerful (and more complicated), the design of the user interface becomes more important. In these matters, the practical operation of both the software and hardware must be facilitated. In most work environments, the presentation of the computer in the workplace has not been a major concern. In the typical office setting, this lackadaisical design philosophy has generated some problems; however, those issues are minor when they are compared with the introduction of computer systems in more complex work settings (such as the operating room). In the latter case, the computer can actually be disruptive to the performance of the requisite tasks. As a result, the integration of the computer workstation into the work environment is of paramount importance. In this regard, head-mounted displays for the surgical team—if implemented appropriately—may be an important advance.

Ergonomic designs that enhance usability are desirable in all computer systems; however, they are especially important for CAS systems for facial fracture reduction. Surgeons who have used these systems have universally commented that the systems are so cumbersome that they are almost unusable. The use of CAS for facial fracture reduction by surgeons other than those self-described "early adopters" will require substantial and meaningful changes in CAS system design.

The ways in which surgeons use preoperative images (i.e., CT scans) will likely be substantially updated. The standard use of preoperative images is "uncoupled" from the actual surgery; the surgeon must relate remote preoperative imaging data and the actual intraoperative anatomy. In contrast, in CAS surgical navigation, the surgeon utilizes a CAS system that integrates preoperative images, planning, simulation, and actual surgery; in this way, all aspects of the procedure are "coupled" [19].

Although CAS holds considerable promise, it would be foolish to assume that other alternatives would not be explored. For instance, intraoperative CT scans would permit direct assessment of operative reductions. In this regard, the intraoperative CT scanner would be analogous to intraoperative fluoroscopy. In fact, one report has noted that direct intraoperative CT scan confirmation of postreduction relationships is of value in cases of facial fracture reduction [20]. Despite this favorable report, it is unlikely that intraoperative CT scans will become the standard for immediate confirmation of adequate reduction, since intraoperative CT scanners are expensive, cumbersome devices. Obviously, these scanners are expensive, even when compared with CAS. All intraoperative CT scanners require laborious, impractical patient positioning. They also require additional radiation exposure for the patient and staff. Because of the risk of radiation-induced cataracts at relatively low levels of exposure, it has long been considered reasonable to minimize radiation exposure to the orbits. It should also be noted that intraoperative CT scanners provide only static images. In contract, CAS surgical navigation provides dynamic point localizations. In theory, the integration of active virtual modeling with real-time surgical navigation would permit the construction of virtual three-dimensional models of the operative reduction during the actual procedure. Computer-aided design (CAD) and computer-aided manufacturing (CAM) software, which has gained widespread use for its industrial applications, may guide the design of software for the real-time construction of detailed three-dimensional models.

It is important that surgeons with an interest in CAS and its extended applications (including facial fracture reduction) continue to test new systems; their feedback will provide guidance to the CAS engineering teams at the CAS companies. Meaningful progress will require collaboration among surgeons and engineers, who together will mold technological advances into practical, powerful CAS systems. As these new platforms are introduced, further clinical evaluation of CAS systems will be necessary to confirm that CAS implementation improves the functional and cosmetic results of the operative repair of facial fractures and decreases the morbidity of these procedures.

REFERENCES

1. Chen CT, Lai JP, Chen YR, Tung TC, Chen ZC, Rohrich RJ. Application of endoscope in zygomatic fracture repair. Br J Plast Surg 53:100–105, 2000.
2. Lee C, Stiebel M, Young DM. Cranial nerve VII region of the traumatized facial skeleton: optimizing fracture repair with the endoscope. J Trauma 48:423–431, 2000.
3. Manson PN. Computed tomography use and repair of orbitozygomatic factures. Arch Facial Plastic Surg 1:25–26, 1999.
4. Marentette LJ, Maisel RH. Three-dimensional CT reconstruction in midfacial surgery. Otolaryngol Head Neck Surg, 98:48–52, 1988.
5. Hardeman S, Kokoska MS, Stack BC, Citardi MJ. Stereotactic image assessment of malar projection in facial fractures. Abstract presented at American Academy of

Facial Plastic and Reconstructive Surgery fall meeting, New Orleans, LA, September 23, 1999.
6. Kokoska MS, Hardeman S, Cooper M, McNeil W, Bucholz R, Citardi MJ. Computer-aided sequential reduction of zygomatic fractures. Presented at American Academy of Facial Plastic Surgery spring meeting, Orlando, FL, May 13, 2000.
7. Altobelli DE, Kikins R, Mulliken JB, Cline H, Lorensen W, Jolesz F. Computer-assisted three-dimensional planning in craniofacial surgery. Plast Reconstr Surg 92: 576–585, 1993.
8. Cutting C, Grayson G, McCarthy JG, Thorne C, Khorramabadi D, Haddad B, Taylor R. A virtual reality system for bone fragment positioning in craniofacial surgical procedures. Plast Reconstr Surg 102:2436–2443, 1998.
9. Cutting C, Grayson B, Kim H. Precision multi-segment bone positioning using computer-aided methods in craniofacial surgical applications. IEEE Eng Med Biol Soc 12:1926, 1990.
10. Bettega G, Dessenne V, Raphael B, Cinquin P. Computer-assisted mandibular condyle positioning during orthognathic surgery. J Oral Maxillofac Surg 54:553, 1996.
11. Santler G, Karcher H, Gaggl A, Kern R. Stereolithography versus milled three-dimensional models: comparison of production method, indication and accuracy. Comput Aid Surg 3:248–256, 1998.
12. Kragskov J, Sindet-Pedersen S, Gyldensted C, Jensen KL. A comparison of three-dimensional computed tomography scans and stereolithographic models for evaluation of cranofacial anomalies. J Oral Maxillofac Surg 54:402–411, 1996.
13. Sailer HF, Haers PE, Zollikofer CP, Warnke T, Carls FR, Stucki P. The value of stereolithographic models for preoperative diagnosis of craniofacial deformities and planning of surgical corrections. Int J Oral Maxillofac Surg 27:327–333, 1998.
14. Holck DE, Boyd EM Jr, Ng J, Mauffray RO. Benefits of stereolithography in orbital reconstruction. Ophthalmology 106:1214–1218, 1999.
15. Bill JS, Reuther JF, Dittmann W, Kubler N, Meier, JL, Pistner H, Wittenberg G. Stereolithography in oral and maxillofacial surgery planning. Int J Oral Maxillofac Surg 24:98–103, 1995.
16. Marmulla R, Niederellmann. Computer-assisted bone segment navigation. J Craniomaxillofac Surg 26:347–359, 1998.
17. Enislidis G, Wagner A, Ploder O, Ewers R. Computed intraoperative navigation guidance—a preliminary report on a new technique. Br J Oral Maxillofac Surg 35: 271–274, 1997.
18. Blackwell M, Morgan F, DiGioia AM. Augmented reality and its future in orthopaedics. Clin Orthop Relat Res 354:111–122, 1998.
19. DiGioia AM, Jaramaz B, Colgan BD. Computer-assisted orthopedia surgery. Clin Orthop Relat Res 354:8–16, 1998.
20. Stanley RB. Use of intraoperative computed tomography during repair of orbitozygomatic fractures. Arch Facial Plastic Surg 1:19–24, 1999.

25
Future Directions

Martin J. Citardi, M.D., F.A.C.S.
Cleveland Clinic Foundation, Cleveland, Ohio

25.1 INTRODUCTION

A chapter filled with prognostications about future technological developments and applications may seem to be an appropriate conclusion to a book about new technology; however, such an approach is fraught with problems. At the very best, the time interval between completion of the manuscript and distribution of the printed text may be so long that the rapid pace of technological improvements may eclipse the printed predictions. At worst, such predictions may appear almost laughable within a relatively short time as future developments unfold in patterns that were unforeseen.

Despite these problems, this book requires a final look forward. Rather than present a vision of the future, this chapter will present several (but certainly not all) emerging technologies, which may (or may not) have a positive impact on computer-aided surgery (CAS). This presentation will describe current engineering efforts, which are a response to perceptions of current need. As a result, these developmental technologies also reflect the current state of CAS.

The book's CD-ROM includes four movies (Movie 25-1, Movie 25-2, Movie 25-3, Movie 25-4) that illustrate important principles discussed in this chapter. All movies are in AVI format and can be viewed with an appropriate multimedia reader (such as Windows Media Player 6 or greater, Microsoft Corporation, Redmond WA, http://www.microsoft.com/windows/windowsmedia/EN/default.asp).

The specific technologies in this chapter represent a wide range of technological development. Although all of them are in the engineering phase, some of them are beginning to enter the clinical arena. These technologies, which are still in their early stages, will doubtlessly undergo significant refinement.

Again, it must be emphasized that the point of this chapter is not to project a vision of the future of CAS within otorhinolaryngology–head and neck surgeries. Instead, the emphasis is upon developmental technologies, which offer significant promise, but have not yet been widely accepted.

25.2 VOLUME RENDERING TECHNOLOGY AND PERSPECTIVE VOLUMETRIC NAVIGATION

Computer-based, three-dimensional modeling based on raw axial magnetic resonance imaging (MRI) or computed tomography (CT) data has become widely available. Current systems offer volume-rendering protocols that can build three-dimensional (3D) models with a high degree of fidelity. Models based on volume rendering offer maximal opportunities for creating multiple views of the same data set, since more of the initial data is incorporated into the model. The major limitation has been that these models are much more complex to create and manipulate, since the amount of incorporated data is so great. Fortunately, speedier and less costly microprocessors, computer memory, graphics cards, and display systems have made volume-rendered models a feasible option.

The CBYON Suite™ (CBYON, Palo Alto, CA; www.cbyon.com) incorporates sophisticated volume rendering protocols (known as Dynamic Data Filtering™) into a CAS package that also includes standard surgical navigation features. This software offers enhanced options for viewing the models. Surgeons can melt away various tissue layers and fly through the area of interest (Figure 25.1). The CBYON Suite also permits the creation of short "movies" of fly-through paths of the models (Figure 25.2) (Movie 25-1, Movie 25-2, Movie 25-3). The models are sharp and clear, and the system performance (i.e., frame refresh rate) is remarkably fast. The CBYON CAS platform, which was introduced in 2000, offers capabilities that were previously only attainable in specialized computer laboratories for routine use in the operating room.

The CBYON software also can display the three-dimensional volume renderings from the perspective of a surgical instrument so that the view of the model from the tip of the instrument during actual surgery can be visualized. This technique, called Perspective Volumetric Navigation™ (PVN), incorporates positional information obtained from standard surgical navigation with features of virtual endoscopy. Finally, virtual endoscopic view provided by PVN can be temporally and spacially synchronized with intraoperative endoscopic images through Image-Enhanced Endoscopy™ (IEE). IEE combines so-called virtual endoscopy based upon perspective volume rendering with the real world endoscopic

Future Directions 465

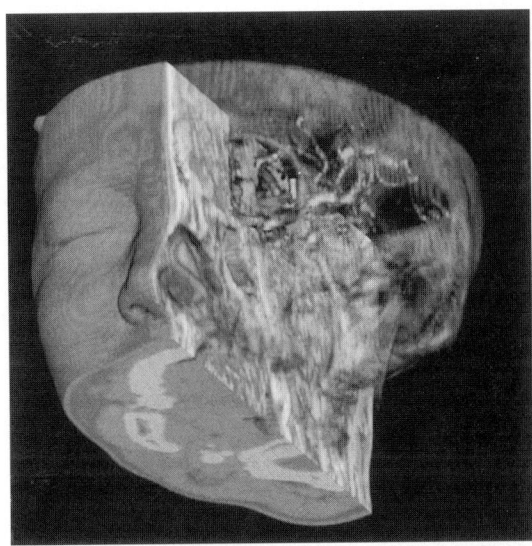

FIGURE 25.1 The CBYON Suite™ (CBYON, Palo Alto, CA) uses volume rendering for the creation of three-dimensional models. Surgeons may melt away layers through Dynamic Data Filtering™, which uses image data filters. In this still image, the overlying soft tissue has been rendered transparent in the left half of the model, the corresponding bone has been rendered partially transparent, and the intracranial vasculature has been rendered in red. (Courtesy of CBYON, Palo Alto, CA.)

view (Figure 25.3) (Movie 25-4). In order to accomplish this, the CBYON system tracks the position of the rigid endoscope tip, and can reconstruct the virtual view (from the preoperative CT or MRI data) that corresponds to the view through the endoscope. The net result is that the real world endoscopic view and the virtual endoscopic view are coregistered.

PVN and IEE can provide significant orientation information. Although the rigid endoscope provides offers a bright view, blood and other surgical debris can obscure that view. Furthermore, the endoscopic view is only a two-dimensional representation of complex three-dimensional anatomy; as a result, perceptual distortion is common. To the extent that the PVN provides additional information about orientation and localization, it will simplify endoscopic visualization. In doing so, PVN may permit the development of endoscopic techniques for procedures that currently require open approaches for the maintenance of surgical orientation.

PVN adaptations also may have significant impact on endoscopic sinonasal surgery for inflammatory sinonasal diseases. In these procedures, surgical naviga-

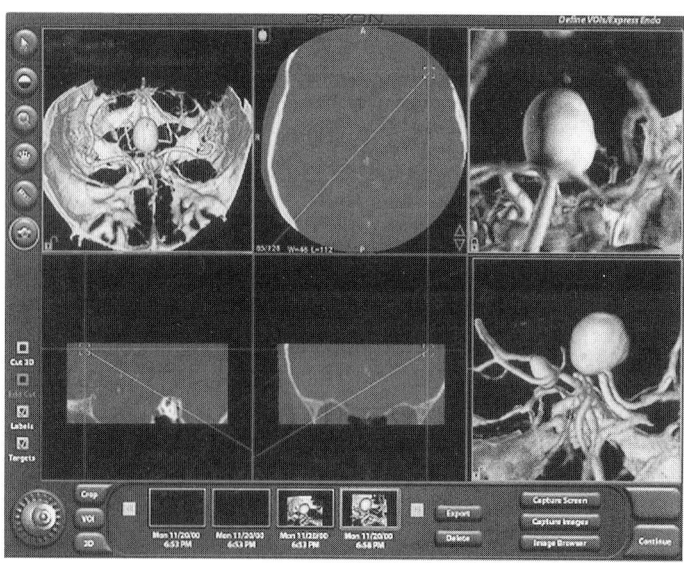

FIGURE 25.2 This CBYON Suite™ (CBYON, Palo Alto, CA) supports the creation of "fly-by" and "fly-through" movies of three-dimensional models created from CT and MR images. This still image capture depicts a snap shot of the trajectory of a movie of an intracranial aneurysm. (Courtesy of CBYON, Palo Alto, CA.)

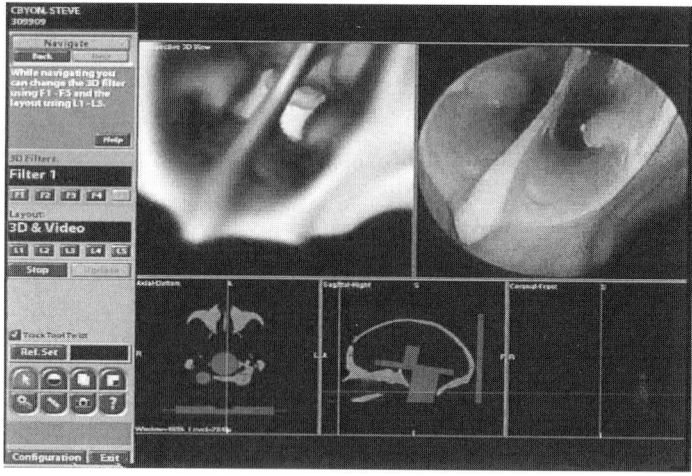

FIGURE 25.3 In Image-Enhanced Endoscopy™, the CBYON Suite (CBYON, Palo Alto, CA) matches the corresponding views of the real surgical anatomy (i.e., the view provided by the endoscope) and the virtual three-dimensional model (created by the computer software). This still image capture shows the synchronization between the virtual (upper left panel) and real view (upper right panel). (Courtesy of CBYON, Inc., Palo Alto, CA.)

Future Directions

tion often provides information about the boundaries of the paranasal sinuses. In this way, the computer system guides the surgeon away from the intracranial space, the orbital space, the optic nerve, etc. In contrast, surgical navigation more commonly provides guidance to reach a target. For most sinus surgery, the objective is target avoidance, which helps the surgeon avoid potentially catastrophic complications. Although PVN clearly supports targeting capabilities, it can also support antitargeting; that is, the CBYON system can highlight specific structures that must be avoided (Figure 25.4). This information can be displayed on the perspective volumetric reconstruction (the virtual view), which actively correlated with the real view provided by the telescope.

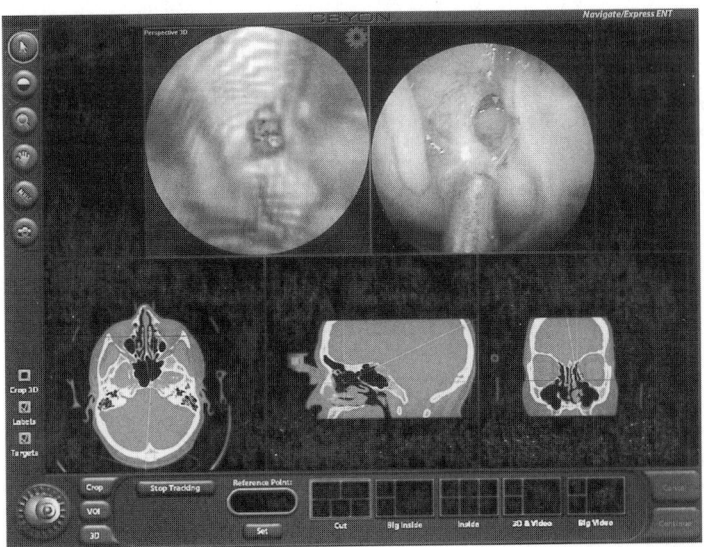

FIGURE 25.4 The CBYON Suite™'s Image-Enhanced Endoscopy (IEE) may provide better appreciation of three-dimensional anatomy and can support both tracking to a target as well as tracking away from a critical structure. In this instance, volume-rendering protocols were used to create a three-dimensional model of the optic nerves of a patient, whose sphenoid sinuses had pneumatized around the optic nerves. In this case, the optic nerves were not a surgical objective. The patient was undergoing revision image-guided functional endoscopic sinus surgery for recurrent acute rhinosinusitis of the frontal, ethmoid, and maxillary sinuses; as a result, entry into the sphenoid sinuses was not deemed necessary. This still image capture depicts the view provided by the telescope (upper right panel) and the corresponding view of the virtual model (upper left panel). The virtual model shows the optic nerve (in green in the image on the CD-ROM), but the optic nerve cannot be seen in the standard telescopic view. In this way, IEE provided anatomical information that was supplementary to the view afforded by the nasal telescope. The lower panels depict the relative position of the tip of the suction (seen in the real endoscopic image).

The clinical success of PVN will require robust system performance. The computer-generated views must update rapidly, and the view must be sufficiently detailed. In addition, the registration of the view of virtual space (created by the computer) with the view of real space (created by the telescope and camera system) must be very tight. Small discrepancies will introduce unacceptable errors that will degrade surgical safety and efficacy.

25.3 SURGICAL ROBOTICS

Over the past several decades, practical robotics has moved from the realm of science fiction to the commercial sector, where robotics are commonly employed in manufacturing tasks that require a high level of precision. More recently, robotics has been adapted for use in the operating suite. Although the technology for manufacturing robotics and surgical robotics is quite similar, important differences are also apparent. In factories, robots perform rote functions with relatively little human oversight and intervention. In contrast, surgical robotics requires a skilled human operator (the surgeon) at all times. A surgical robot does not perform its tasks as an automaton. Instead, the surgical robot operates at the interface between the surgeon and the patient.

In operating rooms equipped with surgical robotics, the surgeon controls each action of the robot, which can perform the maneuvers with greater precision than a human surgeon alone. Robots do not have tremors, and they do not fatigue. Furthermore, they can maintain uncomfortable postures indefinitely, unlike even the most ardent human surgeon and assistants. Robots can also be programmed to compensate for patient movements such as respiration and circulation. Without robotics, the surgeons must take compensatory actions; with robotics, the surgeon focuses on only those actions that are necessary for achieving the surgical objective, while the robot can add or subtract additional movements that reflect the inevitable motion of the operative field (due to factors such as respiration and circulation).

Computer Motion (Santa Barbara, CA; www.computermotion.com) has designed three surgical robotic systems. HERMES provides a voice-activated interface that can control medical devices that have been connected to the system. AESOP, which is also voice-activated, uses a robotic arm to position laparoscopic instruments, such as the rigid endoscope. This robot replaces the human assistant who "drives" the camera during laparoscopic procedures. AESOP reduces the personnel needed for these cases, and it can hold the instrument indefinitely in the position selected by the operative surgeon. Finally, the ZEUS robot can perform laparoscopic procedures under the surgeon's immediate control (Figure 25.5). For this system, the surgeon sits at a console, from which he or she can direct three robotic arms, which execute the commands entered by the surgeon (Figure 25.6). The ZEUS arms can perform precise movements without fatigue, tremor, etc.

Future Directions

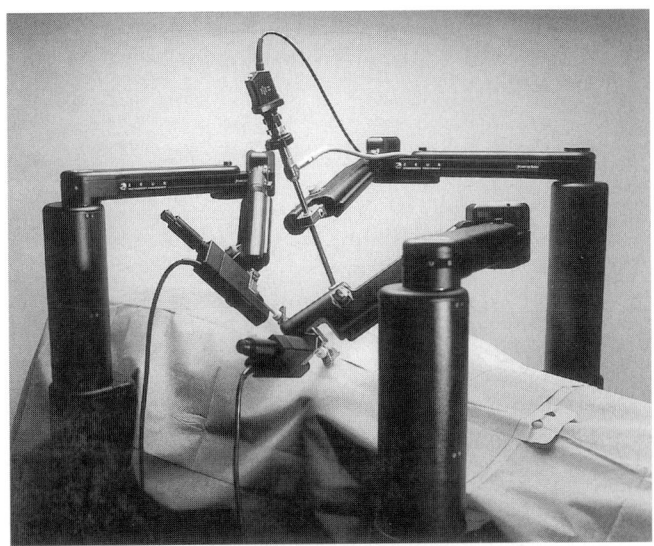

FIGURE 25.5 The ZEUS system from Computer Motion (Santa Barbara, CA) includes three robotic arms for the manipulation of surgical instruments. (© 2001 Computer Motion. Photograph by Bobbi Bennett.)

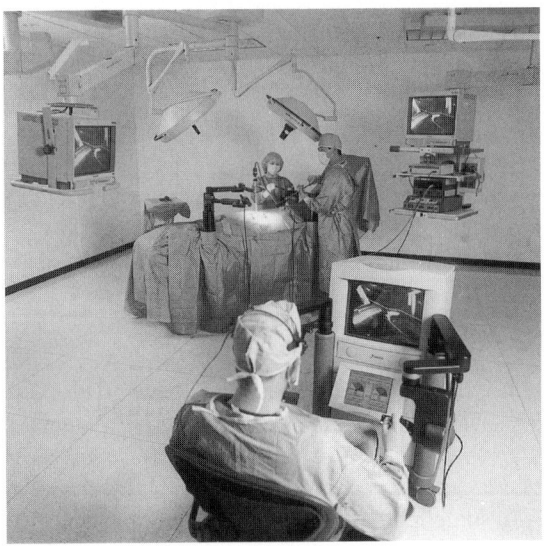

FIGURE 25.6 In surgical robotics, the surgeon directs the actions of the robot from a control panel that is separate from the immediate operating field. (© 2001 Computer Motion. Photograph by Bobbi Bennett.)

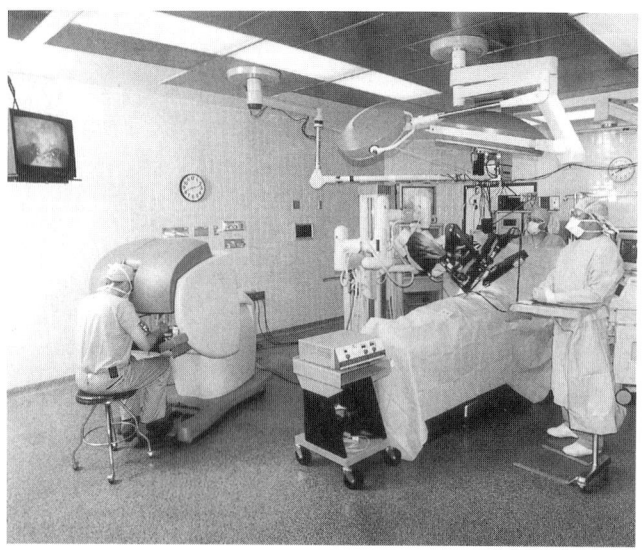

FIGURE 25.7 Surgical robotics requires placement of the robotic arms so that they have the direct access to the surgical field, and the surgeon's control station is placed out of the sterile field. In this example, da Vinci™ Robotic Surgical System (Intuitive Surgical, Inc., Mountain View, CA) is shown. The typical set-up for an operating room equipped for surgical robotics is shown. (© 1999 Intuitive Surgical, Inc.)

Other venders have also introduced robots for the operating suite. Intuitive Surgical (Mountain View, CA; www.intusurg.com) produces da Vinci™ Robotic Surgical System (Figure 25.7). Like ZEUS, da Vinci includes a surgeon's console from which the surgeon can control the movements of the robotic arms. Surgeons are using both ZEUS and da Vinci in operating rooms throughout the world.

25.4 AUGMENTED REALITY

Several years ago, the concept of virtual reality (VR) was introduced to the general public. In VR systems, users enter a completely synthetic experience generated by computers. In true VR, computers create visual, audio, and haptic stimuli and cues that together emulate a real world experience, and users cannot perceive any elements from the real world. Although VR technology has enormous potential for entertainment applications, its medical usefulness may be limited, since VR creates a substitute reality. Surgeons are more interested in accurate and precise representations of real world anatomy. As a result, the surgical importance of VR rests upon the integration of its core components with relevant physical

Future Directions

features. Augmented reality or tele-immersion seeks to superimpose three-dimensional computer-rendered images upon the actual surgical field. The objective of this approach is to eliminate the need for standard view boxes and cathode ray tube (CRT) displays; instead, all relevant imaging data will be presented directly to the surgeon in the operative field.

How can this be achieved? One approach is to move from CRTs that are remote from the operative field; rather, the display system may be directly incorporated into the equipment in the operative field. Of course, standard CRTs are large and cumbersome, and even liquid crystal displays (LCD), LCD projectors, and plasma screens are probably too large to be successfully integrated into the operative field.

Head-mounted display (HMD) units may represent a potential solution. Current HMDs incorporate traditional LCD displays into a headset that the surgeon wears during the procedure. Since HMDs provide binocular information, they can be used to created stereovision. Unfortunately, early HMD units have been less than optimal. Some surgeons have noted perceptual distortion and disorientation, and these sensations may even lead to eyestrain, headaches, and nausea. In addition, the HMD resolution has been poor and the image sizes are typically small. These factors create the impression of viewing a grainy image at a distance through a narrow tube—clearly not an optimal image for surgical applications.

Retinal scanning display (RSD) technology, which incorporates a small, low-power image to directly "paint" an image on the user's retina, may overcome the limitations of current HMD systems. Monocular, monochromatic RSD technology has been used to convey relevant information to pilots who fly certain military helicopters. In this military application, pilots can perceive targeting and other data while viewing the real scene through the cockpit window. The incorporation of binocular, full color RSDs into an HMD may represent a viable approach for clinically useful augmented reality and tele-immersion. Microvision, Inc. (Bothell, WA; www.mvis.com) is actively developing RSD-based HMD units.

25.5 FINAL COMMENTS

The final direction of the paths created by volume-rendering protocols, surgical robotics, augmented reality, and other technologies cannot be fully anticipated. New technology will inevitably grow and evolve in ways that are impossible to predict, and surgeons will creatively apply these new tools to solve relevant surgical challenges. The only safe assumption in this process is that CAS technologies will provide a means for greater surgical precision and decreased morbidity. In this way, surgeons will utilize CAS so that better patient outcomes can be achieved.

Index

3D Navigator, 335

A

Aachen group, 20–22, 187
AESOP, 468
Agger nasi cell, 247–249
ANALYZE, 405
Anterior cranial base surgery (*see* Sinonasal tumors and anterior cranial base)
Augmented reality, 425–427, 470–471

B

BrainLab (*see* VectorVision)

C

Calibration, 9, 32, 54–55
CAPS, 424–425
CAS (*see* Computer-aided surgery)
CAVE, 435–436
CBYON (*see also* SAVANT), 67–68, 197, 464
Cephalometrics, 377–380
Computer-aided surgery (*see also* Craniofacial surgery, Facial plastic surgery, Maxillofacial fractures, Soft tissue surgery, Software-enabled cephalometrics, Surgical navigation, Surgical simulation, Registration, Tumor modeling, Virtual endoscopy, Virtual reality)
  accuracy, 152–153
  advantages, 191–192, 283–284, 346–349
  anterior cranial skull base, 277–292
  augmented reality, 425–427, 470–471
  CAS systems, 446–449
  CT, 145–148
  cost, 196
  definition, 4

473

[Computer-aided surgery]
  disadvantages, 192, 283–284, 346–349
  endoscopy, 145
  error, 69–71, 153
  FESS (*see also* IG-FESS), 185–198, 226–227
  frontal sinus mucocele, 257–260
  frontal sinus surgery, 243–261
  future developments, 273, 349–353, 431–438, 458–460, 463–471
  history, 15–28, 136–137, 187–188, 226–227
  image-enhanced endoscopy, 464–470
  image resolution, 151–152
  imaging modalities, 143–150
  indications, 188, 219–220
  lateral frontal sinus lesions, 260
  limitations, 220–221, 240, 456–458
  MRI, 148–151
  new paradigm for, 11–13
  otology and neurotology, 297–309
  osteoplastic flap, 260–261
  perspective volumetric navigation, 464–468
  revision sinus surgery, 223–241
  scope of, 5
  sinonasal tumors, 277–292
  surgical robotics, 468–470
  terminology, 4–5, 28
  transsphenoidal hypophysectomy, 263–273
  ultrasound, 145
  x-ray fluoroscopy, 145
Computer Motion (*see* AESOP, HERMES, ZEUS)
Craniofacial surgery, 395–420
  case examples, 410–416
  data acquisition and processing, 396–397
  philosophy, 407
  preoperative planning, 404–407
  rapid prototyping, 401–404
  rendering, 398–399
  segmentation, 399–401
  surgical navigation, 416–419
  techniques, 408–410

D

da Vinci Robotic Surgical System, 470
Digital imaging, 117–133
  advantages, 126–127
  clinical applications, 128–131
  color printers, 124–125
  compression, 118–119
  computer, 122
  digital cameras, 119–122
  digital video, 124
  disadvantages, 127
  facial plastic surgery, 363–366
  fundamentals, 118
  image capture systems, 131–133
  LCD projectors, 125–126
  presentations, 366–368
  software, 122
  storage media, 122–123
  techniques, 119
Dynamic Data Filtering, 52, 451, 464

E

Electromagnetic tracking, 32, 39–42
  accuracy, 45
  expense, 45
  operating room time, 44–45
  patient headset, 44
  patient selection, 46
  signal distortion, 43–44
  surgical instrumentation, 45
  vs. electromagnetic tracking, 31–46
Encephalocele, 290
Endoscopic sinus surgical simulator, 107–113
Expert systems, 103–107, 423–424

F

Facial plastic surgery, 361–375
  applications, 372–374
  digital imaging, 363–366

Index

[Facial plastic surgery]
  future developments, 374–375
  internet applications, 369–371
  medical education, 368–369
  office software, 362–363
  outcomes research, 371–372
  presentations, 366–368
FEM (*see* Finite element mesh)
FESS (*see also* Computer-aided surgery, IG-FESS, Surgical navigation), 223–241
  overview, 223–224
  frontal sinus surgery, 243–261
  revision surgery examples, 229–240
  surgical failures, 224–226
  technique, 227–229
Finite element mesh, 424
Flashpoint system, 23, 31
Framed stereotaxy, 15–16, 162
Frameless stereotaxy, 16–20, 163
Frontal cells, 249–252
Frontal sinus
  agger nasi cell, 247–249
  anatomy, 245–256
  frontal cells, 249–252
  frontal recess concept, 243
  frontal recess dissection, 245–247
  frontal sinus mucocele, 257–260
  integrated approach, 244
  interfrontal sinus cell, 253–255
  lateral frontal sinus lesions, 260
  osteoplastic flap, 260–261
  physiology, 245
  recessus terminalis, 256
  sinusitis, 243
  stents, 259
  suprabullar cell, 255–256
  supraorbital ethmoid cell, 252–253
Fused deposition modeling, 404

G

Gamma knife, 179–180
GE Medical Systems (*see* 3D Navigator)

H

Head-mounted display (*see* HMD)
HERMES, 468
HMD, 422, 425, 471

I

IG-FESS (*see also* FESS), 201–222
  cases, 212–219
  computer-aided CT review, 206–208
  indications, 219–220
  limitations, 220–221
  paradigm, 204–206
  rationale, 202–203
  registration, 209–212
ILD, 51–52
Image coordinate, 17, 18
Image-enhanced endoscopy, 67–68, 464–470
Image fusion, 67
Image-guided functional endoscopic sinus surgery (*see* IG-FESS)
Image-guided surgery (*see also* Computer-aided surgery, Surgical navigation), 4, 5, 28, 205–206
InstaTrak, 24, 39–42, 194–195
International Society for Computer-Aided Surgery (*see* ISCAS)
Internet-enabled surgery, 91–98, 369–371
Intraoperative MRI, 73–87
  advantages, 85–86
  anesthesia considerations, 77–78
  applications, 80–84
  disadvantages, 86–87
  open MRI unit, 74–75
  optical tracking, 78
  personnel, 79–80
  real-time MRI, 78–79
  surgical instrumentation, 78
Intraoperative multiplanar imaging (*see also* Intraoperative MRI), 74

Intuitive Surgical (*see* da Vinci Robotic Surgical System)
Inverted papilloma, 286
ISCAS, 3–4, 28, 206
ISG (*see* Viewing Wand)

J

Juvenile angiofibroma, 288

L

LandmarX, 26–27, 34, 195–196, 450
LINAC, 178–179

M

Malar point, 386–390
Marconi Medical Systems (*see* Voyager)
Mayo Biomedical Imaging Resource (*see* ANALYZE)
Maxillofacial fractures, 443–460
 CT issues, 445–446
 future developments, 458–459
 ideal system, 444–445
 limitations, 456–458
 models, 455
 projection, 455
 rationale, 443–444
 techniques, 449–458
Medtronic Surgical Navigation Technology (*see* StealthStation)
Medtronic Xomed (*see* LandmarX)
Meningocele, 290
Microelectromechanical systems, 434–435
Microvision, 471
Middle cranial fossa surgery, 298–301
MP (*see* Malar point)
Mucociliary clearance, 245

N

Natural language processing, 105
Neuronavigator, 17
Neurotology (*see* Otology and neurotology)

O

Optical tracking, 32, 34–39
 accuracy, 45
 expense, 45
 operating room time, 44–45
 patient headset, 44
 patient selection, 46
 signal blocking, 43–44
 surgical instrumentation, 45
 vs. electromagnetic tracking, 31–46
ORTHODOC, 426–427
Osteoplastic flap, 260–261
Otology (*see* Otology and neurotology)
Otology and neurotology, 297–309
 instrumentation, 305–308
 middle cranial fossa surgery, 298–301
 petrous apex, 301–305
Outcomes research, 371–372

P

Patient care model, 2–4
Performance Machines, 426
Perspective rendering (*see* Rendering)
Perspective volumetric navigation, 464–468
Petrous apex, 301–305
Preoperative planning, 279–282, 404–407

R

Recessus terminalis, 256
Registration, 9, 33, 49–71, 137–139, 164–167

Index

[Registration]
  automatic, 59–64, 209
  contour methods, 64–67, 165–167
  DRF, 52
  dynamic, 52–53
  error, 53–54, 69–71, 201–211
  ILD, 51–52
  manual, 55–59, 209
  paired point methods, 164–165
  RMS, 53, 62
  semi-automatic, 62–63
  sinus surgery, 208–212
  vs. calibration, 54–55
Rendering, 319–321, 331–334, 336, 398–399, 464–468
Retinal scanning display, 471
RMS, 53, 62, 138–139
Root means square (see RMS)
RSD (see Retinal scanning display)

S

SAVANT (see also CBYON), 35
SBR (see Skull base reference)
Segmentation, 317–319, 335–336, 399–401
Selective laser sintering, 404
Shaded surface display, 335–336
SIMCAST, 314–317
Sinonasal tumors (see Sinonasal tumors and anterior cranial base)
Sinonasal tumors and anterior cranial base, 277–292
  advantages and disadvantages, 283–284
  anatomic landmarks, 279–282
  benign tumors, 290
  challenges, 277–278
  encephalocele, 290
  endoscopic resection, 285–292
  inverted papilloma, 286
  juvenile angiofibroma, 288
  malignant tumors, 291–292
  maxillofacial reconstruction, 282–283
  meningocele, 290
  preoperative planning, 279–282

Sinus surgery (see FESS, IG-FESS)
Skull base reference, 386–389, 450
Soft tissue surgery, 421–439
  applications, 427–431
  augmented reality, 427
  CAPS, 424–425
  expert system, 423–424
  finite element mesh, 424
  future developments, 431–438
Software-enabled cephalometrics, 377–394
  applications, 383–392
  challenges, 393–394
  definition, 380–383
  traditional cephalometrics, 377–380
SSD (see Shaded surface display)
StealthStation, 167
Stereolithography, 404, 455
Stereotactic radiosurgery, 178–180
Stereotaxis, 162
Surface rendering (see Rendering)
Surgical navigation (see also Electromagnetic tracking, Optical tracking, Registration)
  accuracy, 152–153, 211–212
  advantages, 283–284
  anterior cranial skull base, 277–292
  atlases, 174–175
  components, 6–9, 136–137
  craniofacial surgery, 395–419
  disadvantages, 283–284
  effectors, 170–172
  error, 69–71, 153, 210–211
  digitizers, 168–170
  FESS (see also IG-FESS), 185–198, 226–227
  frames, 167–168
  frontal sinus mucocele, 257–260
  frontal sinus surgery, 243–261
  image-enhanced endoscopy, 464–470
  image resolution, 151–152
  indications, 219–220
  lateral frontal sinus lesions, 260
  limitations, 220–221, 240
  neurosurgery applications, 175–180
  osteoplastic flap, 260–261

[Surgical navigation]
  otology and neurotology, 297–309
  perspective volumetric navigation, 464–468
  reference systems, 170
  revision sinus surgery, 223–241
  sensors, 139–143
  sinonasal tumors, 277–292
  transsphenoidal hypophysectomy, 263–273
Surgical simulation, 99–114, 433
  endoscopic sinus surgical simulator, 107–113
  expert systems, 103–107
  haptic sensations, 102–103
  immersive simulators, 101, 103
  maxillofacial surgery, 454–455
  nonimmersive simulators, 101–102
Sustained accuracy, 33

T

Telemedicine, 436–437
Transsphenoidal hypophysectomy, 263–273
  anatomy, 266–270
  history, 263–264
  technique, 266–273
Tumor modeling, 311–326
  data acquisition, 312–317
  future directions, 324–326
  interface, 322–324
  multimodal data merge, 319
  rationale, 311–312
  rendering, 319–321
  segmentation, 317–319

V

Vector Vision, 24, 35, 196
Viewing Wand, 18, 22, 23, 137
Virtual endoscopy, 329–354
  advantages, 346–349
  airway obstruction, 346
  applications, 338–353
  data acquisition, 334–335
  data processing, 335–336
  definition, 329
  flight path, 336–338
  future developments, 349–353
  larynx, 340–346
  limitations, 346–349
  middle ear, 338–339
  nasal cavity, 339–340
  paranasal sinuses, 339–340
  pharynx, 340–346
  perspective rendering, 331–334, 336
  temporal bone, 338–339
  tumor assessment, 343–345
Virtual reality (*see also* Surgical simulation, Virtual endoscopy), 431–433, 434, 436, 437–438, 470
Visible Human Project, 434
Visualization technology (*see* InstaTrak)
Volume rendering (*see* Rendering)
Voyager, 335
Vital Images (*see* VoxelView/Vitrea)
VoxelView/Vitrea, 335
VTI (*see* InstaTrak)

Z

ZEUS, 468

About the Editor

Martin J. Citardi, M.D., F.A.C.S., is a Staff Member in the Department of Otolaryngology and Communicative Disorders at the Cleveland Clinic Foundation, Ohio. The author or coauthor of more than 40 journal articles, book chapters, and books, he is a Fellow of the American College of Surgeons, the American Rhinologic Society, and the American Academy of Otolaryngology–Head and Neck Surgery. Dr. Citardi also coordinates the Internet efforts for the American Rhinologic Society. He received the B.A. degree (1987) in biology from The Johns Hopkins University, Baltimore, Maryland. After receiving his M.D. degree (1991) from The Johns Hopkins University School of Medicine, Baltimore, Maryland, he completed his otorhinolaryngology–head and neck surgery residency at Yale University and a rhinology fellowship at the Georgia Rhinology & Sinus Center, Savannah, Georgia.

ISBN 0-8247-0641-2

90000